Vocal Rehabilitation for Medical Speech–Language Pathology

For Clinicians by Clinicians

Deanie Vogel and Michael P. Cannito, Series Editors

This book, *Vocal Rehabilitation for Medical Speech–Language Pathology*, is the 13th book in the For Clinicians by Clinicians series of texts on the diagnosis and clinical management of speech, language, and voice disorders. Each text provides a contemporary perspective on one major disorder or clinical area and is designed for use in clinical methodology courses and continuing education programs. Authors have been selected who represent a broad spectrum of clinical interests and theoretical positions and who hold the common belief that their viewpoints, experiences, and successes should be shared in order to provide a forum for clinicians by clinicians.

The idea for this series came from Dr. Harris Winitz, who served as editor of the series until 1997. During Dr. Winitz's tenure as series editor, many important titles were added to the series, including the following volumes: *Treating Language Disorders, Treating Articulation Disorders, Case Studies in Aphasia Rehabilitation, Treating Cerebral Palsy, Alaryngeal Speech Rehabilitation, Treating Disordered Speech Motor Control, Cleft Palate,* and *Language Intervention: Beyond the Primary Grades.*

The last five additions to the series, *Aging and Communication, Alaryngeal Speech Rehabilitation, Evaluation of Dysphagia in Adults, Treating Disordered Motor Speech Control,* and this book, have been guided by the new series co-editors, Deanie Vogel and Michael P. Cannito. Their intent is to continue the rich tradition of this important series that was established many years ago by Dr. Winitz.

Vocal Rehabilitation for Medical Speech–Language Pathology

Edited by

Christine M. Sapienza
Janina K. Casper

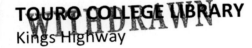
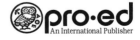
pro·ed
An International Publisher

8700 Shoal Creek Boulevard
Austin, Texas 78757-6897
800/897-3202   Fax 800/397-7633
www.proedinc.com

MW

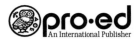
An International Publisher

© 2004 by PRO-ED, Inc.
8700 Shoal Creek Boulevard
Austin, Texas 78757-6897
800/897-3202   Fax 800/397-7633
www.proedinc.com

Library of Congress Cataloging-in-Publicaton Data
Vocal rehabilitation for medical speech-language pathology/edited by Christine
M. Sapienza & Janina Casper.
    p. ; cm. — (For clinicians by clinicians)
  Includes bibliographical references and index.
  ISBN 0-89079-924-5 (hard cover)
1. Voice disorders—Patients—Rehabilitation.
  [DNLM: 1. Voice Disorders—diagnosis.   2. Voice Disorders—therapy.
3. Speech–Language Pathology—methods.   WV 500 V8718   2004]
I. Sapienza, Christine M.   II. Casper, Janina K.   III. Series.
  RF510.V635   2004
  616.85'506—dc22   2003066421

Art Director: Jason Crosier
Designer: Nancy McKinney-Point
This book is designed in Palatino and Eras.

Printed in the United States of America

1 2 3 4 5 6 7 8 9 10   08 07 06 05 04

5/10/05

To my son, Frankie, and my daughter, Kim, my two shining stars. You are wonderful, supportive, and the fun in my life.

—*Christine M. Sapienza*

To my many friends and colleagues around the globe whose work in the "world of voice" has stimulated me and whose support has sustained me.

—*Janina K. Casper*

Dedication

This book is dedicated to Dr. G. Paul Moore in recognition of his years of contributions to voice management and treatment. Dr. Moore is a legacy to the field, a model researcher and clinician who conducted scientific inquiry into how the voice worked and how disease affected its function. He taught us which tools and instrumentation are best used to examine the voice and is famous for his work in laryngeal imaging. His published works were on the forefront of research findings that shaped what we know today about vocal fold movement. Dr. Moore taught countless students and clinicians how to manage patients and differentially diagnose voice problems. A professional in the field for more than 60 years, he continues to stimulate young minds. Now retired, he continues to invent ideas, stimulate programs of education for young clinicians and researchers, and reinforce young clinicians' dreams through dialogue. Dr. Moore truly is an inspiration and has proven his dedication to the field. His accolades are too numerous to list here, but his impact will always be remembered and treasured.

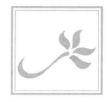

Contents

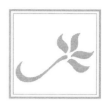

Contributors

Mary Andrianopoulos, PhD
Department of Communication
    Disorders
Arnold House, Box 34610
University of Massachusetts
Amherst, MA 01003-4610

Julie Barkmeier-Kraemer, PhD
Department of Speech and Hearing
    Sciences
University of Arizona, Tucson
PO Box 210071
1131 E. 2nd Street
Tucson, AZ 85721-0071

Mitchell F. Brin, MD
Movement Disorders Center
One Gustave L. Levy Place, Box 1052
Mount Sinai School of Medicine
New York, NY 10029

Janina K. Casper, PhD
Department of Otolaryngology and
    Communication Sciences
SUNY Upstate Medical University
241 Campus West, 750 East Adams
    Street
Syracuse, NY 13210

Savita Collins, MD
Department of Otolaryngology
University of Florida
Gainesville, FL 32611

Paul Davenport, PhD
Department of Physiological Sciences
PO Box 100144 Health Science Center
University of Florida
Gainesville, FL 32610-0144

Pamela Davis, PhD
The University of Sydney
G10–Raglan Street Building
Sydney, NSW 2006 Australia

Cynthia Fox, PhD
Department of Speech and Hearing
    Sciences
University of Arizona, Tucson
PO Box 210071
Tucson, AZ 85721

Gregory Gallivan, MD
Thoracic Surgery and Voice Care
Noble Hospital
299 Carew Sreet, Suite 404
Springfield, MA 01104-2361

Glendon M. Gardner, MD
Department of Otolaryngology
Henry Ford Hospital
2799 West Grand Boulevard
Detroit, MI 48202

Leslie Glaze, PhD
Department of Communication
    Disorders
University of Minnesota Twin Cities
115 Shev H.
164 Pillsbury Drive SE
Minneapolis, MN 55455

Steven Gray, MD
Department of Surgery
Division of Otolaryngology
University Hospital 3C120
50 North Medical Drive
University of Utah
Salt Lake City, UT 84132

Bari Hoffman Ruddy, PhD
Department of Communicative
    Disorders
University of Central Florida
PO Box 162215, HPA 2, Room 101 K
Orlando, FL 32826-2215

Barbara Jacobson, PhD
Speech–Language Sciences Disorders
Henry Ford Hospital
2799 West Grand Boulevard
Detroit, MI 48202

Timothy D. Lee, PhD
Department of Kinesiology
McMaster University
Hamilton, Ontario L8S 4K1 Canada

Michael Lyon, PhD
Department of Otolaryngology
Upstate Medical University
750 East Adams Street
Syracuse, NY 13210

Leslie T. Malmgren, PhD
Department of Otolaryngology and
    Communication Sciences
Room 156 WSK
SUNY Upstate Medical University
750 East Adams Street
Syracuse, NY 13210

Thomas Murry, PhD
Department of Otolaryngology/Head
    and Neck Surgery
Columbia University at New York
    Presbyterian Hospital
New York, NY 10032

Lorraine Olson Ramig, PhD
Department of Speech, Language and
    Hearing Sciences
University of Colorado at Boulder
Boulder, CO 80309

Robin Samlan, MS
Department of Otolaryngology/Head
    and Neck Surgery
Johns Hopkins Outpatient Center
601 North Caroline Street, 6th floor
Baltimore, MD 21287

Christine M. Sapienza, PhD
Communication Sciences and
    Disorders Department
University of Florida
PO Box 117420
Gainesville, FL 32611-7420

Edythe A. Strand, PhD
Division of Speech–Language
    Pathology
Mayo Clinic Rochester
200 First Street SW
Rochester, MN 55905

Susan L. Thibeault, PhD
1201 Behavioral Sciences Building
390 South 1530 East
University of Utah
Salt Lake City, UT 84112-0252

**Monica Nindra Tipirneni, RPh, and
    Kiran Tipirneni, MD, FACS**
The Ear Nose Throat and Plastic
    Surgery Associates
201 N. Lakemont Avenue, Suite 100
Winter Park, FL 32792

Miodrag Velickovic, MD
Movement Disorders Center
One Gustave L. Levy Place, Box 1052
Mount Sinai School of Medicine
New York, NY 10029

Katherine Verdolini, PhD
Department of Communication
    Science and Disorders
School of Health and Rehabilitation
    Sciences
University of Pittsburgh
4033 Forbes Tower
Pittsburgh, PA 15260

Gayle E. Woodson, MD
Division of Otolaryngology/
    Department of Surgery
Southern Illinois University
Springfield, IL 62794-9638

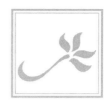

List of Figures and Tables

Figures

Tables

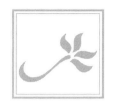

Foreword

Vocal Rehabilitation in Medical Speech–Language Pathology is an outstanding addition to the literature. It combines the insights of some of the field's most distinguished scholars with a wealth of practical, expert clinical experience. In the rapidly evolving world of voice care, a book that organizes state-of-the-art information and presents it with the mature perspective of world-class clinician–scientists should prove to be an invaluable resource for voice-care professionals.

To introduce the book, Sapienza and Casper provide a broad perspective on the evolution of vocal rehabilitation. The following chapter by Thibeault and Gray summarizes elegantly Gray's classic discoveries about the body's response to trauma, as well as the work of other authors. This information crystalizes the scientific basis of phonotraumatic injury, which underlies many of the behaviors that require the intervention of a speech–language pathologist. Chapter 3, Neurophysiology of Vocal Rehabilitation, reviews this complex subject well, with a particularly insightful discussion of the central components of phonatory neuroanatomy and neurophysiology. Chapter 4, Vascular Supply of the Larynx, and Chapter 13, Optimizing Motor Learning in Speech Interventions, provide similarly erudite syntheses of complex material. Malmgren and Glaze integrate basic science into their clinical approaches for the management of vocal fold atrophy, bowing, and immobility in Chapter 5 and provide a particularly good overview of relevant muscle research. Chapters 6, 7, and 8, which deal with spasmodic dysphonia, paradoxical vocal fold movement, and Parkinson's disease, respectively, are definitive, as would be expected from the authors who were selected to write them. Chapters 9 and 10, which discuss laryngeal manifestations of systemic illness and reflux disease, respectively, provide overviews that should be of practical value to speech–language pathologists. In Chapter 11, Davenport and Sapienza provide the expected and elegant review of pulmonary function and its relation to phonation and voice rehabilitation. The chapter on medications is also expertly written and of immediate value to the practicing clinician. Finally, Chapter 13 offers a cogent analysis of motor learning theory. This new book combines into one convenient volume the scientific insights and clinical perspectives of many of the finest experts in the field of voice. It is an invaluable addition to the literature and should be in the library of every voice-care professional.

Robert Thayer Sataloff, MD, DMA
Professor of Otolaryngology—Head and Neck Surgery
Thomas Jefferson University
Chairman, Department of Otolaryngology—
Head and Neck Surgery
Graduate Hospital
Philadelphia, Pennsylvania

Chapter 1

Evolving Perspectives of Voice Assessment and Treatment

Christine M. Sapienza and Janina K. Casper

Sapienza and Casper discuss a philosophical rationale for this text on voice and voice disorders, outlining the general and specific medical issues that affect the practicing speech–language pathologist (SLP). These issues have evolved as the discipline of speech pathology has changed in response to modifications in health-care delivery, such as multidisciplinary care and enhancements in medical technologies and medical care. The importance of the clinician's role and response to the changing environment is presented.

1. *What are the changes in the medical profession that suggest that professionals working with voice and voice disorders must be involved in continuing education processes directed at enhancing the field of medical speech–language pathology?*

2. *How might professionals prepare for current and future challenges involving multidisciplinary care of the voice?*

3. *Are there examples that we can provide of advances in medical technology that have influenced our clinical care of the voice?*

A number of years ago, Special Interest Division 3, The Voice and Its Disorders, of the American Speech-Language-Hearing Association (ASHA) sponsored a consensus conference on medical speech pathology. It became clear during this 2-day conference that medical speech pathology is not based solely on, nor can it be defined by, place of employment. The world of speech–language pathology has undergone incredible changes in all settings. Due to major changes in educational philosophy and the recognized need to educate all children in the least restrictive environment, speech–language pathologists in the public schools now have to treat children with severe medical problems and disabilities that have major effects on speech, voice, language, swallowing, and respiration.

Johnson and Jacobson (1998) dedicated an entire book to the general medical issues that affect the speech–language pathologist and reviewed the current issues in health-care delivery. They also reviewed the various perspectives concerning differentiating medical speech–pathology practices from more traditional speech–pathology practices. Regardless of the perspective one holds, and regardless of the setting in which one practices, science plays an integral role in shaping clinical practice. In addition, because of the human ability to produce voice, shape it into meaningful tones and sounds, and use it for so many varied purposes, our science depends on—and must be partnered with—a variety of medical disciplines. When members of various disciplines join in an effort to successfully assess and treat patients, we witness a true relationship between knowledge and practice.

Indeed, our field is constantly growing and changing, and we must be highly knowledgeable in the medical aspects of voice care. For the SLP, the emphasis has shifted from a purely educational, developmental, linguistic, or pragmatic role to one that increasingly includes medical practice sites. Patient issues require the clinician to have more skills and fluid knowledge in human anatomy and physiology, neuroanatomy and physiology, instrumentation, computer applications, and multitudes of other topics in the medical management area. Sometimes the changes to which we, as clinicians, must adapt are radical, and sometimes they occur slowly, over time.

As a discipline within the field of communication disorders, the field of voice has changed its direction slowly, evolving from a behaviorally oriented discipline to one that has responsibilities within the medical domain. The role of the speech–voice pathologist has broadened and includes vocal imaging specialist, researcher, therapist guiding recovery and restoration of healthy voice, trainer guiding effective voice use, counsel, and more. We have broadened our scope, yet maintained specificity, working hard to enhance our knowledge base so that we are better able to communicate effectively with the medical management team and with our patients.

The educational foundation of voice care is now a multidisciplinary, cooperative effort. The study of voice encompasses a large number of disciplines, ranging from molecular biology to psychiatry (see Figure 1.1). We attend many conferences in order to keep ourselves informed and current in our approaches. Issues surrounding specialty training have surfaced, and we find other areas within speech–language pathology requiring skill-based training, such as fluency or neurogenic disorders. In the field of voice, we have developed ad hoc position statements defining the role of the speech–language pathologist and teacher of singing in the remediation of singers with voice disorders (American Speech-Language-Hearing Association and National Association of Teachers of Singing, 1992). We have guidelines for training in endoscopy and videostroboscopy and guidelines for the role of the SLP with respect to the evaluation and treatment of tracheoesophageal fistulization/puncture and prosthesis. These position statements indicate that a certain level of skill must be obtained prior to administering particular assessment and treatment techniques.

In the areas of the assessment and treatment of voice, we find ourselves challenged by cases involving syndromic complexities and are asked to delve into histories involving multiple disease processes or polypharmacies. Our training programs must reflect these changes and increasing complexities of practice. Fortunately, enhancement of programs is taking place. Curricula have been modified to accommodate the faster pace of an ever-changing health-care industry. Increased and improved fieldwork education must be a priority. Further requirements must be made so that the student and practicing clinician can engage with others from the contributory sciences involved in the care of the voice (see Figure 1.1). Electronic learning is a new educational component in which on-line programs for enhancing skill-based theory can be developed.

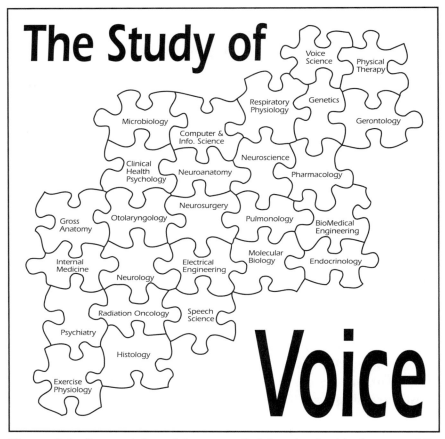

Figure 1.1. Representation of the many disciplines involved in the care of the voice.

Multiple choice questions that test retention of information, and bulletin boards and live chat areas that provide opportunities to discuss information with instructors and peers, are available. Conspicuously absent from electronic learning, however, is a key ingredient: authentic interactive practice activities with tracking and analysis of performance patterns, diagnosis of misconceptions and faulty reasoning, and individualized feedback or coaching. Individuals conducting transfer research have consistently concluded that a critical element to the transfer of learning is the opportunity to practice skills in varied contexts with monitoring and feedback that identifies and corrects misconceptions and faulty reasoning. To date, we have had very little opportunity to train our currently practicing clinicians in this type of domain, although it appears there is discussion by ASHA's Special Interest Division 3 about exploring how these possibilities could work.

In addition, the reorganization of the health-care industry has dealt us an extensive array of changes in the organization, ownership, and regulation of health-care providers and in the delivery of services. Cost concerns, increasing competition, influence of investor priorities, technological advances, changing social attitudes, and an aging and increasingly diverse population are factors that sustain this dynamic condition. Among the primary organizational changes in health care are less reliance on hospital-based care, more reliance on care provided in outpatient settings and in long-term-care nursing facilities, and a shift to managed care. As with any corporation or industry, health-care systems desire efficiency. Internal organizations seek to save money while at the same time trying to improve patient (customer) satisfaction. Typically, this results in the employee's working harder and longer to meet the internal organization's goals. The result is increasing physical and emotional stress levels for the provider (Pindus & Greiner, 1997) and the administrator who is heading the department.

Another requirement is objectively documenting the outcomes of specific treatments in order to provide hard evidence that can be analyzed, data based, studied, and modeled. The most immediate and pronounced effect of these changes has been a closer examination of the nature, frequency, necessity, and costs of services. In response to this call, ASHA's executive board responded by appointing an ad hoc committee in 1998–1999 on the changing role of the speech–language pathologist across the health-care continuum. The charge of the committee was to provide current, relevant information about the rapidly changing arena of speech–language pathology service delivery across the broad spectrum of health care. The committee members prepared a series of issue briefs on four different settings: acute care in a medical setting, inpatient rehabilitation hospitals, long-term care, and home care (American Speech-Language-Hearing Association Ad Hoc Committee, 1998). One area that deserves attention here is related to patient factors.

These factors, along with the evolving responsibilities of the speech–voice pathologist, have prompted the development of this book, which is meant to bring together science and practice in hopes of presenting advanced material on topics of interest to the voice community and particularly to researchers in voice. The topics of interest were developed largely from observation of communications that occurred among researchers and clinicians on the Special Interest Division 3 listserv. Often these persons were searching for information about topics or problems encountered in practice they could not find in available texts.

The patient factors that are creating a need to tie science to practice are due in part to changes in the nation's demographics and in part to the expectations of patients concerning their care. First, the population as a whole is living longer. Science has made many advancements and has managed to slow down the disease processes associated with aging. Second, when patients do develop illnesses, treatment is sustaining them, sometimes in an acute stage of their illness, sometimes in a more chronic state. The provider's treatment regimen has to be expanded, the duration of time the patient is seen becomes longer, and the plan of care needs to be adapted to meet the patient's current and future needs. Third, as technology advances and research yields improved surgical techniques with minimal morbidity, there is a reduced need for certain behavioral methods of therapy. For example, treatment of vocal fold paralysis previously may have relied on behavioral intervention focused on vocal adduction exercises or other compensatory voicing strategies, such as amplification. Now we have sophisticated surgical interventions that often reduce the degree of behavioral voice therapy needed to produce a positive outcome. Fourth, the patient population has become increasingly culturally diverse. Basic science has directed attention to studying gender, age, race, regional differences, and other cultural differences in order to place a value on these differences and understand how they may influence assessment and treatment choices or outcomes. Fifth, our patients are better informed. They come to their assessment with information from support groups and through Internet access to medical sites that explain their disease process or their symptoms. Patients' expectations are high, and patients have access to many treatment places.

Consumers are becoming activists in their health care rather than passively allowing health-care plans or providers to dictate the destiny of their health. They are well aware of reimbursement issues and are acutely aware of the financial burdens of what may be prescribed for them. ASHA's ad hoc committee summarized the impact of all of these changes on the patient delivery model, and we find that we are acting more as consultants as well as rehabilitation specialists with regard to some disease processes. We also are becoming increasingly responsible for collaborating and communicating with all members of a patient's health-care team, and we need to familiarize ourselves with the ever-changing medical models. We must continue to educate ourselves so we may keep up with the advances in technology. This need may be due not only to a rapidity of change in our discipline but also to the rapidity of change in other disciplines (e.g., imaging, molecular biology, surgery).

Numerous technological advances cross over into the field of voice. In 1999 the Council on the Economic Impact of Health Care Change addressed the impact technology has had on the health-care system and on disease management. The Council predicted that in the next 20 years, more computer-assisted biological science and pharmaceutical and clinical lab innovations will be transforming our clinical capabilities and the assessment and treatment of disease. According to the Council report, it may not be unusual to see treatments for some diseases being conducted prior to birth. This will have an impact on our field as current treatment regimes for certain congenital conditions become obsolete or vastly altered.

The National Institutes of Health, a major force behind technological development, has received substantial increases in funding. Since 1998, there have been significant advances in the following areas of medicine, all of which have an impact on the care of the voice:

- pharmacogenomics
- brain damage and spinal cord injury
- cancer therapy and viruses
- antibiotics and resistant infections
- autoimmune disease
- the aging process

Within our discipline, technological advances include functional magnetic resonance imaging, high-speed video image analysis, computer-assisted biofeedback techniques, advanced animal modeling techniques, and enhanced surgical procedures. It was not that long ago that we witnessed the first laryngeal transplant, which was performed in 1999 at the Cleveland Clinic by Dr. Marshall Strome and his team of physicians.

In order to appreciate such groundbreaking events, we need to acknowledge the fact that advances in the core science of our discipline are being made nationally and internationally at facilities dedicated to the advancement of science and medical practice. For example, one area of voice research was begun in the late 1940s in Groningen at the Institute of Physiology of the Faculty of Medicine by Van den Berg. His fundamental 1958 article on the myoelastic–aerodynamic theory of voice production forever shaped our perceptions concerning the function of the vocal folds. There are many important contributors to research on the voice, voice care, and voice science. The contributors to this book, as well as all of our contemporary colleagues dedicated to the study of voice, are among that group.

Our mission over the next 10 to 20 years will be to continue to enhance our knowledge of the literature, conduct open discussion and debate regarding specialization, promote continuing education, develop distance-learning programs, and offer workshops to prepare practicing clinicians in the medically based practice issues previously discussed. We have promoted mentoring as a means to organize the training of professionals who want advanced educational experiences. Professionals in the field are making videotapes and offering organized experiences outside of the traditional academic setting. In the development of these venues, we must always consider the pragmatics of time, costs, and geographic region so that everyone in need of skills enhancement can participate.

Finally, our national organization (ASHA) is requiring that academic programs change curricula so that clinical skills will be assessed. It appears that there will be new freedoms in defining curricula, although documenting knowledge and skills will still be required. Some individuals believe that curricular changes should address the areas of the physical and biological sciences to increase the abilities of graduate students and prepare them to deal with the technological advances that will occur throughout their careers. In addition to curricular changes, more practicum hours at the graduate level, with an emphasis on developing skills across the life span and addressing diverse populations, will be required.

For persons practicing in the area of voice and its disorders, we expect the following academic preparation: understanding of the normal and physiologic processes of voice production; understanding of the etiological bases of voice disorders; the ability to examine and interpret laryngeal structure and function; understanding of the instrumentation used to examine laryngeal structure and function; understanding of the principles of diagnosis; understanding of the structural and functional differences across the life span; the ability to assist in differentially diagnosing the disorder and classifying it as functional, organic, or neurological; and the ability to develop a treatment plan that considers the patient's functional outcome goals. Additional courses might include issues surrounding continuum of care, interdisciplinary approaches, pharmacology, medical terminology, patient advocacy, and accreditations. This is not an exhaustive list, but rather one that suggests that our literature, as well as academic coursework, must accommodate our needs more fully.

The For Clinicians by Clinicians series is associated with clinical practice, and the authors of the chapters in this book worked together to interpret how scientific knowledge and findings influence assessment and treatment. They exchanged their ideas and communicated with each other, blending their areas of interest. For this book, we asked individuals in the fields of basic science, medicine, and clinical practice to help bridge the gap between science and practice, to help us understand the complexity of certain disease processes, to update us on the current literature, and to discuss entities related to voice and disease that are not broached in the routine classroom textbook. As the various knowledge bases continue to grow, it is imperative that we use this approach of combined learning to inform our practice.

References

American Speech-Language-Hearing Association Ad Hoc Committee. (1998). *Health care issues brief: Acute care.* Retrieved September 15, 2001, from http://professional.asha.org/community/slp/acute_care.cfm

American Speech-Language-Hearing Association and National Association of Teachers of Singing. (1992, November/December). The role of the speech–language pathologist and teacher of singing in remediation of singers with voice disorders: ASHA and NATS joint statement [Position paper]. *The NATS Journal,* p. 3.

Council on the Economic Impact of Health Care Change. (1999). *Summary.* Retrieved September 15, 2001, from http://sihp.brandeis.edu/council/html/technology_summary.htm

Johnson, A. F., & Jacobson, B. H. (Eds.). (1998). *Medical speech–language pathology: A practitioner's guide.* New York: Thieme.

Pindus, N. M., & Greiner, A. (1997). *The effects of health care industry changes on health care workers and quality of patient care: Summary of literature and research.* Retrieved September 15, 2001, from http://www.urban.org/health/pindus.htm#2

Van den Berg, J. (1958). Myoelastic-aerodynamic theory of voice production. *Journal of Speech and Hearing Research, 1,* 227–244.

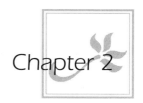

Chapter 2

Response of the Vocal Mechanism to Trauma

Susan L. Thibeault and Steven Gray

Thibeault and Gray point out that an improved insight into the etiology of vocal fold lesions provides a better understanding of treatment. The authors note that knowledge of predisposing factors to tissue injury and poor wound repair allows improved management that will, in turn, minimize or eliminate subsequent dysphonia. In this chapter, Thibeault and Gray discuss the wound-healing paradigm and describe the cellular response of the larynx to various traumas.

1. *What are the main elements of wound repair?*

2. *How can the information presented in this chapter be integrated into clinical care from the perspectives of the speech–language pathologist, the otolaryngologist, and the patient?*

3. *How can we predict the vocal fold tissue's reaction to phono-trauma, and will it be the same in every case?*

Trauma of the vocal mechanism is a consequence of a wide variety of etiologies, including excessive vocal use, that lead to phonotrauma, intubation, intentional or incidental resection of laryngeal tissue, inflammation caused by infection or physical irritants, and laryngeal injury secondary to acute or blunt accident. Trauma can be the cause of dysphonias related to benign lesions, scarring, and hyperfunctional voice usage. Histologically, the majority of injuries are limited to the superficial lamina propria, and pathogenesis abides by a wound-healing paradigm. Knowledge of the wound repair process allows clinicians to better understand the altered tissue composition and its relationship to vocal tissue mobility.

Wound Repair

Wound repair is a highly organized biologic process that can fluctuate to some extent, depending on the tissue type and wound injury. Wound repair of the larynx involves complex processes and is similar to wound repair for other parts of the body. The major stages of repair are hemostasis/coagulation, inflammation, mesenchymal (or matrix) cell migration and proliferation, angiogenesis, epithelization, protein and proteoglycan synthesis, and wound contraction and remodeling. Most reports regarding wound healing are based on research performed on humans and animals. The research models usually use skin and dermis and underlying connective tissue. Because few wound healing studies have been conducted on the vocal folds, the timeline discussed in this chapter is based on commonly accepted research on wound healing in general (see Figure 2.1). Some specific items may be different, however, in regard to the vocal folds. Most surgeons believe that wound healing occurs more rapidly in the vocal folds than in soft tissue or skin wounds.

Hemostasis/Coagulation

The stoppage of the flow or circulation of blood is *hemostasis*. This is accomplished by the formation of a blood clot to plug the damaged blood vessels. Hemostasis is the first step in most wound healing

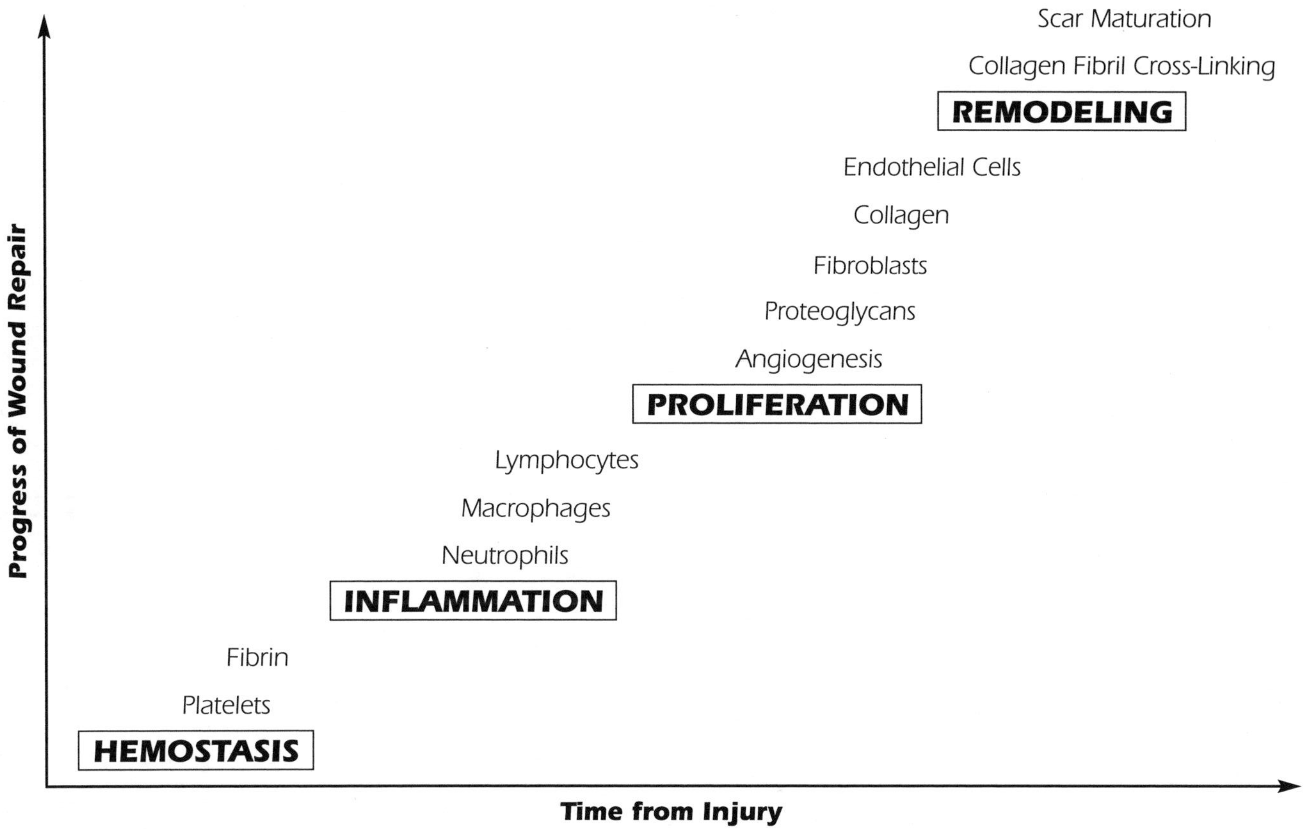

Figure 2.1. Timeline of the biological process involved in wound healing.

following tissue injury. The intrinsic pathway of the coagulation cascade is activated when blood is exposed to a negatively charged foreign surface or wound site. As a result of the coagulation cascade, a fibrin clot is formed in platelet aggregates. Fibrin becomes the primary component of the provision matrix that forms in the wound during the early healing period. This matrix provides a scaffold for future migration of inflammatory and mesenchymal cells. The coagulation cascade also releases chemical messages that tell the body that tissue injury has occurred so that the body will send cells to help with the wound healing. Consequently, a large blood clot will stimulate more aggressive wound repair than a small clot. For this reason, surgeons try to minimize bleeding and blood clots.

Inflammation

Inflammation is defined as the reaction of vascularized living tissue to local injury, and it elicits a series of events that have implications for the entire healing process. Inflammation is initiated through intense local vasoconstriction (to help stop bleeding and promote hemostasis) that is replaced by vasodilation after approximately 10 to 15 minutes (Lawrence, 1998). Plasma leaks into the extravascular compartment via newly formed gaps between the endothelial cells of the capillaries, generating edema. Large numbers of neutrophils in the matrix serve to engulf foreign material and absorb it by using hydrolytic enzymes and oxygen radicals. Approximately 48 to 84 hours after injury (Lawrence, 1998), neutrophils are phagocytosed and destroyed by macrophages. These macrophages also break down damaged matrix during remodeling.

Inflammation plays a necessary and important role in wound healing. However, because inflammation is mostly involved with destroying damaged proteins, dead tissue, and bacteria, persistent inflammation can lead to excessive tissue damage and subsequent infection, both of which create a less than optimal environment for tissue regeneration.

Matrix Cell Migration and Proliferation

Matrix cell migration and proliferation are mediated by the fibroblasts. These connective tissue cells migrate from surrounding undamaged tissue into the wounded matrix. The presence of fibroblasts is important for subsequent synthesis of extracellular matrix components, such as proteins, lipids, and carbohydrates. Fibroblasts are generally considered to be cells of maintenance. During wound repair, fibroblasts undergo a change that allows them to be more effective at both maintaining and actually repairing the tissue. These changed fibroblasts are called *myofibroblasts*. The presence of myofibroblasts in any tissue indicates injury has occurred recently at that location. One of the important studies on vocal injury involved finding and counting myofibroblasts in normal human vocal folds. Catten, Gray, Hammond, Zhou, and Hammond (1998) reported that a majority of the normal adult vocal folds they studied had myofibroblasts and that most of them were located in the superficial layer of the lamina propria. This study partially answered questions concerning whether average daily phonation is associated with some level of tissue injury and the areas of the vocal fold most likely to experience actual tissue injury. Catten et al.'s work indicated that most daily phonation does cause mild tissue injury, generally in the superficial layer, and that this injury is associated with matrix repair. This probably is a chronic condition and process that occurs throughout life in all humans. In some people, this chronic, low-grade tissue injury eventually becomes pathologic, leading to dysphonia.

Angiogenesis
New vasculature is formed by small capillary sprouts that develop on the venules at the periphery of the devascularized area. Through proliferation and organization of endothelial cells into capillary tubes, fewer larger vessels are present in the healed wound.

Epithelization
Epithelization begins within hours of injury and is initiated by thickening of the basal cell layer at the wound edge. If the basement membrane is intact, the epithelial cells migrate over it. If the basement membrane is not intact, the cells migrate over a provisional matrix. Cells at the edge of the wound begin to divide approximately 48 to 72 hours after injury (Lawrence, 1998). In vocal fold

injuries, this time frame is probably shorter and faster. This proliferation contributes new cells to the advancing epithelial monolayer. Once contact inhibition (cells come in contact with other cells) is achieved, the epithelial cells differentiate into more basal-like cells. In comparison to normal epithelia, the newly differentiated basal cells are fewer, and the interface between the dermis and epidermis—the basement membrane zone (BMZ)—is atypical. Preserving epithelia and the BMZ seems to improve wound-healing. The reasons for this are not entirely known, but an epithelial covering reduces infection and inflammation. By minimizing these, the body can move to the subsequent steps of the wound-healing process faster. Surgeons therefore try to preserve the epithelium and the BMZ to allow total coverage of the vocal fold wound upon completion of the surgery. By minimizing bleeding, preserving epithelia, and containing surgical injury, surgeons can influence selected aspects of wound repair.

Proteoglycan Synthesis

The fibroblasts that migrate into the wound produce fibrous and interstitial proteins. This cellular activity generally begins about 3 to 5 days after injury. The major protein that is synthesized is collagen, which makes up 50% of the protein found in a scar. Collagen synthesis reaches its maximum about 2 to 4 weeks after injury. In a wound, a collagen matrix eventually takes the place of the earlier fibrin scaffold.

Proteoglycans are also produced by fibroblasts in the wound site. High levels of hyaluronic acid are found in the wound area in the early stages, and fibronectin is present throughout all stages of wound healing. Elastin is not synthesized in response to injury (Martins-Green, 1997); subsequently, scar tissue lacks the normal amount of elastin, decreasing the elastic properties of the repaired tissue.

Wound Contraction and Remodeling

Wound contraction, which begins about 4 to 5 days after injury, denotes centripetal movement of the wound edge toward the center of the wound. Scar remodeling is the final phase of wound healing.

It has been found that the net accumulation of collagen becomes stable at approximately 21 days postinjury (Lawrence, 1998; Martins-Green, 1997). Scar remodeling can continue up to 12 months, with turnover of collagen in a denser, more organized fashion along lines of stress. Various metalloproteinases, tissue inhibitors of metalloproteinases, and enzymes are involved in remodeling. This remodeling is an important process that has ramifications for tissue mobility. Early immature scar tissue is present during the first 1 month to 3 months following injury and is stiff and thick. More mature scar tissue, which is usually found 1 year after injury, is thinner and more pliable.

Traumatic Vocal Fold Lesions

The vocal mechanism is an intricate system that undergoes repetitive forces—shear, stress, and strain. When the vocal mechanism undergoes excessive forces, it is not uncommon for subsequent phonotrauma to occur. The majority of the trauma is evidenced by the presence of benign lesions, which represent an attempt by the system to repair itself. The large majority of benign pathologies appear as differences in the cellular ultrastructure and the extracellular matrix of the superior lamina propria. Lesions can be acute or chronic in nature; histological analysis will indicate which type the lesions are.

Edema of the vocal folds is a generalized swelling of the vocal folds and represents inflammation and capillary leakage. *Acute edema* is the result of increased vasodilation and the subsequent leakage of plasma into the extravascular compartment. *Chronic edema*, also known as *Reinke's edema* or *polypoid degeneration*, indicates hemorrhage, the presence of fibrin and edematous lakes, thickening of the BMZ, and increased vessel wall thickness. Recurrent inflammation may induce an acute edema into a chronic state. The histological characterization of Reinke's edema may represent a recurring injury or repair paradigm that never completely heals.

Repetitive vocal trauma, as seen in vocal fold nodules, may represent changes in the BMZ indicating a separation of the epithelium from the underlying dermis. It has been proposed that this represents an area of stress when the tissue is put into vibration (Gray,

Hammond, & Hanson, 1995). Electron microscopy studies by Gray, Pignatari, and Harding (1994) and Moussallam, Kotby, Ghaly, Nassar, and Barakah (1986) demonstrated thickening of the BMZ, and Courey, Shohet, Scott, and Ossoff (1996) found increased fibronectin, which may represent tearing forces in the subepithelium (see Figures 2.2A–2.2F). Kotby, Nassar, Seif, Helal, and Saleh (1988) described nodular lesions with gaps at the intercellular junctions, disruption and duplication of the BMZ, and collagen fiber depositions. The presence of increased fibronectin corresponds to all stages of wound healing; fibronectin is ubiquitous throughout the process. Gray et al. (1995) suggested that the disorganized BMZ (particularly in injury to the anchoring fibers) may leave the vocal fold in a predisposed state for repetitious injury and that the fibronectin deposition may lead to increased stiffening of that part of the membranous fold.

Polyps have been found to have less fibronectin deposition, less BMZ injury, and more vascular injury (Courey et al., 1996), indicating a primarily acute vascular injury. This injury would correlate with capillary damage and leakage with hemorrhage. Dikkers and Nikkels (1995) described hemorrhage, fibrin and iron deposition, and thrombosis as the components of a "clinical diagnosis" of a polyp. Kotby et al. suggested that edema nodules and polyps may represent a continuum of vocal fold injury. The differences depend on chronicity and whether the tissue injury was focal or diffuse.

Vocal fold cysts are often associated with increased vocal trauma, either as a direct cause or by increasing vocal forces because of their interruption of the glottic vibratory cycle, producing a more forceful vocal closure pattern. Cysts can be lined with columnar or squamous epithelia (Shvero et al., 2000), with a BMZ thickness that falls between the thickness of polyps and that of nodules (Courey et al., 1996).

In most of these lesions, the fibroblasts produce proteins that suggest they are maintaining the tissue in an abnormal state. Whether the fibroblasts are doing this abnormal maintenance in response to ongoing trauma or as a result of past trauma is unclear. Figure 2.3 shows profiles from a normal fold, a laryngeal granuloma, and a left vocal fold polyp. There are differences in protein

(text continues on p. 24)

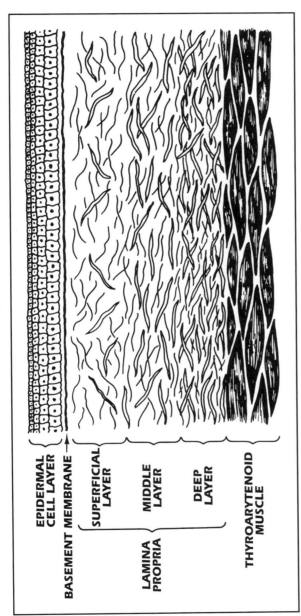

Figure 2.2A. Schematic drawing of the vocal folds. The basement membrane zone is the junction between the epithelial layer and the lamina propria. Phonotraumatic injury generally occurs at the basement membrane zone or in the superficial layer. Capillaries and small blood vessels are not present in the epithelial layer or the basement membrane zone; therefore, any hemorrhage or bleeding into the tissue implies injury to the superficial layer of the lamina propria. Copyright by Steven Gray.

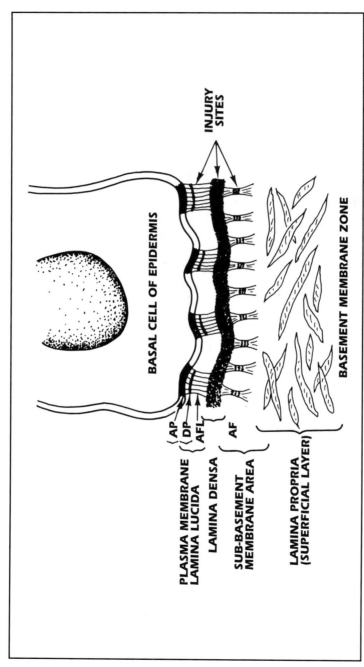

Figure 2.2B. Schematic drawing of the basement membrane zone. This shows how cells of the epithelial layer of the vocal folds attach or secure themselves to the soft, pliable tissue of the lamina propria. The basement membrane zone is composed of a number of proteins to accomplish this. AP = attachment plaques (part of the cell membrane); AFL = anchoring filaments (these attach the cell membrane to the lamina densa, which is collagen Type 4 and is a tough layer of collagen); AF = anchoring fibers made of collagen Type 7 (these fibers loop into the superficial layer of the lamina propria and attach to the lamina densa). Note that injury can occur at many of these areas. Copyright by Steven Gray.

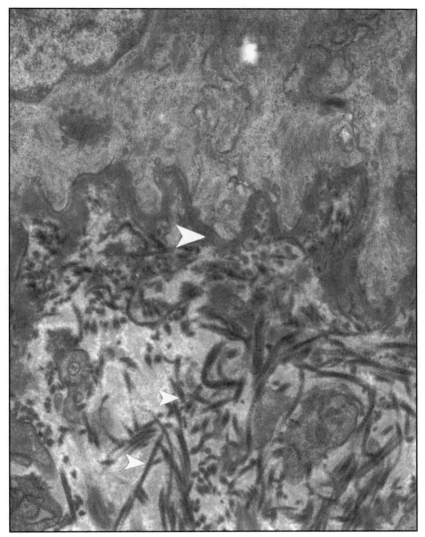

Figure 2.2C. Electron micrograph of a cell from a normal human vocal fold in the top half and the superficial layer in the bottom half. The top white arrow points to the junction of the two and the continuous gray line across the middle, called the lamina densa. Note in the lamina propria the collagen fibers (small arrows) that look like long spindles with a hint of periodic banding. The normal lamina propria should look like this, which shows collagen and some elastin fibers interspersed with a matrix or "soup" of other proteins such as fibronectin, hyaluronic acid, and decorin. Magnification = 50,000 X.

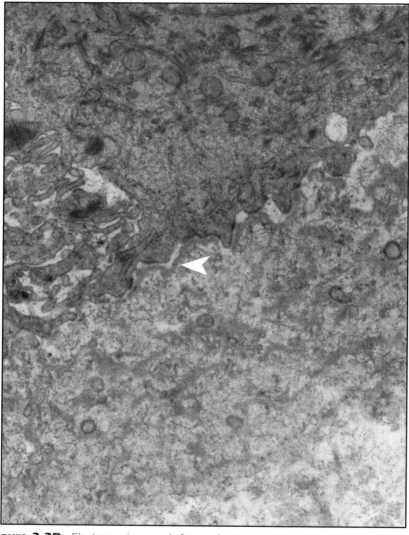

Figure 2.2D. Electron micrograph from a human vocal nodule. The epithelial cell is in the top half and the nodule is in the bottom half. The white arrow points to the junction of the two, which is in the middle of the micrograph. The arrow points exactly to the lamina densa. Note that in this case the lamina densa is discontinuous and there are no collagen fibers below the lamina densa. Instead, the lamina propria area is filled up with "junk" that is poorly organized. Compare this with Figure 2.2C. Magnification = 40,000 X.

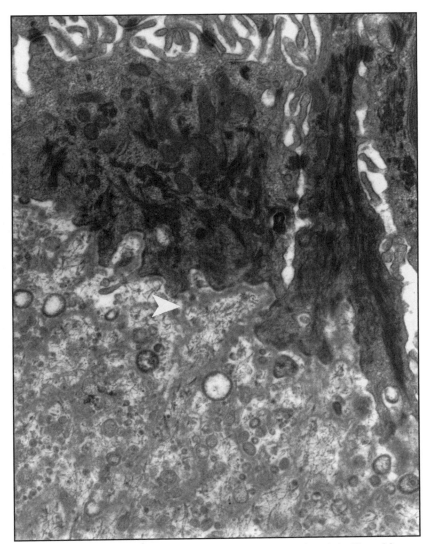

Figure 2.2E. Electron micrograph of another human vocal nodule. The white arrow again points to the junction between the cells and the lamina propria. Note that the lamina densa is again discontinuous and occasionally reduplicates and heads off into the lamina propria. The reduplicated lamina densa is seen as the grayish bands that convolute through the area that should be the lamina propria. A closer inspection of Figure 2.2D also shows this. In this micrograph you can also see many round structures (called extracellular organelles) in the lamina propria area. These probably are proteins that are incompletely organized or assembled due to persistent trauma and injury of the tissue. Magnification = 40,000 X.

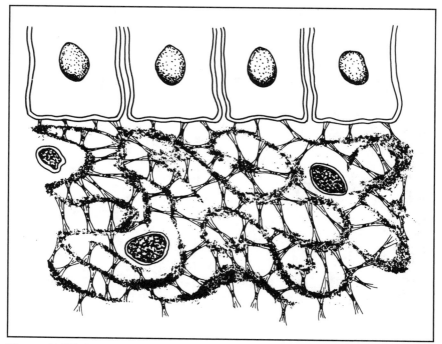

Figure 2.2F. Schematic of a vocal nodule at the cell/lamina propria junction. This illustration shows a discontinuous lamina densa that reduplicates. Normal lamina propria structures, such as collagen and elastin fibers, are absent. Anchoring fibers are unorganized and dispersed throughout the area. Round extracellular organelles, which usually are not found in the superficial layer, are present. These changes probably are the result of repetitive injury and incomplete healing before the next injury occurred.

production among the three. Clearly the fibroblasts are behaving differently in each lesion.

Vocal fold scarring can occur after surgery or injury. Vocal fold scarring represents completed wound healing with resultant disorganized collagen, decreased procollagen, decreased elastin, and changes in the proportion of other interstitial proteins. The altered relationship between the fibrous and interstitial proteins is probably responsible for the negative effect on the propagation of the mucosal wave and the considerable stiffness seen in vocal fold scarring. In fetal wounds, healing occurs without the occurrence of a scar because the environment is rich in hyaluronic acid and fibro-

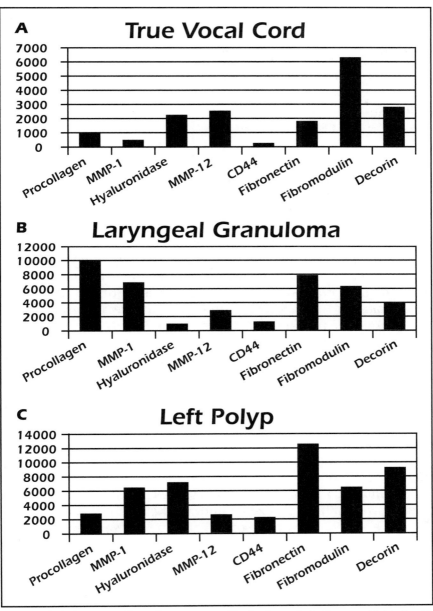

Figure 2.3. Three profiles of gene expression by the cells in the vocal folds for (A) normal vocal folds, (B) vocal process granuloma, and (C) vocal polyp. Note that the profiles of which proteins are being produced or enzymatically destroyed is different for each condition. This is the state-of-the art method for researching benign conditions of the vocal folds. *Note.* MMP-1 = matrix metalloproteinase 1; MMP-12 = matrix metalloproteinase 2; CD44 = recyclable surface cell receptor for hyaluronic acid.

nectin (Mackool, Gittes, & Longaker, 1998). Future research investigating the effects of hyaluronic acid and fibronectin on a vocal fold scar may provide information that will lead to promising treatment options.

Treatment

Physical mucosal irritants—gastroesophageal reflux disease (GERD), smoking, and allergies—predispose tissue to be less than optimum, which can hinder healing due to prolonged inflammation and edema. Catten et al. (1998) demonstrated that in normal larynges there is a significant macrophage presence in the superficial 20% of the lamina propria and suggested that this indicates mediation of inflammation in response to mucosal irritants. Prior to surgical intervention, management may include smoking cessation and medical treatment for GERD. If vocal tissue is not at its optimum at the time of surgery, more serious scarring effects can occur.

Iatrogenic trauma can be minimized during surgical intervention by limiting, whenever possible, dissection in the superficial lamina propria. The superficial lamina propria ultrastructurally has increased decorin (Pawlak, Hammond, Hammond, & Gray, 1996), which has been hypothesized to play a role in minimizing scarring and promoting wound healing in other parts of the body. In addition, excision of the lesion without excessive tissue removal is recommended to promote wound healing.

A gender effect that predisposes women to increased vocal fold injury has been hypothesized. In normal histological studies, Gray, Titze, Alipour, and Hammond (2000) found a gender effect concerning hyaluronic acid, in that the women had less hyaluronic acid than did the men. Gray et al. suggested that perhaps the presence of more hyaluronic acid in men allows for withstanding increased phonotrauma and the subsequent occurrence of fewer nodules.

Intubation may cause granulomas along the arytenoids via prolonged intubation, use of too large a tube, or incorrect placement or removal of the tube. GERD has also been implicated as a significant cause of granulomas. Medical or surgical treatment is a probable treatment route for elimination of granulomas.

Postoperatively, a period of vocal rest may help reduce vibratory forces and allow prompt and undisturbed tissue healing. The exact length of this rest period has not been determined, because of a paucity of research in this area. What research has been done has been largely anecdotal. All researchers and clinicians do agree, however, that some period of rest is appropriate. Voice rest may consist of limited, easy onset, and soft vocalizations. This reduces the possibility of placing excess forces on the tissue, which will maximize healing and minimize inflammation.

Conclusion

When exposed to trauma, the vocal mechanism attempts to repair itself through the pathophysiological process of wound healing. Studies that have looked at markers of wound healing in the vocal mechanism have demonstrated that the phases of wound repair vary according to the type of traumatic lesion. These different representations of wound repair mostly likely have concomitant varied effects on the mucosal wave and vibratory pattern. Better understanding of the biology of the effects of trauma will help the clinician improve his or her management of the healing process.

References

Catten, M., Gray, S. D., Hammond, T. H., Zhou, R., & Hammond, E. (1998). Analysis of cellular location and concentration in vocal fold lamina propria. *Archives of Otolaryngology—Head & Neck Surgery, 118,* 663–666.

Courey, M., Shohet, T. A., Scott, M. A., & Ossoff, R. H. (1996). Immunohistochemical characterization of benign lesions. *Annals of Otology, Rhinology & Laryngology, 105,* 525–531.

Dikkers, F., & Nikkels, P. (1995). Benign lesions of the vocal folds: Histopathology and phonotrauma. *Annals of Otology, Rhinology & Laryngology, 104,* 698–703.

Gray, S. D., Hammond, E., & Hanson, D. F. (1995). Benign pathologic responses of the larynx. *Annals of Otology, Rhinology & Laryngology, 104,* 13–18.

Gray, S. D., Pignatari, S., & Harding, P. (1994). Morphologic ultrastructure of anchoring fibers in normal vocal fold basement membrane zone. *Journal of Voice, 8*(1), 48–52.

Gray, S. D., Titze, I. R., Alipour, F., & Hammond, T. H. (2000). Biomechanical and histologic observations of vocal fold fibrous proteins. *Annals of Otology, Rhinology & Laryngology, 109,* 77–85.

Kotby, M. N., Nassar, A. M., Seif, E. I., Helal, E. H., & Saleh, M. M. (1988). Ultrastructural features of vocal fold nodules and polyps. *Acta Otolaryngology, 105,* 477–482.

Lawrence, W. T. (1998). Physiology of the acute wound. *Clinics in Plastic Surgery, 25,* 321–340.

Mackool, R. J., Gittes, G. K., & Longaker, M. T. (1998). Scarless healing: The fetal wound. *Clinics in Plastic Surgery, 25,* 357–365.

Martins-Green, M. (1997). The dynamics of cell–ECM interactions with implications for tissue engineering. In R. Lanza, R. Langer, & W. Chick (Eds.), *Principles of tissue engineering* (pp. 33–56). New York: R. G. Landes.

Moussallam, I., Kotby, M., Ghaly, A., Nassar, A., & Barakah, M. (1986). Histopathological aspects of benign vocal fold lesions associated with dysphonia. In J. Kierchner (Ed.), *Vocal fold histopathology: A symposium* (pp. 65–80). San Diego, CA: College Hill Press.

Pawlak, A. S., Hammond, T., Hammond, E., & Gray, S. D. (1996). Immunocytochemical study of proteoglycans in vocal folds. *Annals of Otology, Rhinology & Laryngology, 105,* 6–11.

Shvero, J., Koren, R., Hadar, T., Yaniv, E., Sandbank, J., Feinmesser, R., et al. (2000). Clinicopathologic study and classification of vocal cord cysts. *Pathology, Research and Practice, 196*(2), 95–98.

Chapter 3

Neurophysiology of Vocal Rehabilitation

Pamela Davis and Edythe A. Strand

Davis and Strand approach human speech and singing as a precise neural integration of a large number of muscle groups. They define vocalization as a highly complex motor skill involving the respiratory system, larynx, and supralaryngeal structures. The authors present a summary of new developments in the fields of neuroanatomy and neurophysiology while considering possible implications for vocal rehabilitation following impairment of the central nervous system (CNS).

1. *Discuss the significance of the periaqueductal gray in the production of both simple and complex vocalization. Provide support from experimental research.*

2. *What is the role of the sensory component of the respiratory system in producing and modifying voice production?*

3. *Numerous phonatory conditions that arise from neuro-anatomical or neurophysiological impairment(s) pose challenges in treatment and assessment. Discuss at least three clinical conditions addressed in this chapter and list the anatomical and physiological changes associated with the disease process.*

The lower brain stem and spinal cord structures essential for life also contain the motoneuronal pools for vocalization. From the caudal, or tail end, upward from the spinal cord junction, the brain stem consists of the medulla, the pons, and the midbrain. The thalamus and hypothalamus are also usually included in definitions of the brain stem. The medulla, pons, and midbrain contain neuronal networks responsible for generating the respiratory rhythm and for maintaining consciousness. Lesions to these regions often result in death. All the major medullary and pontine respiratory structures are probably involved in the patterning of breathing for speech and song, which is no less complex than the integration of the normal respiratory rhythm. We do not know whether breathing and vocalization are integrated by different neural mechanisms. If they are, this may explain why patients who have had traumatic brain injury may adduct their vocal folds for speech out of synchronization with the respiratory system's generation of expiratory abdominal effort.

The cell bodies of the motoneurons that innervate the laryngeal muscles are located in the nucleus ambiguus in the medulla with the cricothyroid (CT) motoneurons rostrally (toward the head), immediately caudal to the facial nucleus, followed by the internal laryngeal muscle representation, thyroarytenoid (TA), lateral cricoarytenoid (LCA), and posterior cricoarytenoid (PCA) in overlapping pools (P. J. Davis & Nail, 1984; Yoshida, Miyazaki, Hirano, Shin, & Kanaseki, 1982). The illustration in Figure 3.1 shows laryngeal TA, PCA, and CT motoneurons labeled by a neurochemical marker. They are labeled on separate sides of the medulla so that the representation of each can be appreciated, but the TA and PCA motoneurons appear to be largely overlapping because they are each located on both sides. The LCA motoneurons (not shown) are essentially co-located in the most caudal half of the TA representation, and the same is considered likely for the interarytenoid motoneurons (Yoshida et al., 1983). Although these motoneurons have been studied only in experimental animals, the principles of arrangement are similar to those in humans. The pharyngeal and palatal motoneurons are located at a similar level to the CT motoneurons (Yoshida et al., 1983), reflecting the different embryonic development of these muscles compared to the other internal laryngeal muscles (TA, LCA, and PCA). This distribution of motoneurons

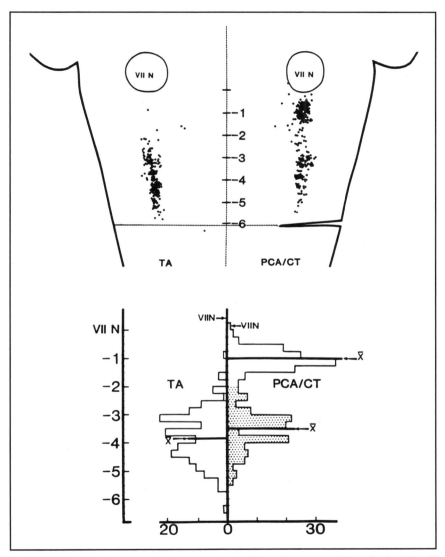

Figure 3.1. Laryngeal thyroarytenoid, posterior cricoarytenoid, and cricothyroid motoneurons labeled by a neurochemical marker.

suggests that a lesion to the nucleus ambiguus would affect all the structures within it, but a small focal lesion would be more likely to affect the TA, LCA, and PCA motoneurons as a group or the CT, pharyngeal, and palatal motoneurons by a more rostrally located small focal lesion. It was also shown by P. J. Davis and Nail (1984) that the size of the laryngeal motoneurons reflects their activity profile, with the PCA and CT muscles, which act to dilate the laryngeal aperture with each breath, having smaller motoneurons than the TA and LCA muscles, which innervate the constrictor muscles. The latter are known to be very fast muscles, whereas the PCA and CT muscles are somewhat slower.

Other important motoneuronal groups for voice production consist of the muscles responsible for opening the mouth and the muscles of the lips, tongue, pharynx, palate, intercostal area, and the abdomen. These extend, almost in a long column, throughout the ventral (toward the belly) and lateral part of the lower brain stem and the spinal cord. The respiratory motoneurons of the diaphragm are located in the cervical spinal cord (C3–C5), with the intercostal and abdominal motoneurons located more caudally in the thoracic and lumbar spinal cord.

Motoneurons are controlled by premotoneurons, or interneurons, and together they form the basic motor unit. Those muscles that have multiple functional roles usually are driven by different premotoneurons. For example, in vocalization, the TA muscle appears to be driven by premotoneurons in the nucleus retroambiguus (NRA), a group of expiratory-related premotoneurons in the caudal part of the medulla. If the medulla is destroyed by medullary transections, which destroy the vocalization motor output, the TA muscle can still be activated by injection of fluid into the mouth via elicitation of the swallowing reflex and via the swallowing premotoneurons located in the pons and medulla, which drive the TA and other muscles for swallowing.

An intact midbrain, and in particular the caudal two thirds of the periaqueductal gray (PAG), is known to be essential for vocalization. An aggregation of neuronal cell bodies, the PAG forms a zone of ventricular gray matter surrounding the cerebral aqueduct. Rostrally the PAG is continuous with the gray matter surrounding the third ventricle in the hypothalamus and thalamus, and caudally it is continuous with the gray matter surrounding the pontine part of the fourth ventricle. In every species studied, vocalization can be evoked by electrical stimulation of the PAG, as well as by electrical stimulation of other sites in the brain (such as the hypothalamus) that stimulate PAG neurons indirectly, because these sites have neuronal connections to the PAG (Bandler, 1982). Studies have shown that destruction of the PAG renders experimental animals and humans mute (Adametz & O'Leary, 1959; Esposito, Demeurisse, Alberti, & Fabbro, 1999; Kelly, Beaton, & Magoun, 1946; Skultety, 1962).

Significantly, a section of the lateral part of the PAG, as described below, is the only brain site from which vocalization can be evoked by injection of chemicals that are excitatory to neuronal cell bodies (Bandler, 1982; Jürgens & Richter, 1986; Lu & Jürgens, 1993). These findings have provided information about the specific neuronal areas that are critical for vocalization. Bandler and Shipley (1994) discovered that (a) the neurons in the PAG are not homogeneous and (b) they form a series of longitudinal columns that are key structures in emotional expression. The columns have different outputs to many voluntary and autonomic body systems, and neurons in these columns are triggered into action by different afferent inputs (Bandler, Keay, Vaughan, & Shipley, 1996). The lateral column is known to mediate vocalization, the fight or flight response through increases in blood pressure and heart rate, a redistribution of blood flow in the body, and the production of nonopioid analgesia (Bandler & Carrive, 1988; Bandler, Carrive, & Zhang, 1991; Bandler et al., 1996; Zhang, Davis, Bandler, & Carrive, 1994).

The PAG neurons that can produce vocalization do not appear to target the motoneurons directly; instead, axons of lateral PAG neurons traverse the midbrain, pons, and medulla to target the NRA. The PAG–NRA pathway has been described in cats (Holstege, 1989) and in primates (Vanderhorst, Terasawa, Ralston, & Holstege, 2000). These NRA premotoneurons in turn project to abdominal, intercostal, pharyngeal, palatal, lingual, facial, and masticatory motoneurons, and probably to laryngeal motoneurons in the nucleus ambiguus (the latter are dispersed and are difficult to identify without specific labeling [P. J. Davis & Nail, 1987]).

There is little doubt that the lateral PAG region plays a key role in the production of emotional vocal sounds produced by animals and humans and in the production of vocal expression by newborns

(P. Davis & Zhang, 1991). What role does the PAG play in more so-phisticated speech and song?

There is extensive input to the PAG from the cortex (Shipley, Ennis, Rizvi, & Behbehani, 1991). It has been suggested that the lateral PAG's sound production circuitry may also be used by cortically evoked vocalization as part of speech and song (P. Davis, Winkworth, Zhang, & Bandler, 1996; P. Davis, Zhang, & Bandler, 1996a, 1996b; H. Holstege & Ehling, 1996), with the emotional expression from the PAG explaining the close links of voice and emotion. It has been suggested that the patterns of human laryngeal and respiratory muscle activation are built upon a neural organization for vowel and voiceless sound production similar to that present in the lateral column of the PAG of subprimate species, such as the cat (P. Davis et al., 1996a, 1996b; Zhang et al., 1994).

Other findings support a role for the PAG in the control of the vocalization underlying speech and song. It has been shown that the laryngeal and vagal afferents provide an important control that is activated during PAG-evoked vocalization so that the duration of vocalization is regulated not only according to the amount of stimulation, and hence probably also to emotional intent, but also according to the amount of air available in the lungs (P. Davis, Bartlett, & Luschei, 1993). This is a fundamental level of control that is present at birth and that rarely becomes impaired. Ambalavanar, Tanaka, Damirjian, and Ludlow (1999) showed a possible pathway for this and other reflex control of vocalization; using c-Fos expression, they demonstrated that internal laryngeal nerve afferents project to the columns of the PAG involved in vocalization. Nonaka, Takahashi, Enomoto, Katada, and Unno (1997) noted that the essential neuronal mechanisms for evoking the Lombard reflex exist within the brain stem. This reflex occurs when a speaker increases his or her vocal effort while speaking during ambient noise. This study showed that the Lombard reflex could be evoked during PAG-evoked vocalization. The studies cited here were conducted with animals, but they offer suggestions as to how some of the basic reflexes underlying vocalization in humans may be organized.

Because the midbrain and the medullary circuitry just described, including the PAG and the structures that it targets (such as the NRA), are essential for generating respiratory patterns specific for vocalization, it is possible that this circuitry plays an important role not only for emotional vocalization but also for the breath-control aspects of voluntary speech and song. These activities are generally perceived as more "natural" if the breathing pattern is not consciously driven, an observation known to actors and singers.

Price (1996) used positron emission tomography (PET) studies in humans to determine that the anterior cingulate cortex and lateral prefrontal cortex were not activated by vocal repetitions and thus are not candidates as a cortical vocal motor pathway to the PAG neurons. He suggested that the anterior cingulate pathway is related to "effortful attention." This speculation led Bandler et al. (1996) to consider an alternative hypothesis for the role of the lateral PAG in speech and song. They suggested that the PAG might not turn laryngeal, respiratory, and orofacial motoneurons on and off during voicing but instead might set a state of emotional and vocal readiness for sound production, with excitation being dependent on control by higher brain centers and afferent input. This proposal was consistent with other evidence, including the cortical inputs to laryngeal motoneurons (Ludlow & Lou, 1996), as described below, and the continuous firing behavior of the PAG neurons during vocalization by primates (Larson, 1991). Bandler et al. (1996) further suggested that cortical voluntary drive to the vocalization motoneurons might be insufficient to generate sound without a parallel level of critical activity in the lateral PAG. This might explain why muteness occurs after a lesion to the part of the brain involving the PAG or the anterior cingulate cortex, even when the voluntary vocal motor system appears to be intact (Boczán, Sorszegi, & Kleininger, 1972; Botez & Barbeau, 1971; Esposito et al., 1999). It may also explain why an injury to the motor cortex does not lead to mutism, because the emotional vocal expression by the lateral PAG is left intact. This was, in fact, suggested earlier by Robinson (1972), following clinical observations on the effects of drugs and emotional state on speech disorders of central origin, which suggested that speech represents a mixture of the neocortical voluntary speech system facilitated by the more primitive emotional vocal system. What is clear is that the hypothesis that both the voluntary and emotional motor systems are needed to speak or sing requires careful testing.

Peripheral Neural Control

The innervation of the internal laryngeal muscles—PCA, TA, LCA, and interarytenoid (IA)—is derived from the axons of the motoneurons in the nucleus ambiguus, which traverse the medulla and exit the CNS in the ipsilateral vagus nerve. The axons of these laryngeal motoneurons make up the recurrent laryngeal branch of the vagus nerve, and they are not segregated into functional groups to the various muscles until the nerve actually enters the larynx. There are relatively few sensory axons in the recurrent laryngeal nerve, and the small number that it contains are from sensory receptors in the tracheal mucosa and smooth muscle, as well as the laryngeal subglottis region.

The CT muscle is innervated by axons from the rostral part of nucleus ambiguus motoneurons that exit via the external laryngeal branch of the superior laryngeal nerve and penetrate the larynx via a foramen, or hole, in the thyroid lamina. The internal laryngeal nerve of the superior laryngeal nerve provides the laryngeal mucosa rostral to the vocal folds with a particularly rich sensory innervation. Many of the sensory axon nerve endings with receptive fields on the aryepiglottic folds, epiglottis, and arytenoid cartilage may be excited by prodding the mucosa with an indentation less than 10 microns, and these neurons are sensitive to movements up to several hundred hertz at these tiny indentations (P. Davis & Nail, 1987). Many of us experience the exquisite nature of laryngeal sensory reflexes such as coughing, which are elicited through stimulation of these nerve endings by, for example, the inhalation of a cake crumb. These nerve endings are ideally designed for this protective function. It has also been shown that these nerve endings discharge during vocalization (Garrett & Luschei, 1987), but the role of this sensory discharge in modulating vocalization remains unclear.

From the respiratory motoneuron cell bodies in the spinal cord, axons exit the CNS in the phrenic, intercostal, subcostal, and thoracoabdominal nerves to innervate the respiratory musculature. The respiratory system is also well endowed with sensory receptors and stretch-sensitive receptors in the smooth muscle lining the trachea and bronchi. They signal the brain that air is filling the lungs, while "irritant" receptors and fine nerve endings located in the respiratory mucosa respond to various irritant and painful stimuli.

The rib cage, abdominal muscles, and abdominal tendons are richly supplied with sensory receptors, including muscle spindles and tendon organs. Gandevia and Macefield (1989) showed that muscle afferents from the parasternal and lateral intercostal and pectoralis major project to the cerebral cortex, and the intercostal muscle afferents appeared to contribute to proprioception and kinesthesia. On the other hand, the diaphragm is poorly supplied with muscle spindles, and projection from the diaphragm to the sensory cortex is weak or unable to be recorded in some humans (Gandevia & Macefield, 1989).

Reflex Control

The reflex control of the structures used for vocalization is a large topic. A great number of reflexes involve the larynx, and many of them are designed to protect the lungs from the ingress of foreign particles. Other reflexes ensure that the laryngeal muscles control the glottic area during breathing, so that breathing is optimized. The key question is which reflexes are facilitated during voice production and which ones are inhibited? P. Davis, Bartlett, and Luschei (1993) summarized some of these respiratory and defensive reflexes and the receptors that are thought to be responsible. They also presented evidence of suppression of protective cough reflexes during vocalization.

Wyke and colleagues (Wyke, 1974, 1983; Wyke & Kirchner, 1975) proposed a theory of "phonatory tuning" that was attractive in that it explained how the laryngeal muscles might be controlled by stretch reflexes originating from laryngeal muscle spindles and laryngeal mucosal and joint receptors. This theory was developed from a fine line of neurophysiological research in which the "servo" hypothesis was used to explain how muscle spindles might work to control muscle activity. Wyke's theory was subsequently shown to be substantially flawed for a number of reasons, including the histological evidence that animal and human laryngeal muscles are poorly endowed with muscle spindles, the negative evidence for stretch reflexes from the larynx (Testerman, 1970), the negative evidence for the fine (gamma) nerves associated with muscle spindles, the lack of evidence for significant recurrent laryngeal nerve afferents, and by physiological testing (Testerman, 1970). The theory had merit, however, in that it stimulated much research, and some aspects require further testing.

Sensory input from the respiratory system, as well as from the larynx, has been shown to be capable of modifying the pattern of activity in laryngeal muscles during vocalization (P. Davis, Bartlett, & Luschei, 1993; P. Davis, Zhang, & Bandler, 1993; Garrett & Luschei, 1987; Testerman, 1970). Even during tracheostomy breathing, it has been shown in experimental animals that altering the air pressure in the lungs and airways, or in the larynx during vocalization, has a profound effect on the motor nerve output to vocalization, the muscle activity, and in particular on the timing of respiration and vocalization. The receptors believed responsible for this reflex lie in the smooth muscle of the tracheobronchial tree (Breuer, 1970; Sant'Ambrogio, 1982) as well as the larynx (P. Davis, Bartlett, & Luschei, 1993). Reflexes from these receptors are naturally elicited by changes in lung volume and air pressure, and they determine the duration of expiration and inspiration. It is thought that these reflexes are utilized in vocalization to interact with the voluntary or emotional intention to determine the duration of the breath group vocalized, according to the availability of air in the lungs.

Higher Brain Control of Voice Production

The human somatic motor system consists of two systems that have evolved separately. Each system can control movement. The older mammalian medial motor system is involved in postural control and the integration of body movements, including orientation of the body and the head. It includes a number of tracts that are concerned with phylogenetically older systems for control of limb movement, such as the red nucleus and rubrospinal tract (G. Holstege, 1996), as well as reticular formation and vestibular structures that are important in facilitation or inhibition of reflex activity controlling muscle tone. This system is also referred to as the *indirect activation pathway of the extrapyramidal system*. The term *extrapyramidal system* is also used to refer to a number of important subcortical structures—the basal ganglia, the subthalamic nucleus, and the substantia nigra (Love & Webb, 2001).

In primates, a lateral voluntary motor system developed that enabled fine and independent control of limb movements, with neurons from the cortex projecting directly to spinal motoneurons controlling limb movement via a corticospinal tract. Some of the cortical neurons project directly to motoneurons; others project via interneurons at the level of the motoneurons, but the pathway is a fast and direct one that is under voluntary control. If the pyramidal system is destroyed, limb movements are retained, although fine control is lost and initiation may be delayed (Lawrence & Kuypers, 1968). The lateral system is also important for human speech movements, with projections from the face region of the motor cortex directly to the motoneurons innervating mouth, tongue, and pharynx/larynx via the corticobulbar tract (Kuypers, 1958).

Because many of the axons cross the midline, the motor control by each hemisphere is contralateral, or to the other side of the body, although the orofacial and laryngeal musculature generally have both ipsilateral (from the same side of the brain) and contralateral motor projections. Ludlow and Lou (1996) used transcranial magnetic stimulation to achieve results that indicated the likelihood that a fast corticobulbar pathway to the larynx existed in each hemisphere. They stated that their data explained why laryngeal motor deficits do not occur following unilateral cortical injury.

The lateral cerebral cortex involving the sensorimotor cortex and Broca's area is considered important in controlling the larynx for vocalization. Penfield and Roberts (1959) determined the function of the various parts of the primary motor area by stimulating the cortex in patients being treated for epilepsy. Vocalization was described as occurring on the lowest part of this cortical strip, in areas that also resulted in activation of muscles in the lips, jaw, and tongue. Close to the primary voice motor area is the premotor cortex (Brodmann's area 6) and the supplementary motor area, which appears to play an important role in speech initiation. Recent research has discovered that much of the subcortical association areas are critical for speech production, but the specific role of these areas in voluntary and emotional vocal control, as opposed to speech and language activities, is not yet clear. Humans are unique in their ability to inhibit emotional sounds, such as to stop or alter the sound of an emotional cry that might lead to some unwanted consequence. This ability has evolved to a high level as the human cortex has evolved, and it probably has played a survival role.

The use of measurement of cerebral blood flow by PET has been significant in developing our understanding of cortical and subcortical activation during vocalization. During singing, cerebral blood flow increases in cortical areas related to motor control were seen in the supplementary motor area, anterior cingulate cortex, precentral gyri, anterior insula (and the adjacent inner face of the precentral operculum), and cerebellum, replicating most of the activated areas previously seen during speech (Perry et al., 1999).

The hypothesis that the organization of prosody in the right hemisphere mirrors that of propositional speech on the left side has followed reports that the anatomical organization of the cortical areas subserving affective speech in the right hemisphere seems to be similar to the organization of cortical areas subserving propositional speech in the left, or "major," hemisphere (Ross & Mesulam, 1979). Recent clinical research has not provided support for this hypothesis (Bradvik et al., 1991), however. The most likely explanation is that the brain utilizes interactive networks over many cortical and subcortical brain regions of both sides of the brain, especially for complex activities such as emotional expression through the vocal patterns of speech and song. The role of higher brain structures in the control of vocalization for speech and song remains less well explored than the role of these structures in language and speech articulation.

Clinical Implications

The previous review of the neuroanatomical and neurophysiologic mechanisms important to phonation points out how extremely complex voice production is. This section will focus on types of phonatory impairment that may result from lesions or damage to the central or peripheral nervous systems and the implications for vocal rehabilitation of neurologic voice disorders.

Voice disorders resulting from neurologic deficits are varied in type and severity. It is sometimes difficult to differentiate a "voice" problem from a more general motor-speech disorder. The voice problem may be among the signs or symptoms of the motor-speech disorder (e.g., the strained vocal quality often seen in spastic dysarthria), or it may be the only manifestation of the disorder (e.g., hypophonia due to Parkinson's disease that is not yet accompanied by other aspects of hypokinetic dysarthria). In either case, it is important to understand the neurophysiologic mechanisms responsible for the dysphonia in order to plan an appropriate intervention.

Neurologic voice problems range from no voice at all (mutism and aphonia) to disorders resulting in hypophonia (too little vocal fold adduction) to hyperphonia (too much vocal fold adduction). Aperiodicity of vocal fold vibration may result from neurologic impairment resulting in changes in (a) the neuromuscular status of the phonatory muscles, (b) respiratory support, or (c) the coordinative control mechanisms that organize the coordination of respiratory/ laryngeal mechanisms. Furthermore, voice production is dependent on respiratory systems for subglottal air pressure and airflow to create and transmit the acoustic signal for speech. Damage to the neural mechanisms important to respiration thus will also affect phonatory function.

The neurophysiologic mechanisms important to voice were reviewed earlier in this chapter. Because of the complexity of those mechanisms essential for vocalization, it sometimes is difficult to isolate the specific neural impairment that is responsible for the voice disorder in a particular patient. It is possible, however, to describe particular phonatory deficits that can be predicted due to damage to specific neural subsystems. In clinical terms, these subsystems include the upper motoneurons (those motoneurons in the cortex and their descending fibers), the lower motoneurons (motor nuclei in the brain stem and their peripheral nerve fibers, which innervate the muscles), the basal ganglia, the cerebellum, and the subcortical and midbrain structures essential for phonation.

A general discussion of the types of phonatory impairment that may result from damage to particular parts of the central and peripheral nervous systems is necessary at this point. This discussion is organized according to neurologic subsystem, with examples of neurologic diseases that impair each subsystem and the associated phonatory characteristics. Mutism is discussed first because it is associated with a number of different neuropathophysiologic etiologies, including the subcortical and midbrain structures essential for phonation. Following will be phonatory deficits resulting from damage to the upper motoneurons, the lower motoneurons, and the basal ganglia and cerebellum. A brief discussion of basic principles of intervention in neurologic voice disorders concludes this chapter.

Subcortical and Midbrain Lesions

The most severe form of neurologic voice impairment is *aphonia,* or loss of phonation. Clinically, an individual with aphonia exhibits an extremely breathy or whispered voice but can execute movement for the production of phonemes, words, and sentences. In contrast, *mutism* is a condition in which the individual has no speech or voice. Although the diagnosis of mutism involves more than just a neurologic problem with phonation, it is relevant to a discussion of neurologic voice deficits. In some mutism cases, there is no phonation at all. In other cases, there may be some reflexive voice, but no voice is used for speech.

Because mutism refers to the absence of speech, there are numerous possible causes. It may be due to loss of consciousness, to structural deficits, to "elected" or volitional causes, to psychiatric disturbance, or to any one of a number of neurologic deficits. Because this chapter focuses on the neurophysiologic mechanisms of voice, only those types of mutism related to central or peripheral nervous systems dysfunctions will be discussed here.

Duffy (1995) noted that mutism may result from the most severe forms of dysarthria, verbal apraxia, aphasia, and other cognitive/affective conditions (see Table 3.1 for a summary of the different types of mutism as described by Duffy).

Mutism resulting from damage to neurophysiologic mechanisms is complex and may relate to a number of interactive neurologic processes, including damage to the bilateral lower motoneurons, the ventral pons and midbrain, the bilateral opercular cortex, the frontal lobe and limbic system, the cerebellum, or the reticular activating system.

A review of the literature indicates that in terms of neurologic deficits, clinical reports of mutism fall into three main categories.

Table 3.1
Major Types of Neurogenic Mutism

Motor speech	Language	Cognitive–Affective	Frontal/Limbic
Anarthria	Aphasia	Decreased arousal	Akinetic mutism
Apraxia of phonation		Persistent vegetative state	
Apraxia of speech			
Cerebellar mutism			

Note. Adapted from the concepts in *Motor Speech Disorders: Substrates, Differential Diagnosis, and Management,* by J. R. Duffy, 1995, St. Louis, MO: Mosby-Yearbook.

A number of researchers reported examples of mutism following corticolimbic damage (Chaudhuri et al., 1999; Cummings, Benson, Houlihan, & Gosenfeld, 1983; Quattrini et al., 1997; Selcuklu, Kurtso, Oktem, Koc, & Kavuncu, 1997). Vascular damage to subcortical areas, including the thalamus and the PAG, have also resulted in mutism (Esposito et al., 1999; Kothare et al., 1998; Nagaratnam, McNeil, & Gilhotra, 1999; Orefice, Fragassi, Lanzillo, Castellano, & Grossi, 1999). The largest body of literature on mutism involves cases following surgery for cerebellar and posterior fossa tumors in adults (Coplin, Kim, Kliot, & Bird, 1997; Dunwoody, Alsagoff, & Yuan, 1997) and, more often, in children (Janssen et al., 1998; Sinha, Rajender, & Dinakar, 1998; Turgut, 1998). Kai, Kuratsu, Suginohara, Marubayashi, and Ushio (1997) noted that the predominance of mutism in children may be due to a relatively high incidence of vermian tumors and the tendency of children to experience personality and behavioral changes after posterior fossa surgery.

Although many researchers have described cases of mutism following posterior fossa surgery, its occurrence is quite rare. Koh, Turkel, and Baram (1997) reported that of 210 children who underwent posterior fossa surgery, only 4 developed mutism. Doxey, Bruce, Sklar, Swift, and Shapiro (1999) reported that the latency for mutism ranged from 1 day to 7 days, and its duration ranged from 6 days to 365 days. Mutism resolved in all cases. Turgut (1998) reviewed 93 cases of mutism following posterior fossa surgery and found that the onset of mutism occurred between postsurgery and 168 hours after and lasted from 1 day to 168 days. Dysarthria was present following mutism in 80% of those cases.

Mutism has also been reported after traumatic brain injury (Dayer, Roulet, Maeder, & Deonna, 1998; Vogel & von Cramon, 1983). Vogel and von Cramon reported on recovery patterns of eight patients with closed-head injury who exhibited mutism. All eight exhibited similar patterns. During the mute stage, phonation occurred only reflexively (e.g., during coughing). In the second stage, nonverbal vocalizations occurred spontaneously or as the result of stimulation. The transition to verbal utterances was accomplished with the onset of a weak whisper. During the next stage, phonation was achieved but usually was dependent on elicitation by the examiner. Spontaneous speech was still whispered. In the final stage, the patient produced phonation in all speaking situations. The authors hypothesized that all patients were affected by compression of the midbrain structures caused by cerebral edema. Computerized tomography scans indicated traumatic midbrain syndrome for all the patients.

Mutism has also been reported to accompany apraxia of speech, especially in the first few days following a cerebral vascular accident (CVA, or stroke; Wertz, LaPointe, & Rosenbek, 1991). This apraxia of phonation often resolves early in treatment. Marshall, Gandour, and Windsor (1988) reported a case study that demonstrated an apraxia of phonation that caused the patient to exhibit what appeared to be aphasia and apraxia of speech. However, when the patient used an electrolarynx, essentially circumventing the larynx, he demonstrated no linguistic deficits, and his supralaryngeal articulation was normal. The authors concluded that the patient did not in fact have an apraxia of speech but rather a selective form of apraxia confined to laryngeal gestures, or apraxia of phonation.

In summary, mutism usually involves much more than just lack of phonation. Neurogenic mutism may result from a variety of neurologic etiologies, and it may be due to deficits in a number of different areas of the nervous system. In many cases, mutism resolves, sometimes leaving the patient with dysarthria.

Upper Motoneuron Damage

There are two major descending motor systems. The pyramidal system (composed of the corticobulbar and corticospinal tracts) is the direct pathway for fine, rapid, and voluntary movement. A number of other tracts (collectively known as the extrapyramidal tracts) affect movement indirectly, primarily by inhibiting excitation of the lower motoneurons. These cell bodies of motoneurons in cortex *and* their descending fibers are clinically referred to as the upper motoneurons (UMNs). The cell bodies of motoneurons in the brain stem and spinal cord (and the peripheral nerve fibers that run from them to muscle) are called lower motoneurons (LMNs).

Lesions of the pyramidal system (corticobulbar tract) result in loss in performance of fine, rapid, and voluntary movement. Lesions to the extrapyramidal descending tracts result in spasticity, or too much muscle tone (*hypertonicity*). Spasticity of the muscles results in weakness, decreased range of motion, and decreased rate of movement. Along with spasticity, the patient will exhibit exaggerated deep muscle reflexes and pathologic oral reflexes, such as suck, snout, and jaw jerk reflexes. Typically, a lesion or disease process affects both pyramidal and extrapyramidal tracts.

Because most of the cranial nerves, including the Xth cranial nerve (the vagus, which supplies the larynx) are bilaterally innervated, unilateral lesions rarely result in laryngeal paralysis. It is important not to confuse two uses of the term *extrapyramidal*, which is used to denote two very different neurologic systems. In this discussion, the term *extrapyramidal* refers to those descending motor pathways, other than the pyramidal tracts, that work to inhibit excitation of the muscles. The term *extrapyramidal* is also used to refer to the basal ganglia, a group of subcortical nuclei that work to facilitate control of movement, including initiation, amplitude, and speed of movement.

When UMNs are damaged bilaterally, however, spasticity will result. Table 3.2 lists the speech and voice characteristics commonly seen in spastic dysarthria. The individual with spasticity in the larynx will exhibit a number of changes in phonatory quality and pitch and in laryngeal flexibility. The most salient sign is a harsh to strained/strangled vocal quality (Duffy, 1995). The reduced inhibition from damaged UMNs causes hyperadduction of the vocal folds and the ventricular folds. The result is increased laryngeal resistance, and the patient must put forth more effort to keep air flowing through the constricted glottis (Aronson, 1990).

The dysphonia resulting from spasticity may also be associated with pitch and phonation breaks. The fundamental frequency is

Table 3.2
Spastic Dysarthria

Phonation	Articulation	Resonance	Prosody
Harsh to strained/strangled phonatory quality	Imprecise consonants	Hypernasality	Slow rate
Reduced fundamental frequency	Vowel distortions		Decreased use of lexical and sentential stress (due to decreased pitch and volume variations)
Tendency for reduced intonational contours			
• Decreased pitch variation (monopitch)			
• Decreased loudness variation (monoloudness)			
Pitch and voice breaks			

often lower. There may be decreased pitch and variation in volume that impedes the individual's ability to mark lexical and sentential stress. This in turn causes a flattening of the overall intonational contours. A bias in laryngeal spasticity toward adduction, with a corresponding difficulty in achieving abduction, often occurs. As a result, patients will frequently voice voiceless sounds.

Etiologies Resulting in Upper Motoneuron Deficits

Table 3.3 lists a number of possible different neurologic etiologies for laryngeal spasticity. The most common is the CVA that has affected both cerebral hemispheres. More diffuse damage also

Table 3.3

Examples of Neurologic Etiologies Resulting in Spasticity

Etiology	Description	Associated dysarthria
Bilateral upper moto-neuron lesions	Typically bilateral strokes or one stroke in internal capsule	Spastic
Pseudobulbar palsy	Neurologists use this term to refer to bilateral paralysis or weakness of the bulbar muscles due to spasticity	Spastic
	Speech–language pathologists may use this term to denote spastic dysarthria	
Traumatic brain injury		Spastic or mixed
Degenerative disease Amyotrophic lateral sclerosis	Motoneuron disease that affects both upper motoneurons and lower motoneurons in both bulbar and spinal systems	Mixed—flaccid/ spastic
Primary lateral sclerosis	Motoneuron disease that affects only upper motoneurons in both spinal and bulbar systems	Spastic
Progressive supranuclear palsy	The most common among the parkinsonian-plus syndromes	Mixed— Hypokinetic and/or spastic; may also see ataxia
	Usually involvement of the subthalamic nucleus, globus pallidus, superior colliculus, pretectal area, and substantia nigra; may also be involvement of a number of brain stem cranial nuclei	
	Usually no cortical involvement, except for frontal lobe	

frequently results in spasticity. This diffuse damage may be caused by traumatic brain injury, anoxia, or a degenerative disease (e.g., amyotrophic lateral sclerosis [ALS], also known as Lou Gehrig's disease). The laryngeal spasticity observed in these disorders results in a strained phonatory quality. This type of dysphonia is often considered a salient sign of spastic dysarthria.

Neurologists often use *pseudobulbar palsy* as a descriptive term for a number of associated characteristics that result from bilateral UMN damage to the corticobulbar system. Individuals will present with spasticity that results in coordinated, but slow, movement and a decreased range of motion. Typically, the orofacial muscles will exhibit UMN signs, such as snout, suck, and jaw jerk reflexes. The patient frequently exhibits a pseudobulbar affect (sometimes called *emotional lability*) in which he or she has difficulty suppressing laughter and tears. The term *pseudobulbar palsy* has also been used in the speech pathology literature as another term for spastic dysarthria (Colton & Casper, 1996). The phonatory quality is harsh to strained/strangled, with all of the laryngeal characteristics frequently cited for spastic dysarthria.

Some degenerative processes also include laryngeal spasticity among the salient signs and symptoms. ALS is a degenerative motoneuron disease. Although the disease results in both spasticity (due to degeneration of UMNs) and flaccidity (due to degeneration of LMNs), the laryngeal muscles typically exhibit more spasticity than flaccidity. This results in a strained phonatory quality, with reduced intonational contours (Strand, Buder, Yorkston, & Ramig, 1994). Carrow, Rivera, Mauldin, and Shamblin (1974) reported that a large percentage of their patients with ALS exhibited strained/strangled or harsh voice qualities. The patient with ALS may exhibit laryngeal stridor due to difficulty with laryngeal abduction. Increased laryngeal resistance due to spasticity is frequently further compromised by reduced respiratory drive. The individual with ALS thus often sounds strained, seems to exhibit a great deal of effort to phonate, uses short phrase lengths, and typically has difficulty devoicing.

Primary lateral sclerosis (PLS) is another category of motoneuron disease. In PLS, the individual exhibits deficits only in UMNs in the spinal or bulbar system (Gastaut, Figarella-Branger, & Somma-Mauvais, 1988; Pringle et al., 1992). The phonatory characteristics will be strained/strangled, accompanied by a decreased ability to vary pitch and intensity. Individuals will exhibit phonatory effort, have difficulty devoicing, and often use very short phrase lengths.

Progressive supranuclear palsy (PSP) is the most common of the parkinsonian-type syndromes (Goetz & Pappert, 1999). Usually, the subthalamic nucleus, globus pallidus, superior colliculus, pretectal area, and substantia nigra are involved. Except for the frontal lobe, there is no cortical involvement. Individuals with PSP share some clinical features with Parkinson's disease, including bradykinesia, rigidity, dysarthria, dysphagia, and dementia. Frequently, bilateral frontal lobe dysfunction (e.g., pseudobulbar affect) occurs. These patients frequently present with a mixed dysarthria. Hypokinetic and spastic dysarthria are most frequently noted. Patients with PSP who have a spastic component to their dysarthria may present with a strained phonatory quality and reduced intonation contours.

Lower Motoneuron and Peripheral Nerve Damage

The clinical manifestations of damage to the LMNs and peripheral nerves are quite different from those seen in cases of UMN damage. In contrast to the spasticity that results from UMN deficits, LMN deficits result in flaccidity, atrophy, and fasciculations. There will be weakness in voluntary and involuntary movements, diminished reflexes, and sometimes paralysis. Phonatory quality is often breathy, hoarse, and reduced in volume. There may also be stridor, or audible inspiration, due to weakness of the laryngeal abductors.

The peripheral nerve includes the LMNs and the efferent peripheral nerve fiber that leaves the motoneuron pool to innervate muscle. As described earlier in this chapter, the Xth cranial nerve, or vagus, is responsible for phonation. The LMNs lie in the nucleus ambiguus in the medulla on each side of the brain stem. Bilaterally, the peripheral nerve fibers divide into three main branches: pharyngeal, superior laryngeal, and recurrent laryngeal. The clinical implications of lesions to the vagus nerve depend on which of its branches are damaged and whether the damage is unilateral or bilateral.

Lesions to the motor nuclei of the vagus in the nucleus ambiguus will affect all peripheral nerve fibers of all three branches (Aronson, 1990). All muscles supplied by the motor component of this nerve therefore will be affected. If the lesion is bilateral, the individual will have little or no movement of the vocal folds, which will be in the abducted position. The patient will exhibit severe hypernasality and loss of pitch range. The voice will be whispered, and the patient will exhibit dysphagia. If the lesion is unilateral, the patient may have mild to moderate hypernasality and a breathy to whispered voice, with some reduced volume and loss of pitch range. The vocal fold will be fixed in the abducted position on the side of the lesion.

Because the pharyngeal branch is responsible for pharyngeal constriction and palatal elevation, lesions that affect only this branch will not have an effect on vocal fold function. The patient will have difficulty with elevation of the soft palate, which will deviate toward the unaffected side when it elevates upon phonation (due to the pulling action of the unimpaired side as it elevates). The individual will have mild to moderate hypernasality.

The superior laryngeal nerve (SLN) has two main branches, the internal branch and the external branch. Isolated damage to the SLN often occurs postviral, with some individuals regaining function within 9 to 12 months. The internal branch of the vagus contains afferent fibers, and damage to it may result in patient complaints of "I always have to clear my throat," or "It feels like something is in there." Because the external branch supplies the cricothyroid muscle, damage to it will result in reduced pitch range and difficulty with pitch control. Patients with superior laryngeal nerve weakness often report slight breathiness and vocal fatigue. The most common symptoms reported are an inability to elevate, maintain, and vary pitch and loss of the upper vocal register. Typical findings on medical examination include a posterior glottal shift toward the weak side, an asymmetric vocal fold level, and mild vocal fold bowing (Nasseri & Maragos, 2000). Acoustic findings vary, depending on whether the recurrent laryngeal nerve is also affected; however, Nasseri and Maragos reported decreased acoustic power and decreased pitch range with superior laryngeal nerve deficits.

The recurrent laryngeal nerve supplies all the other intrinsic muscles of the larynx. Lesions to this branch of the vagus will result in paralysis of the vocal fold. Aronson (1990) noted that if a lesion is isolated to the recurrent laryngeal nerve, the vocal fold will be fixed in the paramedian position. Because the cricothyroid muscle is still able to stretch the vocal fold, it acts as an adductor, pulling th cal fold closer to the midline. If the lesion is higher and includes superior laryngeal nerve, the fold will be fixated more laterally. A unilateral lesion to the recurrent laryngeal nerve will result in a breathy, hoarse voice with reduced volume and possible diplophonia. Bilateral lesions will result in a breathy, hoarse voice and reduced volume.

The type of dysphonia resulting from peripheral nerve damage will vary, depending on the etiology and whether there is bilateral or unilateral involvement. Many neurologic etiologies result in damage to all or part of the vagus. These include trauma, damage due to surgery, inflammation, vascular problems, and degenerative diseases. For example, a vascular problem or trauma due to surgery may cause a unilateral deficit. Unlike UMN deficits due to unilateral lesions, where there may be little consequence to the voice, a unilateral lesion to the vagus will result in phonatory weakness, increased breathiness, and reduced volume (see Chapter 5 for a detailed discussion of vocal fold atrophy and immobility).

Etiologies Resulting in Lower Motoneuron Deficits

Trauma may result in damage to the motor nuclei or to the peripheral nerve. Traumatic brain injury may cause damage to the nuclei in the brain stem. Accidents (automobile accidents, falls where there is a blow to the larynx or neck) may cut or damage the peripheral nerve. Trauma to the nerves supplying the larynx can also occur during some surgical procedures, especially thyroid surgery, cardiac/thoracic surgeries, and some neurosurgical procedures.

Myasthenia gravis is an autoimmune disease in which the acetylcholine (ACh) receptors on the muscle are not able to take up the ACh that makes muscles contract (Goetz & Pappert, 1999). Antibodies are formed against the ACh receptors in the postsynaptic membrane. The number of receptor sites at the motor end plate is reduced, resulting in a decrease in the response of the muscle fiber. Myasthenia gravis is characterized by weakness that is caused by or increased by movement of the muscle and improved by rest. Muscle contraction gets weaker and weaker with repeated use. Individuals with myasthenia gravis may exhibit a normal voice with rest but will exhibit a breathy, hoarse voice with reduced volume

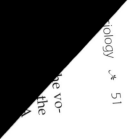

:al assessment, fatiguing the laryngeal mus-
or oral reading) will result in a progressively
lthough, as noted, the voice will improve
get weaker again with continuous use.

ative disease can also affect lower moto-
as discussed earlier because it can result in
..,...geal spasticity due to UMN involvement. Because this is a disease that affects both UMNs and LMNs, the individual may exhibit
phonation more characteristic of LMN deficits. Although most patients with ALS exhibit laryngeal spasticity, especially as the disease progresses, some patients may develop significant atrophy
and weakness of the vocal folds and therefore exhibit a weak,
breathy voice with very low volume (Strand et al., 1994). Patients
with ALS also demonstrate changes in long-term phonatory instability. Aronson, Ramig, Winholtz, and Silber (1992) examined acoustic characteristics of sustained phonation in patients with ALS and
found flutter, which is a fast (9–12 Hz) and rhythmic fluctuation in
pitch and intensity. Flutter is characteristic of the LMN involvement in ALS. Ramig, Scherer, Klasner, Titze, and Horii (1990) examined short-term phonatory instability and found that *shimmer*
(cycle to cycle variability in peak amplitude) and *jitter* (cycle to cycle
variability in the fundamental frequency) increased over time for
one patient during disease progression. Maximum phonation time,
as well as frequency range, decreased over time as the individual's
disease progressed and the phonatory aspects of the dysarthria
became more involved.

Another form of motoneuron disease is progressive bulbar
palsy. Unlike ALS, in which both UMNs and LMNs are involved,
progressive bulbar palsy is the term used when only the LMNs in the
brain stem are affected. The typical LMN deficit of atrophy may occur, resulting in hypophonia. The individual may exhibit a soft
voice with low volume, a weak and breathy voice, and perhaps
flutter. Because of the breathy air escape, he or she may use short
phrase lengths due to reduced subglottal air pressure.

Basal Ganglia and Cerebellar Involvement
The basal ganglia and the cerebellum both work to regulate movement and therefore have an impact on phonatory performance. The

two systems control different aspects of movement through complicated circuitry. Both systems receive input from widespread areas of the cortex and send information back to it through different thalamic nuclei. The specific connections and functions of the two systems are very different, however.

The basal ganglia consist of a group of subcortical structures (striatum, globus pallidus, subthalamic nucleus, and substantia nigra) that work together, through complex interconnections with motor areas of the cortex, to allow automatic performance of learned movement. The basal ganglia are concerned with selective activation and inhibition of motor programs necessary for performance of learned movements and postural control. In general, when movement is generated by cortical or cerebellar mechanisms, the basal ganglia selectively reinforce the desired movement and inhibit competing motor mechanisms. The cerebellum is concerned with the planning and execution of movements by acting as a comparator between motor plans and their actual execution. It works to control posture, balance, and eye movements that maintain equilibrium.

Basal Ganglia Dysfunction. Two very different types of disorders may result from damage to the basal ganglia, depending on whether the damage causes a lack of dopamine or an excess of dopamine. Lack of dopamine impairs the initiation of motor programs, resulting in hypokinesia, or a reduction in movement. An excess of dopamine impairs the suppression of involuntary or extraneous movement (see Kandel, Schwartz, & Jessell [1991] for a more complete explanation of neurotransmitter function in the basal ganglia). The type of phonatory impairment seen in basal ganglia dysfunction will depend on whether there is hypokinesia or hyperkinesia.

Parkinson's disease, a common neurologic disorder, typically is characterized by hypokinesia. It is a degenerative disease resulting in rigidity, bradykinesia, and resting tremor. Many patients with Parkinson's disease have hypokinetic dysarthria in which there is accelerated rate, decreased range of motion of the articulators, reduced volume, and monopitch (Darley, Aronson, & Brown, 1975). Aronson (1990) noted that monopitch results from the rigidity and reduced range of motion of the intrinsic and extrinsic laryngeal muscles. In addition, there is often bowing, or incomplete closure, of the vocal folds, resulting in a breathy voice quality. Hanson, Gerratt, and Ward (1984) reported a relationship between the amount of breathiness and reduced volume with increasing amounts of glottic gap due to bowing of the vocal folds.

Methods of treatment of the hypophonia noted in Parkinson's disease have been widely reported (Baker, Ramig, Johnson, & Freed, 1997; Ramig, Countryman, O'Brien, Hoehn, & Thompson, 1996; Ramig, Countryman, Thompson, & Horii, 1995; Ramig & Dromey, 1996; Ramig & Verdolini, 1998). Please refer to Chapter 8 for a more complete discussion of the dysphonia accompanying Parkinson's disease.

Disorders of the basal ganglia can also result in hyperkinesia, or too much movement or involuntary movement. People with *chorea*, a common example of hyperkinesia, display brief, rapid, and unexpected movements. *Huntington's disease* is a neurodegenerative disorder characterized primarily by chorea and progressive dementia. Phonation is affected in individuals with chorea because of sudden, unexpected movements of the respiratory and laryngeal musculature. This results in irregular pitch fluctuations, voice breaks, and sudden changes in volume. Sudden forced inspiration or exhalation may also be present. Darley, Aronson, and Brown (1969a, 1969b) reported harsh voice quality, strained/strangled phonation, monopitch and monovolume, excess volume variations, transient breathiness, and voice arrests.

Another type of hyperkinesia is *dystonia*, which is a distorted and involuntary twisting or movement of parts of the body. Dystonia may be either focal or generalized, and the degree of speech and voice impairment depends on the muscle groups affected (Hartman & Abbs, 1988.) Disorders of phonation result from laryngeal dystonias and may be characterized by harshness, strained/strangled voice quality, excess volume variation, and voice arrests. There may also be stridor during inhalation, which is secondary to involuntary vocal fold adduction. Golper, Nutt, Rau, and Coleman (1983) reported that of 10 patients referred with Meige's syndrome (blepharospasm–oromandibular dystonia) more than half had voice abnormalities, including voice arrests, inhalation phonation, strained/strangled phonation, harsh voice, vocal tremor, and audible grunts at the end of phrases.

Spasmodic dysphonia is a type of voice disorder characterized by strained vocal quality resulting from laryngospasms that involve either the laryngeal adductors or abductors. The etiology of spasmodic dysphonia may be psychogenic, idiopathic, or neurogenic. If it is neurogenic, it is often action-induced and may be associated with tremor or with dystonia. (See Chapter 6 for a complete discussion of spasmodic dysphonia.)

Phonatory Deficits Due to Cerebellar Dysfunction

Cerebellar Involvement. In contrast to the basal ganglia, which work with the cortex to facilitate volitional movement and inhibit involuntary movement, the cerebellum works to maintain muscle tone and facilitate smooth, coordinated movement. Although surgery to the posterior fossa and the vermis of the cerebellum may result in mutism (see the discussion of mutism earlier in this chapter), damage to the cerebellum does not usually cause loss of phonation or even isolated phonatory deficits. Cerebellar lesions do result in ataxic dysarthria, however, which can affect phonatory function. The cerebellum receives information from the cortex about intended movement goals for speech and then works to compare the adequacy of the movement, making adjustments as necessary to ensure smooth and coordinated movement. Although the speech deficits in ataxic dysarthria are primarily articulatory and prosodic (due to inaccurate direction and timing of movement), phonatory deficits will be seen. Typically, the individual will have difficulty coordinating the respiratory/phonatory mechanisms for speech. He or she may also exhibit a harsh vocal quality, vocal tremor, monopitch, monovolume, and excess volume variation (Darley et al., 1975; Duffy, 1995).

Neurologic Voice Disorders and Rehabilitation

Neurologic voice disorders vary considerably in type and severity, depending on which parts of the central or peripheral nervous systems are involved, the cause of the neurologic damage, and the prognosis for neurologic recovery. Although some types of neurologic deficits are followed by spontaneous recovery (e.g., CVA), others result in a continuous decline in function (e.g., degenerative diseases such as ALS). The intervention used thus will depend on the type of phonatory deficit and the patient's prognosis for recovery. This section covers a number of issues related to clinical thinking concerning neurologic voice rehabilitation. Because a number of chapters in this book address approaches to rehabilitation of the voice depending on the specific type of neurologic dysfunction, references to those chapters are made, where appropriate.

There is very little discussion in the literature regarding treatment for mutism. Intervention approaches used will vary, depending on the neurologic etiology. For example, patients who are mute and abulic due to frontal or limbic pathology may respond to stimulation strategies focused on attention and intent to vocalize. Strategies for patients who are mute due to anarthria and severe forms of dysarthria may benefit most from augmentative communication. For other patients, mutism may resolve quite quickly, leaving him or her with dysarthria. In such cases, traditional approaches to dysarthria treatment will be appropriate.

Individuals with LMN deficits involving the laryngeal muscles may benefit from surgery to medialize the fold or augment the bulk of the fold. However, otolaryngologists typically delay such surgery until 9 months to a year after onset, because spontaneous recovery may occur. For cases of mild weakness or paralysis in which there is good compensation from the healthy vocal fold, exercises to increase the patient's awareness of efficient glottal adduction, without extraneous supraglottic tension, are helpful. Patients with myasthenia gravis are typically successfully treated with anticholinesterase drugs or with a thymectomy. This medical management usually results in improvement in voice and reduction of vocal fatigue.

Treatment of phonation due to laryngeal spasticity is difficult, and behavioral intervention usually is not successful for patients with this problem. Aronson (1990) noted that "aside from therapy for unilateral and bilateral vocal fold paralysis ... most voice disorders due to central and peripheral nervous system diseases are resistant to modification" (p. 342). Most clinicians find this to be especially true for UMN phonatory deficits. Techniques to facilitate head and neck relaxation, as well as laryngeal relaxation, and strategies to maximize efficiency of the respiratory system and use postural control may be helpful. Patients with phonatory deficits due laryngeal dystonia pose similar problems. (Please refer to Chapters 6 and 7 for a more complete discussion of intervention for these types of phonatory deficits.)

The phonatory deficits associated with Parkinson's disease typically are treated by helping the patient achieve and self-monitor for increased laryngeal adduction. The *Lee Silverman Voice Therapy Program* (Ramig et al., 1995; Ramig et al., 1996) has been shown to be efficacious for patients with Parkinson's disease and is a commonly used therapy technique to improve volume in these patients. (Voice therapy for patients with Parkinson's disease is discussed in detail in Chapter 8.)

Treatment of neurologically based hypophonia, hyperphonia, and uncoordination of respiratory/laryngeal movement is often addressed as part of comprehensive treatment for dysarthria. In these cases, the clinician treats phonation in the context of the associated respiratory, articulatory, and prosodic deficits. The focus of treatment is on the interaction of the physiologic subsystems, and the goal is to improve intelligibility. For patients with degenerative disease such as ALS, early treatment may focus on maintaining intelligibility, and staging and timing of the intervention are important (Yorkston, Miller, & Strand, 1995). Later in the disease's progression, the treatment focus is less on respiratory/laryngeal function and more on helping the patient convey more information, even with a degraded acoustic system. This treatment focuses on comprehensibility rather than intelligibility (Yorkston, 1996) and often allows the patient to continue to use speech for a much longer period of time before having to use augmentative or alternative communication systems.

Conclusion

Voice disorders resulting from neurological disease or trauma pose a large set of diagnostic and treatment challenges for the clinician. Neurogenic phonatory impairment varies considerably in type and severity, depending on what neural subsystems are affected. Furthermore, neurologic voice problems often occur as part of a more general motor-speech disorder. Differential diagnosis thus focuses not only on the neurologic etiology but also on the type of phonatory impairment and how the laryngeal impairments interact with respiratory and supralaryngeal movement to impede intelligibility. The phonatory impairments are treated in the context of the phonatory contribution to the dysarthria.

It is clear that phonation plays an important role in intelligibility of speech (Ramig, 1992). Clinicians who assess and treat patients with neurologic communicative disorders must have a broad knowledge base concerning the basic neurophysiology of phonation and an understanding of how neurologic impairment affects laryngeal function. Assessment and management of neurologic voice disorders requires that the clinician consider the interaction of phonatory impairment with respiratory and supralaryngeal movement, which may also be impaired. Although there is a large literature describing the phonatory deficits resulting from neurologic disorders, less has been written about treatment for neurologic voice impairment. Additional clinical research focusing on treatment efficacy in neurologic voice disorders is needed.

References

Adametz, J., & O'Leary, J. L. (1959). Experimental mutism resulting from periaqueductal lesions in cats. *Neurology, 9,* 636–642.

Ambalavanar, R., Tanaka, Y., Damirjian, M., & Ludlow, C. L. (1999). Laryngeal afferent stimulation enhances Fos immunoreactivity in periaqueductal gray in the cat. *Journal of Comparative Neurology, 409,* 411–423.

Aronson, A. E. (1990). *Clinical voice disorders.* New York: Thieme.

Aronson, A. E., Ramig, L. O., Winholtz, W. S., & Silber, S. R. (1992). Rapid voice tremor, or "flutter," in amyotrophic lateral sclerosis. *Annals of Otorhinolaryngology, 101,* 511–518.

Baker, K. K., Ramig, L. O., Johnson, A. B., & Freed, C. R. (1997). Preliminary voice and speech analysis following fetal dopamine transplants in five individuals with Parkinson's disease. *Journal of Speech, Language, and Hearing Research, 40,* 615–626.

Bandler, R. (1982). Induction of rage following microinjections of glutamate into midbrain but not hypothalamus of cats. *Neuroscience Letters, 30,* 183–188.

Bandler, R., & Carrive, P. (1988). Integrated defence reaction elicited by excitatory amino acid injection in the midbrain periaqueductal grey region of the unrestrained cat. *Brain Research, 439,* 95–106.

Bandler, R., Carrive, P., & Zhang, S. P. (1991). Integration of somatic and autonomic reactions within the midbrain periaqueductal grey: Viscerotopic, somatotopic and functional organization. In G. Holstege (Ed.), *Progress in brain research* (Vol. 87, pp. 269–305). Amsterdam: Elsevier.

Bandler, R., Keay, K., Vaughan, C., & Shipley, M. T. (1996). Columnar organization of PAG neurons regulating emotional and vocal expression. In N. Fletcher & P. Davis (Eds.), *Vocal fold physiology: Controlling complexity and chaos* (pp. 137–153). San Diego, CA: Singular.

Bandler, R., & Shipley, M. T. (1994). Columnar organization in the midbrain periaqueductal gray: Modules for emotional expression? *Trends in Neuroscience, 17,* 379–389.

Boczán, G., Sorszegi, P., & Kleininger, O. (1972). Clinical and pathological study of mutism following operations of pinealoma and medulloblastomas. In J. Hirschberg, Gy. Szépe, & E. Vass-Kovács (Eds.), *Papers in interdisciplinary speech research.* Budapest: Akadémiai Kiadó.

Botez, M. I., & Barbeau, A. (1971). Role of subcortical structures, and particularly of the thalamus, in the mechanisms of speech and language. *International Journal of Neurology, 8,* 300–320.

Bradvik, B., Dravins, C., Holtas, S., Rosen, I., Ryding, E., & Ingvar, D. H. (1991). Disturbances of speech prosody following right hemisphere infarcts. *Acta Neurologica Scandinavica, 84,* 114–126.

Breuer, J. (1970). Self-steering of respiration through the nervous vagus. In R. Porter & E. Ullman (Ed. & Trans.), *Breathing: Hering-Breuer centenary symposium* (pp. 365–394). London: Churchill.

Carrow, E., Rivera, V., Mauldin, M., & Shamblin, L. (1974). Deviant speech characteristics in motor neuron disease. *Archives of Otorhinolaryngology, 100,* 212–218.

Chaudhuri, J. R., Anand, J., Shivshankar, N., Jaykumar, P. N., Murali, S. A., & Taly, A. B. (1999). Right parietal infarction with concomitant mutism. *Acta Neurologica Scandinavica, 99,* 77–79.

Colton, R., & Casper, J. L. (1996). *Understanding voice problems: A physiological perspective for diagnosis and treatment.* Baltimore: Williams & Wilkins.

Coplin, W. M., Kim, D. K., Kliot, M., & Bird, T. D. (1997). Mutism in an adult following hypertensive cerebellar hemorrhage: Nosological discussion and illustrative case. *Brain and Language, 59,* 476–493.

Cummings, J. L., Benson, D. F., Houlihan, J. P., & Gosenfeld, L. F. (1983). Mutism: Loss of neocortical and limbic vocalization. *The Journal of Nervous and Mental Disease, 171,* 255–259.

Darley, F. L., Aronson, A. E., & Brown, J. R. (1969a). Clusters of deviant speech dimensions in the dysarthrias. *Journal of Speech and Hearing Research, 12,* 462–496.

Darley, F. L., Aronson, A. E., & Brown, J. R. (1969b). Differential diagnostic patterns of dysarthria. *Journal of Speech and Hearing Research, 12,* 246–269.

Darley, F. L., Aronson, A. E., & Brown, J. R. (1975). *Motor speech disorders.* Philadelphia: W. B. Saunders.

Davis, P., Bartlett, Jr., D., & Luschei, E. (1993). Coordination of the respiratory and laryngeal systems in breathing and vocalization. In I. Titze (Vol. Ed.), *Vocal fold physiology: Vol. 7. Frontiers in basic science* (pp. 189–226). San Diego, CA: Singular.

Davis, P., & Nail, B. S. (1987). Quantitative analysis of laryngeal mechanosensitivity in the cat and rabbit. *Journal of Physiology, 388,* 467–485.

Davis, P., Winkworth, A., Zhang, S. P., & Bandler, R. (1996). The neural control of vocalization: Respiratory and emotional influences. *The Journal of Voice, 10*(1), 23–38.

Davis, P., & Zhang, S. P. (1991). What is the role of the midbrain periaqueductal gray in respiration and vocalization? In A. Depaulis & R. Bandler (Eds.), *The midbrain periaqueductal gray matter: Functional, anatomical, and immunohistochemical organization* (pp. 57–66). New York: Plenum Press.

Davis, P., Zhang, S. P., & Bandler, R. (1993). Pulmonary and upper airway afferent influences on the motor pattern of vocalization evoked by excitation of the midbrain periaqueductal gray of the cat. *Brain Research, 607,* 61–80.

Davis, P., Zhang, S. P., & Bandler, R. (1996a). Midbrain and medullary control of respiration and vocalization. *Progress in Brain Research, 107,* 315–325.

Davis, P., Zhang, S. P., & Bandler, R. (1996b). Midbrain and medullary regulation of vocalization. In N. Fletcher & P. Davis (Eds.), *Vocal fold physiology: Controlling complexity and chaos* (pp. 121–136). San Diego, CA: Singular.

Davis, P. J., & Nail, B. S. (1987). On the localization of laryngeal motoneurons in the cat and rabbit. *Journal of Comparative Neurology, 230,* 13–22.

Dayer, A., Roulet, E., Maeder, P., & Deonna, T. (1998). Post-traumatic mutism in children: Clinical characteristics, pattern of recovery and clinicopathological correlations. *European Journal of Paediatric Neurology, 2,* 109–116.

Doxey, D., Bruce, D., Sklar, F., Swift, D., & Shapiro, K. (1999). Posterior fossa syndrome: Identifiable risk factors and irreversible complications. *Pediatric Neurosurgery, 31,* 131–136.

Duffy, J. R. (1995). *Motor speech disorders: Substrates, differential diagnosis, and management.* St. Louis, MO: Mosby-Yearbook.

Dunwoody, G. W., Alsagoff, Z. S., & Yuan, S. Y. (1997). Cerebellar mutism with subsequent dysarthria in an adult. *British Journal of Neurosurgery, 11,* 161–163.

Esposito, A., Demeurisse, G., Alberti, B., & Fabbro, F. (1999). Complete mutism after midbrain periaqueductal gray lesion. *Neuroreport, 10,* 681–685.

Gandevia, S. C., & Macefield, G. (1989). Projection of low-threshold afferents from human intercostal muscles to the cerebral cortex. *Respiration Physiology, 77,* 203–214.

Garrett, J. D., & Luschei, E. S. (1987). Subglottic pressure modulation during evoked phonation in the anaesthetized cat. In T. Baer, C. Sasaki, & K. Harris (Eds.), *Laryngeal function in phonation and respiration* (pp. 139–153). Boston: College-Hill Press.

Gastaut, J. L., Figarella-Branger, D., & Somma-Mauvais, H. (1988). Chronic progressive spinobulbar spasticity: A rare form of lateral sclerosis. *Archives of Neurology, 45,* 509–513.

Goetz, C. G., & Pappert, E. J. (1999). *Textbook of clinical neurology.* Philadelphia: W. B. Saunders.

Golper, L. A., Nutt, J. G., Rau, M., & Coleman, R. O. (1983). Focal cranial dystonia. *Journal of Speech and Hearing Disorders, 48,* 128–134.

Hanson, D., Gerratt, B. R., & Ward, P. H. (1984). Cinegraphic observations of laryngeal function in Parkinson's disease. *Laryngoscope, 94,* 348–353.

Hartman, D. E., & Abbs, J. H. (1988). Dysarthrias of movement disorders. *Advances in Neurology, 49,* 289–306.

Holstege, G. (1996). The somatic motor system. *Progress in Brain Research, 107,* 9–28.

Holstege, H., & Ehling, T. (1996). Two motor systems involved in the production of speech. In N. Fletcher & P. Davis (Eds.), *Vocal fold physiology: Controlling complexity and chaos* (pp. 121–136). San Diego, CA: Singular.

Janssen, G., Messing-Junger, A. M., Engelbrecht, V., Gobel, U., Bock, W. J., & Lenard, H. G. (1998). Cerebellar mutism syndrome. *Klinische Padiatrie, 210,* 243, 247.

Jürgens, U., & Richter, K. (1986). Glutamate-induced vocalization in the squirrel monkey. *Brain Research, 373,* 349–358.

Kai, Y., Kuratsu, J., Suginohara, K., Marubayashi, T., & Ushio, Y. (1997). Cerebellar mutism after posterior fossa surgery—Two cases. *Neurologia Medico-Chirurgica, 37,* 929–933.

Kandel, E. R., Schwartz, J. H., & Jessell, T. M. (1991). *Principles of neural science.* New York: Elsevier.

Kelly, A. H., Beaton, L. E., & Magoun, H. W. (1946). A midbrain mechanism for facio-vocal activity. *Journal of Neurophysiology, 9,* 181–189.

Koh, S., Turkel, S. B., & Baram, T. Z. (1997). Cerebellar mutism in children: Report of six cases and potential mechanisms. *Pediatric Neurology, 16,* 18–19.

Kothare, S. V., Ebb, D. H., Rosenberger, P. B., Buonanno, F., Schaefer, P. W., & Krishnamoorthy, K. S. (1998). Acute confusion and mutism as a presentation of thalamic strokes secondary to deep cerebral venous thrombosis. *Journal of Child Neurology, 13,* 300–303.

Kuypers, H. G. J. M. (1958). Corticobulbar connections to the pons and lower brain stem in man. *Brain, 81,* 364–388.

Larson, C. R. (1991). Activity of PAG neurons during conditioned vocalization in the macaque monkey. In A. Depaulis & R. Bandler (Eds.), *The midbrain periaqueductal gray matter: Functional, anatomical and neurochemical organization* (pp. 23–40). New York: Plenum Press.

Lawrence, D. G., & Kuypers, H. G. (1968). The functional organization of the motor system in the monkey: II. The effects of lesions of the descending brain-stem pathways. *Brain, 91,* 15–36.

Love, R. J., & Webb, W. G. (2001). *Neurology for the speech language pathologist.* Boston: Butterworth-Heinemann.

Lu, C. L., & Jürgens, U. (1993). Effects of chemical stimulation in the periaqueductal gray on vocalization in the squirrel monkey. *Brain Research Bulletin, 32,* 143–151.

Ludlow, C., & Lou, G. (1996). Observations on human laryngeal muscle control. In N. Fletcher & P. Davis (Eds.), *Vocal fold physiology: Controlling complexity and chaos* (pp. 201–219). San Diego, CA: Singular.

Marshall, R. C., Gandour, J., & Windsor, J. (1988). Selective impairment of phonation: A case study. *Brain and Language, 35,* 313–339.

Nagaratnam, N., McNeil, C., & Gilhotra, J. S. (1999). Akinetic mutism and mixed transcortical aphasia following left thalamomesencephalic infarction. *Journal of the Neurological Sciences, 163,* 70–73.

Nasseri, S. S., & Maragos, N. E. (2000). Combination thyroplasty and the "twisted larynx" combined type IV and type I thyroplasty for superior laryngeal nerve weakness. *Journal of Voice, 14,* 104–111.

Nonaka, S., Takahashi, R., Enomoto, K., Katada, A., & Unno, T. (1997). Lombard reflex during PAG-induced vocalization in decerebrate cats. *Neuroscience Research* (Suppl. 29), 283–289.

Orefice, G., Fragassi, N. A., Lanzillo, R., Castellano, A., & Grossi, D. (1999). Transient muteness followed by dysarthria in patients with pontomesencephalic stroke: Report of two cases. *Cerebrovascular Diseases, 9,* 124–126.

Penfield, W., & Roberts, L. (1959). *Speech and brain mechanisms.* Princeton, NJ: Princeton University Press.

Perry, D. W., Zatorre, R. J., Petrides, M., Alivisatos, B., Meyer, E., & Evans, A. C. (1999). Localization of cerebral activity during simple singing. *Neuroreport, 10,* 3979–3984.

Price, J. (1996). Vocalization and the orbital and medial prefrontal cortex. In N. Fletcher & P. Davis (Eds.), *Vocal fold physiology: Controlling complexity and chaos* (pp. 171–186). San Diego, CA: Singular.

Pringle, C. E., Hudson, A. J., Munoz, D. G., Kiernan, J. A., Brown, W. F., & Ebers, G. C. (1992). Primary lateral sclerosis: Clinical features, neuropathology and diagnostic criteria. *Brain, 115,* 495–520.

Quattrini, A., Del Pesce, M., Provinciali, L., Cesarano, R., Ortenzi, A., Paggi, A., et al. (1997). Mutism in 36 patients who underwent callosotomy for drug-resistant epilepsy. *Journal of Neurosurgical Sciences, 41,* 93–96.

Ramig, L. O. (1992). The role of phonation in speech intelligibility: A review and preliminary data from patients with Parkinson's disease. In R. D. Kent (Ed.), *Intelligibility in speech disorders* (pp. 119–156). Philadelphia: John Benjamins.

Ramig, L. O., Countryman, S., O'Brien, C., Hoehn, M., & Thompson, L. (1996). Intensive speech treatment for patients with Parkinson's disease: Short- and long-term comparison of two techniques. *Neurology, 47,* 1496–1504.

Ramig, L. O., Countryman, S., Thompson, L. L., & Horii, Y. (1995). Comparison of two forms of intensive speech treatment for Parkinson disease. *Journal of Speech and Hearing Research, 38,* 1232–1251.

Ramig, L. O., & Dromey, C. (1996). Aerodynamic mechanisms underlying treatment-related changes in vocal intensity in patients with Parkinson's disease. *Journal of Speech and Hearing Research, 39,* 798–807.

Ramig, L. O., Scherer, R. C., Klasner, E. R., Titze, I. R., & Horii, Y. (1990). Acoustic analysis of voice in amyotrophic lateral sclerosis: A longitudinal case study. *Journal of Speech and Hearing Research, 55,* 2–14.

Ramig, L. O., & Verdolini, K. (1998). Treatment efficacy: Voice disorders. *Journal of Speech, Language, and Hearing Research, 41,* S101–S116.

Robinson, B. W. (1972). Anatomical and physiological contrasts between human and other primate vocalizations. In P. Dolhinow & S. L. Washburn (Eds.), *Perspectives on human evolution* (pp. 438–443). New York: Holt, Rinehart & Winston.

Ross, E. D., & Mesulam, M. M. (1979). Dominant language functions of the right hemisphere? Prosody and emotional gesturing. *Archives of Neurology, 36,* 144–148.

Sant'Ambrogio, G. (1982). Information arising from the tracheobronchial tree of mammals. *Physiological Reviews, 62,* 531–569.

Selcuklu, A., Kurtso, A., Oktem, I. S., Koc, R. K., & Kavuncu, I. A. (1997). Postoperative mutism after the clipping of a distal anterior cerebral artery aneurysm: A case report. *Neurosurgical Review, 20,* 214–216.

Shipley, M. T., Ennis, M., Rizvi, T. A., & Behbehani, M. M. (1991). Topographical specificity of forebrain inputs to the midbrain periaqueductal gray: Evidence for discrete longitudinally organized input columns. In A. Depaulis & R. Bandler (Eds.), *The midbrain periaqueductal gray matter: Functional, anatomical and immunohistochemical organization* (pp. 417–448). New York: Plenum Press.

Sinha, A. K., Rajender, Y., & Dinakar, I. (1998). Transient cerebellar mutism after evacuation of a spontaneous vermian haematoma. *Child's Nervous System, 14*, 460–462.

Skultety, F. M. (1962). Experimental mutism in dogs. *Archives of Neurology, 6*, 235–241.

Strand, E. A., Buder, E. H., Yorkston, K. M., & Ramig, L. O. (1994). Differential phonatory characteristics of four women with amyotrophic lateral sclerosis. *Journal of Voice, 8*, 327–339.

Testerman, R. L. (1970). Modulation of laryngeal activity by pulmonary changes during vocalization in cats. *Experimental Neurology, 29*, 281–297.

Turgut, M. (1998). Transient "cerebellar" mutism. *Child's Nervous System, 14*, 161–166.

Vanderhorst, V., Terasawa, E., Ralston, H., & Holstege, G. (2000). Monosynaptic projections from the lateral periaqueductal gray to the nucleus retroambiguus in the rhesus monkey: Implications for vocalization and reproductive behavior. *Journal of Comparative Neurology, 424*, 251–268.

Vogel, M., & von Cramon, D. (1983). Articulatory recovery after traumatic mutism. *Folia Phoniatrica, 35*, 294–309.

Wertz, R. T., LaPointe, L. L., & Rosenbek, J. C. (1991). *Apraxia of speech in adults: The disorder and its management.* San Diego, CA: Singular.

Wyke, B. (1974). Laryngeal neuromuscular control systems in singing. *Folia Phoniatrica, 26*, 295–306.

Wyke, B. (1983). Reflexogenic contributions to vocal fold control systems. In I. Titze & R. Scherer (Eds.), *Vocal fold physiology: Bio-*

mechanics, acoustics and phonatory control (pp. 138–144). Denver, CO: The Voice Foundation.

Wyke, B. D., & Kirchner, J. A. (1975). The neurology of the larynx. *Scientific Foundations of Otolaryngology, 546–574.*

Yorkston, K. M. (1996). Treatment efficacy: Dysarthria. *Journal of Speech and Hearing Research, 39,* 546–547.

Yorkston, K. M., Miller, R. M., & Strand, E. A. (1995). *Management of speech and swallowing in degenerative diseases.* Tucson, AZ: Communication Skill Builders.

Yoshida, Y., Miyazaki, O., Hirano, M., Shin, T., & Kanaseki, T. (1982). Arrangement of motoneurons innervating the intrinsic laryngeal muscles of cats as demonstrated by horseradish peroxidase. *Acta Otolaryngologica, 94*(3–4), 329–334.

Yoshida, Y., Miyazaki, T., Yamada, M., Mitsumasu, T., Hirano, M., & Kanaseki, T. (1983). Central location of motoneurons supplying the muscles which partake of swallowing and phonation. *Journal of the Japan Bronchoesophagological Society, 34,* 84–92.

Zhang, S. P., Davis, P. J., Bandler, R., & Carrive, P. (1994). Brain stem integration of vocalization: Role of the midbrain periaqueductal gray. *Journal of Neurophysiology, 72,* 1337–1356.

Chapter 4

Vascular Supply of the Larynx

Michael Lyon and Julie Barkmeier-Kraemer

Lyon and Barkmeier provide an overview of the vascular supply of the larynx, its impact on normal function, and its relationship to disease processes. Although textbooks on the voice contain basic information about laryngeal vascular anatomy, and discussion of it is scattered among otolaryngology publications, the authors provide a detailed review and discuss the impact of laryngeal vascular disorders on voice production.

1. *List at least three factors associated with the control of blood flow.*

2. *What is the relationship between metabolic factors and blood flow?*

3. *Name the two primary factors associated with the management of microvascular lesions.*

4. *In addition to speaking techniques, what other behaviors should be modified to avoid phonotrauma?*

In humans, the larynx is generally supplied via three main feed-ing arteries (see Figure 4.1): the superior laryngeal, cricothyroid, and inferior laryngeal arteries. The superior laryngeal and cricothyroid arteries are usually branches of the superior thyroid artery, which is a division of the external carotid artery. One com-mon deviation is for the superior laryngeal artery to branch directly from the external carotid artery. The inferior laryngeal artery is de-rived from the inferior thyroid artery, a part of the subclavian ar-terial system. This anatomical organization suggests not only dif-ferences in embryonic origin but also possible differences in the mechanisms controlling blood flow to the various regions of the larynx. Although there are some variations, this arrangement of three main feeding arteries is fairly similar in the rat (Lyon, 2000b), rabbit (Ichev, 1968; Nakai, Masutani, Moriguchi, Matsunaga, & Sugita, 1991), guinea pig (Franz & Aharinejad, 1994; Nakai et al., 1991), monkey (Freeland, 1975), and human (Claassen & Klaws,

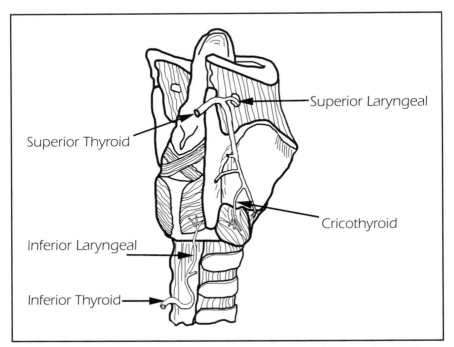

Figure 4.1. The laryngeal arterial supply (after Armstrong & Netterville, 1995).

1992; Lasjaunias, Halimi, & Choi, 1983). The areas supplied by the superior laryngeal artery are above the cricoid cartilage. After piercing the lateral aspect of the thyrohyoid membrane, this artery divides to supply the epiglottis, the aryepiglottic fold, the more superior intrinsic laryngeal muscles (thyroarytenoid [TA], lateral cricoarytenoid [LCA], the vocal folds, and the mucosa). Branches from these divisions anastomose with vessels from the contralateral side, as well as with the more inferior cricothyroid artery. The cricothyroid artery delivers blood to the cricothyroid muscle and membrane as well as to the connective tissue, some of the overlying extrinsic laryngeal muscles, and—after penetrating the cricothyroid membrane—the lower portion of the larynx. The main target of the inferior laryngeal artery is the posterior cricoarytenoid muscle (PCA). Corrosion cast and latex injection studies in humans, as well as in some animals, have shown that there are extensive anastomoses between the ipsilateral and contralateral laryngeal arteries (Claassen & Klaws, 1992; Freeland, 1975; Sokjer & Olofsson, 1979) such that perfusion of a single superior laryngeal artery can reach most laryngeal structures, provided that there is no significant positive pressure in the other laryngeal arteries.

Some studies of laryngeal vascular morphology have focused on the specific pattern of the blood supply in attempts to define anatomical boundaries of the intrinsic laryngeal muscles (Kahane, 1983). Nevertheless, the majority of researchers in this area have concentrated on the vocal folds. The main objective of these investigations has been to gain some understanding of the etiology of voice disorders, paths of tumor spread, formation and reduction of edema, and vascular changes. These have been qualitative descriptions, however, with few or no comparisons to vasculature from other laryngeal or nonlaryngeal regions. Unfortunately, the result has been data with limited impact. No systematic structural studies of the laryngeal microvasculature have been conducted. In the few studies that have examined the capillaries within the larynx, researchers have reported that they are of the nonfenestrated or continuous type (see Figure 4.2A), the most common form of capillary. This includes the capillaries within the vocal folds, as well as the intrinsic musculature. Nonfenestrated capillaries are characterized by a single layer of mesothelial-derived endothelial cells enveloped in a continuous basement membrane that encompasses adhering pericytes (a cell type associated with endothelial cells but whose functional significance is not well understood). The junctions between endothelial cells may be simple or elaborate interdigitations, and frequently the cells overlap. In nonlaryngeal muscles, this junctional gap that separates plasma membranes is usually very small (<10 nm) and filled with electron-dense material. For more details on capillary structure, see Simionescu and Simionescu (1984). These vessels form a continuous, semipermeable barrier that allows movement of water, certain ions, and small proteins to gain access to the surrounding tissue and vice versa. Movement of these substances involves passive mechanisms based on the relationship between hydrostatic and osmotic pressures—known as the Starling hypothesis (Starling, 1896)—as well as active transport systems within the endothelial cell. For example, there are glucose transporters and energy-dependent ion transporters, such as the sodium–potassium "pump," which actively moves sodium and potassium across the plasma membrane, dragging along water. This pump frequently works against large diffusion gradients. In addition, some of the active transport mechanisms involve the formation of pinocytotic vesicles (transcytosis) at the endothelial cell's surfaces for the selective transport of materials. Myocardial capillaries appear to have the highest frequency of vesicles, whereas brain capillaries have very few (Simionescu & Simionescu, 1984). This gap is highly specialized, containing various adhesion molecules, such as platelet endothelial cell adhesion molecules and connexins, as well as actin and myosin filaments (Drenckhahn & Ness, 1997; Michel & Curry, 1999) that can change the geometry of the gap and thus its permeability. Inflammation, injury, disease, or pharmacological agents leading to the extravasation of large proteins and water, with the subsequent development of edema, can also alter the integrity of this region.

Another type of capillary that is occasionally found within muscle is the fenestrated or perforated type (see Figure 4.2B; Korneliussen, 1975). Since data are limited, it is not known whether fenestrated capillaries are normally present within laryngeal muscle or mucosa. Desaki, Kawakita, and Yamagata (1997) reported that fenestrated capillaries were not present in normal rat PCA or arytenoid muscle. However, 3 days following transection of the recurrent and superior laryngeal nerves, approximately 10% of the

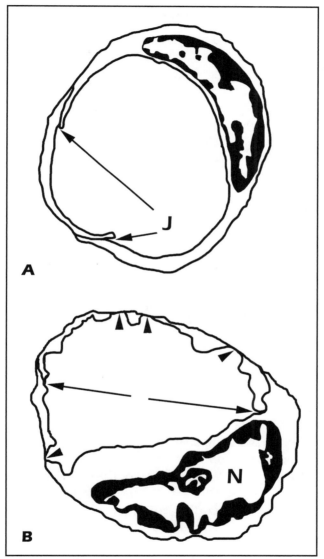

Figure 4.2. Schematics of the capillary types found within skeletal muscle. A = nonfenestrated; B = fenestrated; J = intercellular junctions; N = nucleus; arrowheads in B = fenestrae.

capillaries adjacent to denervated neuromuscular junctions were of this type. This transition has also been reported to occur in other muscles during muscle fiber regeneration (McKinney, Singh, & Brewer, 1977) or limb immobilization (Desaki, Oki, Matsuda, & Sakanaka, 2000; Oki, Desaki, Matsuda, Okumura, & Shibata, 1995). These experiments demonstrate an important aspect of capillary physiology; that is, capillaries are not static structures. Instead, they respond to hemodynamic forces and to pathophysiological stimuli from their environment, which can initiate vascular morphological changes, new capillary growth (angiogenesis), or regression. Fenestrated capillaries are structurally similar to nonfenestrated capillaries, with the exception of pores across the endothelial cell. These fenestrae vary in frequency and size. For example, in the intestine they have a density of 2 to 5 per micron squared, with a radius of 50 to 60 nm, whereas in the renal vasculature (with the exception of the glomerulus) they have a higher density, 20 to 30 per micron squared, and radius, 60 to 88 nm (Levick & Smaje, 1987). The fenestrae are closed by a thin diaphragm (3–5 nm). The permeability to large molecules, such as plasma proteins, is approximately the same for both fenestrated and nonfenestrated capillaries (Granger, Perry, & Kvietys, 1983; Levick & Smaje, 1987; Renkin, 1977); however, fenestrated capillaries are far more permeable to water and solutes. The latter are normally found in the kidney, intestine, and endocrine glands—tissues where the rapid exchange of substances occurs between the blood and surrounding tissues. When fenestrated capillaries are found within muscle, as previously discussed, it is probably as a response to denervation or injury. Muscle fibers frequently remodel due to disuse or injury. They also go through cycles of denervation–reinnervation and regeneration that have been shown to increase during aging of the human thyroarytenoid (Malmgren, Lovice, & Kaufman, 2000). The transition of capillaries to the fenestrated type could aid in muscle remodeling because their permeability characteristic would allow a more facilitated transport of necessary materials. In mice, microvascular remodeling has recently been shown to be produced by airway inflammation (Thurston, Maas, LaBarbara, McLean, & McDonald, 2000). It is possible that capillary transition, or at least changes in permeability, could be triggered by voice disuse or irritants and could be one possible mechanism for the formation of vocal fold edema. As can be seen, the mechanisms of microvascular permeability are extremely complex, involving not only signaling within the endothelial cell but from the surrounding environment as well. A recent review by Michel and Curry (1999) provided further details of microvascular permeability.

The regulation of muscle blood flow is extremely complex, and the following discussion is meant to serve only as a general overview and to provide some insight into these complexities. The majority of this article will deal with some of the local control mechanisms, rather than systemic factors (e.g., angiotensin, endothelin) of vasodilation and vasoconstriction. A number of recent reviews offer more details in this area (Delp & Laughlin, 1998; Janicki, Sheriff, Robotham, & Wise, 1996; Laughlin, Korthuis, Duncker, & Bache, 1996; Rowell, O'Leary, & Kellogg, 1996; Saltin, Radegran, Koskolou, & Roach, 1998).

Vasodilation

Muscle blood flow is heterogeneous within and among muscles, such that it is distributed based on fiber type; the more oxidative the muscle fiber, the higher its blood flow both at rest and during exercise. Blood flow is tightly coupled to the level of skeletal muscle activity (oxygen demand), and there is a near linear increase in relation to work intensity (Andersen & Saltin, 1985; Radegran, 1997). Changes are regulated by the dynamic integration of central neural and cardiovascular mechanisms, circulating and locally produced vasoactive substances, local reflexes, and metabolites. The main action of these regulators is to produce diameter changes in the vessels that compose resistance networks to either increase or decrease blood flow. The cardiovascular changes (i.e., heart rate, stroke volume) that occur during exercise can be considered to be mainly for the maintenance of systemic blood pressure in response to peripheral changes and will not be discussed. For details on this subject, see Janicki et al. (1996). In humans at rest, skeletal muscle blood flow is usually relatively low, in the range of 2 to 5 ml per minute per 100 g, and there is a balance between myogenic tone (vasoconstriction) and endothelial-mediated flow-induced vasodilatory responses. During intense exercise, blood flow can increase nearly 100-fold, to approximately 200 to 300 ml per minute per 100 g (Radegran & Saltin, 1998; Saltin et al., 1998), reflecting increases in cardiac output in combination with increases of vascular conductance in the exercising muscle. At the onset of exercise, blood flow increases rapidly (hyperemia) to more than double that of the resting muscle, usually occurring within 2 to 10 seconds, and it is distributed within the active muscles according to motor unit recruitment. Due to the speed of the initial increase, it is thought to be mainly the result of local factors.

When vasodilation occurs, there is coordination between the capillary and arteriolar networks within the muscle, as well as with the upstream feeding arteries from which these arterioles originate. It has been known for some time that vasomotor responses initiated at distinct vascular sites can spread to include multiple branches of the vascular network (Krogh, Harrop, & Rehberg, 1922). Studies have demonstrated that when various endogenous neurotransmitters are applied to discrete regions of arterioles and cause membrane hyperpolarization, the dilatory responses travel via intracellular connections (gap junctions) between endothelial or smooth muscle cells (Christ, Spray, el-Sabban, Moore, & Brink, 1996; Segal & Duling, 1986b; Welsh & Segal, 1998). In addition, these changes appear to be coordinated responses to recruit previously unperfused capillaries and upstream feeding arteries (Folkow, Sonnenschein, & Wright, 1971; Segal, 1991; Segal & Duling, 1986a). Kurjiaka and Segal (1995), Segal, Welsh, and Kurjiaka (1999), and Welsh and Segal (1997) have suggested that acetylcholine spillover from neuromuscular junctions during motor-nerve muscle-fiber activation is one possible mechanism for this type of conducted vasodilation. Although most of these data come from studies of arteriolar responses, capillaries appear to be just as capable of producing upstream dilation (McCullough, Collins, & Ellsworth, 1997; Song & Tyml, 1993). Vasodilation can be caused by many metabolites that are typically released from muscle fibers and endothelial cells during exercise (e.g., K^+, ATP, ADP, and H^+) as well as by changes in tissue and blood PO_2. There is growing evidence that adenosine, which is released from endothelial cells (Deussen, Moser, & Schrader, 1986), muscle fibers (Hellsten & Frandsen, 1997), and nerves (Cunha & Sebastiao, 1993), may account for as much as 50% of vasodilation during acute hypoxia (Marshall, 2000). In addition to these metabolic factors, mechanical factors, such as the shear stress caused by the flow of red blood cells along the endothelial wall, trigger vasodilation by causing the release of endothelial cell–relaxing factor, which is now known to be the gas nitric oxide.

Besides these local mechanisms, there are a number of central neural components of vasodilation. When stimulated, vasoactive substances, such as vasoactive intestinal peptide (VIP), a potent vasodilator, are released from nerves. VIP can also act as a neuromodulator of noradrenaline (NA) and can upregulate cyclic adenosine monophosphate, thereby influencing metabolic functions; intracellular calcium, which is required for nitric oxide production; and seromucous secretions. Which of these roles VIP serves appears to be dependent on stimulation frequency (Forssmann & Said, 1998). Because many of these transmitters co-localize within nerve fibers, most are not released independently but rather with one or more other peptides. For example, in some laryngeal perivascular nerves, VIP co-localizes with neuropeptide-Y (NPY; Domeij, Dahlqvist, & Forsgren, 1991), substance-P (Tsuda, Shin, & Masuko, 1992), and NA. Each of these can either enhance or inhibit the actions of the others, adding an additional layer of complexity to their actions. In addition, a vasoactive substance might be a vasodilator in one vascular bed but a vasoconstrictor in another (Burnstock, 1990). The effects of vasoactive substances are dependent on their concentrations within the junctional cleft, the width of the cleft, and whether the substances act pre- or postsynaptically (Burnstock, 1987). Furthermore, aging may alter these actions. An age-related reduction in vasodilation is induced by hypercapnia, acetylcholine, adenosine diphosphate, or calcitonin gene-related peptide (Amerini, Mantelli, Filippi, & Ledda, 1994; Lartaud, Bray, Chillon, Atkinson, & Capdeville-Atkinson, 1993; Mayhan, Faraci, Baumbach, & Heistad, 1990). The actions of some of these vasoactive substances may even be reversed, such as occurs with bradykinin, a vasodilator in young animals but a vasoconstrictor in older animals (Mantelli, Amerini, & Ledda, 1995). As noted before, these changes appear to depend on the vascular bed (Marin, 1995). These examples demonstrate the necessity of examining each vascular bed independently and not assuming that what is occurring in one vascular bed is necessarily occurring in another.

Vasoconstriction

In general, vasoconstriction is mediated by the sympathetic nervous system, and skeletal muscle vasculature is richly innervated by sympathetic nerves. Figure 4.3 shows the relationship of sympathetic noradrenergic nerve fibers to the arterial network of the superior laryngeal nerve. Studies have shown that sympathetic nerve discharge and vascular resistance are tightly coupled, and both are contraction intense and time-dependent (Seals, 1989). In quiescent skeletal muscle, myogenic tone, which is important for the maintenance of systemic blood pressure, is maintained by this portion of the autonomic nervous system via the release of vasoactive substances. J. T. Shepherd (1987) observed that patients with autonomic failure couldn't maintain arterial blood pressure, even during light supine exercise. An increase in vasoconstriction can be triggered not only by central neural activation but also by passive muscle stretching, which activates periarteriolar sympathetic nerves (Welsh & Segal, 1996). Although the manner in which this occurs is unclear, it appears to be mechanistically different from the enhanced neuro-

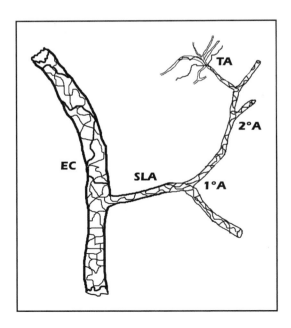

Figure 4.3. Schematic showing the relationship of sympathetic noradrenergic nerve fibers to the arterial network of the superior laryngeal artery. There are fibers extending from the external carotid artery (EC) to the superior laryngeal artery (SLA) and around the primary (1°A) and secondary (2°A) arteries down to the terminal arterioles (TA).

transmitter release from motor nerve terminals in response to similar perturbations, which seems to be due to either elevating internal calcium concentrations or increasing the sensitivity of transmitter release to calcium in the nerve terminal (Chen & Grinnell, 1995).

The major transmitter of sympathetic nerves is NA; however, a number of other transmitters within these nerves are co-released with NA. The most common combination is with NPY, which is a vasoconstrictor when acting alone. NPY also can act in synergy with NA such that NA must be present for NPY to cause vasoconstriction (Cortes et al., 1999). It may be that NPY's main action is as a neuromodulator. Like other transmitters, NPY can be released in response to systemic challenges, such as stress, exercise, or ischemia. For more information on NPY see the review by Hokfelt et al. (1998).

Metabolic factors produced during exercise—such as acidosis, ischemia, and hypoxia—can all attenuate sympathetic tone (functional sympatholysis). These factors act on the signal transduction pathways of the alpha-adrenoceptor–mediated portion of vasoconstriction (McGillivray-Anderson & Faber, 1990) and probably involve ATP-sensitive K^+ channels (Tateishi & Faber, 1995). There are two types of alpha-adrenoceptors, alpha-1 and alpha-2, and they are distributed heterogeneously within the skeletal muscle microcirculation. Both types of receptors are located on the larger resistance arterioles that contribute to the regulation of systemic blood pressure, whereas only alpha-2 adrenoceptors are predominant on the smaller distal nutrient arterioles. Moreover, the alpha-2-adrenoceptors are more sensitive to these metabolites than the alpha-1-adrenoceptors (Anderson & Faber, 1991; McGillivray-Anderson & Faber, 1990). This arrangement allows the preservation of reflex control of upstream resistance arterioles for the regulation of systemic pressure, while the distal nutrient arterioles redistribute the intramuscular blood flow to meet the metabolic demands of the recruited motor units. In rats, this type of contraction-induced attenuation appears to depend on fiber type and muscle contraction intensity, because it is more prevalent during intense contractions of glycolytic (Type 2), but not of oxidative (Type 1), muscles (Thomas, Hansen, & Victor, 1994). In humans, alpha-2-adrenoceptor–mediated vasoconstriction has been reported in skeletal muscle (Nielsen, Hasenkam, Pilegaard, Mortensen, & Mulvany, 1991;

van Brummelen, Jie, Timmermans, & van Zwieten, 1985), but there are also data suggesting that this type of vasoconstriction is mediated primarily via postjunctional alpha-1-adrenoceptors (van Brummelen, Jie, & van Zwieten, 1986). It remains to be determined if similar mechanisms for control of large and small arterioles by alpha adrenoceptors are present in humans.

Another possible mechanism for functional sympatholysis involves nitric oxide. During muscle contraction, it is increased (Balon & Nadler, 1994). Furthermore, this gas has been shown to antagonize alpha-adrenergic vasoconstriction (Habler, Wasner, & Janig, 1997) and to be a more potent antagonist of alpha-2-adrenergic vasoconstriction (Ohyanagi, Nishigaki, & Faber, 1992), thereby eliciting responses similar to metabolites. At present, we know of at least two potential sources for nitric oxide. One obvious source is the endothelial cells, because production of nitric oxide by the enzyme—endothelial nitric oxide synthase—is upregulated when shear stress occurs. The fact that it binds to hemoglobin may limit its effective range, however. The second source is the neuronal isoform of nitric oxide synthase. Recently, it has been found within skeletal muscle perivascular nerves (Hisa et al., 1999; Lyon, 2000b), as well as the sarcolemma (Kobzik, Reid, Bredt, & Stamler, 1994; Nakane, Schmidt, Pollock, Forstermann, & Murad, 1993). Because nitric oxide can readily diffuse up to 200 µm, it can easily reach the distal vasculature. Whether nitric oxide functions to couple microvascular tone to skeletal muscle contraction remains equivocal, however.

In summary, these vasodilatory and vasoconstrictor mechanisms act in synergy so that in active muscles, including cardiac muscle, the resistance vessels relax in response to local changes to provide an increase in blood flow that is adequate to meet their metabolic requirements. There is also an increased release of NA from the sympathetic nerve endings due to an increase of central sympathetic activity. This activates alpha-adrenoceptors, leading to vasoconstriction of both systemic resistance and capacitance vessels outside the active muscles. Beta-receptors are also activated, increasing heart rate, shortening the heart's refractory period, and enhancing myocardial contractility. The result of these changes is increased blood flow to the active muscles, with a corresponding decrease in blood flow to inactive muscles. If the exercise is sufficiently intense, blood is also diverted from internal organs, and if more muscle mass becomes active, there is evidence that sympathetic activity increases, even in the muscle that was previously active, to meet the new demands. There is one exception, however. The maintenance of blood flow to respiratory muscles, including the PCA, appears to have priority.

Laryngeal Blood Flow

Surprisingly few studies have been conducted on laryngeal blood flow. Using dogs as subjects, Shin, Rabuzzi, and Reed (1970) determined "total" laryngeal venous outflow following either vagal or recurrent laryngeal nerve stimulation, reporting a 30% increase. When the dogs were treated with atropine (an anticholinergic) and a similar stimulation paradigm was used, these increases were abolished, suggesting that adrenergic mechanisms were involved. In contrast, when Shin et al. stimulated the superior laryngeal nerve, there was a 20% decrease. This is not surprising, given that this nerve supplies sympathetic innervation to the larynx. It is likely that NPY was also involved. See Figure 4.4 for an example of NPY in the rat superior laryngeal artery. Franco-Cereceda, Matran, Alving, and Lundberg (1995) examined the role of NPY in blood

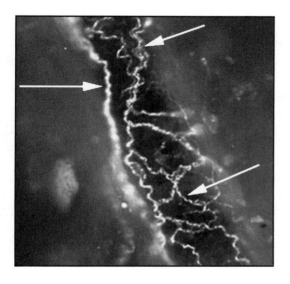

Figure 4.4. A rat superior laryngeal artery that has been immunostained for neuropeptide-Y (arrows). As can be seen, there is an abundance of positive fibers.

flow to the superior laryngeal artery of the pig. Some of the animals in this study were pretreated with reserpine and received a preganglionic sympathetic nerve transection, which results in the depletion of NA without reducing NPY (Lundberg, Franco-Cereceda, Lacroix, & Pernow, 1990). With high-frequency stimulation of the cervical sympathetic nerve, maximal vasoconstriction similar to that in untreated control animals was found, indicating that NPY plays a role in laryngeal vasoconstriction, at least at high-frequency stimulation. Because reserpine treatment can enhance the release of NPY (Lundberg et al., 1990), however, more direct data retrieved under normal physiological conditions are necessary before any conclusions can be drawn as to NPY's role in laryngeal blood flow.

Contrary to the data of Shin et al. (1970), Matsuo et al. (1987) and Tomita, Matsuo, Maehara, Umezaki, and Shin (1988) used needle electrodes to measure intratissue oxygen tension in lightly anesthetized dogs following either painful stimuli, which would produce phonation, or nerve stimulation. They reported ischemic changes in the thyroarytenoid and varying results for the lamina propria. The interpretations of the data from these studies were somewhat flawed. First, the painful stimuli used to produce phonation would have also produced large systemic effects, such as elevations in circulating catecholamines and sympathetic activation, which would have altered systemic blood flow. Second, the reported reductions in oxygen tension were not great enough to be interpreted as ischemia. Instead, they were what might be expected from increased oxygen utilization by muscles during contraction. In a later study, the microsphere technique was used to measure absolute blood flow to the lamina propria and thyroarytenoid at rest and during phonation (Arnstein, Berke, Trapp, & Natividad, 1989). In this technique, an intracardiac microsphere injection is made, and the microspheres become trapped in the distal circulation, based on diameter. Simultaneously with the injection, an arterial blood reference sample is withdrawn at a specific rate (i.e., 1 ml per minute). Counts are made of the number of microspheres within the reference sample and tissues. The blood flow is calculated as a ratio of these results. Arnstein et al. (1989) produced phonation in dogs by passing humidified air across their vocal folds while stimulating the recurrent and superior laryngeal nerves. Although no change occurred in the lamina propria, blood flow increased nearly tenfold to the thyroarytenoid, which supports the more global findings of Shin et al. (1970). This study has provided some valuable information on laryngeal blood flow during phonation, but it does have several weaknesses. Given the results of Shin et al. (1970) and Franco-Cereceda et al. (1995), it is likely that stimulation of the superior laryngeal nerve would have altered blood flow in some manner. Second, although the relative changes may be considered reliable, the absolute flow data may be incorrect. The tissue section thickness used for the microsphere counts was the same as the microsphere diameter. This leads to a complex set of statistical biases (Weibel, 1980) and probably erroneous conclusions.

Some laryngeal blood flow data come from the respiratory physiology literature. These data show that the PCA at rest has the highest blood flow rate not only among laryngeal muscles but also among the other respiratory muscles (Brancatisano, Kelly, Baile, Pare, & Engel, 1993). This is probably due to the higher activity level of the PCA and because it contains a higher proportion of Type I fibers (Malmgren & Gacek, 1981; Teig, Dahl, & Thorkelsen, 1978), a higher volume of mitochondria (Malmgren, Gacek, & Etzler, 1983), and a higher level of oxidative enzyme activity (Brondbo, Dahl, & Teig, 1985). In addition, during increased respiratory load, blood flow in the PCA increases more than in any other respiratory muscle, including the diaphragm (Brancatisano et al., 1993).

One area of interest in laryngeal physiology is age-related laryngeal changes. Recent data have indicated that there are age-related changes to the human thyroarytenoid (Malmgren, Fisher, Bookman, & Uno, 1999; Malmgren et al., 2000). Although muscle fiber remodeling and dropout clearly are occurring, little is known about age-related laryngeal vascular change. Malmgren and Lyon (2000) found a significant age-related reduction in blood flow in the rat, ranging from 42% to 60%, with the greatest decrease occurring in the thyroarytenoid. These changes could be due to one factor or, more likely, to a combination of factors: reduced vasodilatory capacity (Lartaud et al., 1993), loss of vascular elements (Coggan et al., 1992; Degens, 1998), decreased mean capillary diameter (Davis & Lyon, 2000; Lyon & Wanamaker, 1993), and decreased capillary length density (Anversa, Li, Sonnenblick, & Olivetti, 1994). All of these age-related changes have been reported in various systems. These alterations could impair the normal metabolic activity of the laryngeal muscles because there would be a decreased supply of nutrients and oxygen and decreased removal of metabolic by-products. Although it has yet to be determined if similar vascular morphological and blood flow changes occur in the human larynx, preliminary data (Lyon, 2000a) have indicated that endothelial cell apoptosis (programmed cell death) is occurring within the human thyroarytenoid and PCA (see Figure 4.5). Whether this is part of an angiogenic mechanism or vascular regression is not currently known; however, apoptotic endothelial cells become procoagulant, promoting the formation of clots (Bombeli, Schwartz, & Harlan, 1999). This could be a contributing factor to the age-related loss of muscle fibers, the degeneration/regeneration cycle, and fiber-type grouping that occurs in the thyroarytenoid and most likely the PCA. This mechanism of age-related tissue damage represents one potential area for therapeutic intervention. It may be possible to use gene therapy to alter this apoptotic activity, thus preventing or ameliorating the effects of aging on the laryngeal vasculature.

Other age-related changes could influence laryngeal blood flow. During aging, there is an age-related reduction in vasodilation that is induced by hypercapnia, acetylcholine, adenosine diphosphate, or calcitonin gene-related peptide (Amerini et al., 1994; Cook, Wailgum, Vasthare, Mayrovitz, & Tuma, 1992; Lartaud et al., 1993; Mayhan et al., 1990). Sympathetic innervation is also reduced around the cerebral (Andrews & Cowen, 1994) and coronary (Amenta & Mione, 1988) arteries. Data have shown that the superior cervical ganglion neurons are significantly reduced in somal size, dendritic length, arborization, and the number of primary dendrites, and that there are other age-related morphological abnormalities (Andrews, Li, Halliwell, & Cowen, 1994). Because laryngeal sympathetic innervation is derived from the superior cervical ganglion (Domeij et al., 1991; Luts, Uddman, Grunditz, & Sundler, 1990), these data would imply an age-related loss of this important type of innervation. Understanding these mechanisms is essential because a compromise in laryngeal blood flow would affect the quality of life.

As a normal part of our daily physiology, the amount of blood supplied to various tissues can differ with changes in our emotional and physical states, as well as in our level of physical activity and the subsequent changes in metabolic processes. Laryngeal

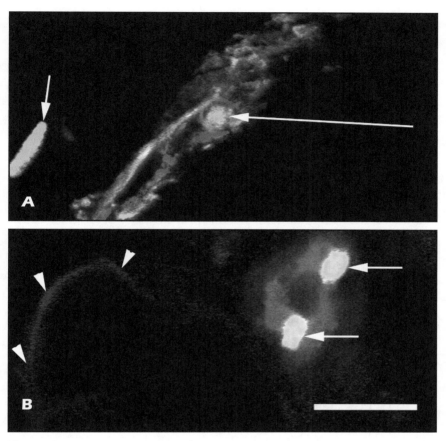

Figure 4.5. Apoptotic endothelial cells in the (A) thyroarytenoid muscle (TA) and (B) the posterior cricoarytenoid muscle (PCA) have been labeled for von Willebrand disease (Factor VIII); TUNEL (terminal deoxynucleotidyl transterase-mediated du TP-biotin nick end labeling) technique was used to tag apoptotic nuclei (damaged DNA); biotinylated lectin, concanavalin A, was labeled to outline cell surfaces. As can be seen, there are apoptotic nuclei within the endothelial cells in both the TA (A, long arrow) and PCA (B, short arrows). There is also an unidentified apoptotic nuclei in the TA section (A, short arrow). The outline of a muscle fiber is indicated by the arrowheads in B. Calibration bar = 20 μm.

blood flow can likewise be affected. As mentioned previously, certain factors are associated with variations in the vascular supply within laryngeal tissues. Some of these are muscle fiber type, muscle activity level, neurotransmitters, metabolites, tissue integrity, and tissue morphology. In addition, the intensity of mental, emotional, or physical activity can affect the vascular supply to the laryngeal tissue. It was discussed previously how blood flow to contracting skeletal muscle increases during activity to meet local tissue metabolic needs as well as in response to neuromuscular factors. Increased blood flow to the vocalis muscle during phonation in the dog has been observed (Arnstein et al., 1989). Interestingly, the vascular supply to the lamina propria and the vocalis muscle did not uniformly increase during phonation (Arnstein et al., 1989). Instead, blood flow to the lamina propria was consistent both at rest and during phonation. Thus, regardless of whether the vocal folds are at rest or vibrating, blood flow to the lamina propria appears to remain constant. Consideration of the morphology of the vascular supply to the lamina propria and vocalis muscle may help in our understanding of observed blood flow patterns during phonation and nonphonation as demonstrated by Arnstein et al. (1989). First, the blood vessels enter the lamina propria of the vocal folds from the anterior and posterior regions and course longitudinally (Nakai et al., 1991). Few blood vessels are found in the external two layers of the mucosa; most are located instead within the intermediate and deep layers of the lamina propria (Hirano, 1975). Blood vessels within the lamina propria branch and connect to create a blood vessel network that disperses the blood supply across the three layers (Nakai et al., 1991). In contrast, the vascular supply within the vocalis muscle courses in a superior-medial direction along the length of the vocal folds and appears separate from the vascular supply within the lamina propria (Hirano, 1975). Both groups of vocal fold blood vessels exhibit an undulating appearance along their course, which probably helps them withstand vocal fold vibratory movements that stretch and compress the vessels (Nakai et al., 1991). Frenzel and Kleinsasser (1982) described the vocal fold blood vessels as consisting primarily of short, intermediate, and thin filaments with lamellate basement membranes. These particular cellular structures are usually identified in blood vessels that reside in physical locations that withstand high levels of stress. The blood vessels within the vocal folds thus appear built to endure mechanical forces such as occur within the larynx during phonation and swallowing. The differential blood distribution to the lamina propria and vocalis muscle reported by Arnstein et al. (1989)

could relate to the separate blood supplies to each region of the vocal folds (Hirano, 1975; Nakai et al., 1991). Another consideration is the significantly greater density noted for the vascular supply to the vocalis muscle than that described within the lamina propria (Nakai et al., 1991). The increased density of blood supply to the muscular portion of the vocal fold could predictably contribute a greater volume of blood flow to that region during phonation, as reported by Arnstein et al. (1989). With the lack of vascular communication between the muscular and mucosal portions of the vocal folds, these two regions could locally regulate blood flow differentially according to their functional differences.

The finding by Arnstein et al. (1989) of increased blood flow to the vocalis muscle during phonation contrasts with that reported by Matsuo et al. (1987) and Tomita et al. (1988). The latter studies indicated a decrease in blood flow to the vocalis muscle during phonation in dogs. The discrepancy between the findings probably relates to (a) differing methods used for measuring blood flow and (b) the manner in which phonation was elicited. Matsuo et al. and Tomita et al. measured intratissue oxygen tension levels under rest and phonation conditions in dogs. In contrast, Arnstein et al. (1989) injected a 15 μm microsphere suspension into the blood supply during rest in a control group and during phonation in the experimental group. In the latter protocol, the quantity of microspheres present in the vocal fold tissues compared to that measured from a referent artery represented the degree of blood flow through the vocal folds. The use of intratissue oxygen tension measurement of regional blood flow did not allow differentiation between local oxygen changes related to blood flow versus oxygen uptake by local tissues during phonation. Matsuo et al. and Tomita et al. did not discuss this possible factor with their findings. Thus, their interpretation of reduced oxygen tension during phonation as indicative of ischemia within the local tissues may not be entirely accurate.

An additional factor for consideration in Matsuo et al.'s study (1987) relates to the elicitation of phonation through use of painful stimuli. The use of pain as a phonation stimulus could have caused the described variations in laryngeal blood flow related to sympathetic regulation of systemic blood flow. Thus, findings reported by Arnstein et al. (1989) may better represent laryngeal blood flow during voicing without overlying systemic sympathetic regulation.

None of the aforementioned studies addressed biomechanical factors associated with vocal fold length changes, or medial compression, and their influence on laryngeal blood flow during phonation. In the studies using nerve stimulation (Arnstein et al., 1989; Tomita et al., 1988), both the superior laryngeal nerve and recurrent laryngeal nerve branches to the larynx were stimulated, although at differing levels of intensity and frequency. Exploration of laryngeal blood flow patterns during phonation at varied pitches and volumes has not been addressed. Blood vessels in the lamina propria and vocalis muscle may constrict as a passive consequence of lengthwise stretching as the vocal folds elongate. This could occur as a result of increased longitudinal tension and reduced cross-sectional mass of the vocal fold. Likewise, shortening of the vocal folds may constrict blood vessels as intratissue pressures increase subsequent to lengthwise compression of the vocal fold tissues. During excessive volume, blood vessels may constrict locally as a protective response to excessive shearing forces in the tissues. Alternatively, constant blood flow to the lamina propria when shearing and impact forces are high may stress blood vessels, leading to rupture.

Individuals suffering from voice disorders subsequent to damage to the vocal fold vascular supply typically report a history of overuse or phonotraumatic vocal habits. Further investigation of changes in laryngeal blood flow with pitch, volume, and prolonged phonation may contribute to our understanding of impaired vocal fold vasculature observed in these voice disorders.

Vocal Fold Vascular Supply and Voice Disorders

Voice disorders involving the vascular supply within the vocal folds typically result from sudden impact forces, such as those associated with sudden loud phonation, or blunt trauma, or from chronic overuse of the voice in ways that wear down or injure the vocal fold tissues where the medial compression forces are greatest. Compromised vocal fold tissues exhibit signs of tissue injury and repair, such as redness and swelling, which are associated with reactive changes in the blood vessels. In mild cases, blood vessels may increase their permeability, allowing excessive fluids to collect in the superficial layer of the lamina propria, leading to Reinke's edema (Frenzel & Kleinsasser, 1982). In more long-term or severe cases, the blood vessels may dilate excessively as they carry increased blood supply to injured areas and rupture or tear, leading to microhematomas or gross-level hemorrhages.

Laryngeal vascular injuries leading to vocal dysfunction entail various levels of hemorrhaging: either localized bleeding associated with pooling of blood from stressed microvasculature or generalized bleeding affecting significant portions, or the entire length, of the superior surface of the vocal fold(s). The vascular supply within the vocal fold can indicate stressed tissue areas by the development of blood vessel networks associated with such vocal fold lesions as polyps, nodules, and cysts. The following laryngeal disorders are the most common forms of injury clinically related to vascular injury within the vocal folds.

Subepithelial Edema

Subepithelial edema arises subsequent to overuse or misuse of the voice, chemical irritation to the mucosa, or inflammation related to viral infection (see Figure 4.6). In a study of vascular responses to inflammation, the venous vessels were the first to exhibit increased leakage, while continued mechanical trauma eventually led to increased capillary leakage (Joris, Cuenoud, Doern, Underwood, & Majno, 1990). In the vocal folds, the onset of subepithelial edema appears linked to changes in the permeability of blood vessels (Frenzel & Kleinsasser, 1982; Sato, Hirano, & Nakashima, 1999) as well as to damage to the endothelium characterized by thinning of

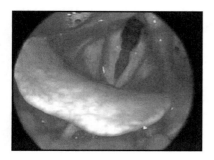

Figure 4.6. Example of bilateral sub-epithelial edema. Courtesy of A. J. Emami, MD, 2001.

the endothelial walls, thickening of the basement membrane, and blood vessel collapse in some cases (Sato et al., 1999; see the example in Figure 4.6). Chronic subepithelial edema can eventually transpire into tissue changes associated with polypoid corditis (Courey & Ossoff, 1996).

Individuals experiencing subepithelial edema may notice changes in their voice quality, the amount of effort needed to voice, and reduced pitch and volume ranges. These symptoms are consistent with the structural and physiologic changes in voice production related to the increased mass of the vocal folds, with possible asymmetry in the distribution of the edema within the affected vocal fold(s). In order to compensate for these changes, individuals may attempt to increase respiratory drive and muscular contraction within and around the larynx.

Vocal Fold Microvascular Lesions: Capillary Ectasias and Varices

Ectasias and varices both indicate excessive dilation and elongation of a blood vessel from the microcirculation of the vocal fold. A *varix* most often arises from a venule (i.e., smallest vein), whereas *capillary ectasias* typically occur at the junction of arterioles and venules within the vocal fold. The occurrence of microvascular vocal fold lesions such as ectasias and varices has been reported to occur most often in women who use their voice professionally (Hochman, Hillman, Sataloff, & Zeitels, 1999; Postma, Courey, & Ossoff, 1998). Bouchayer and Cornut (1988) reported finding capillary varices more frequently in women than in men and in individuals who were older than 40 years. An important clinical consideration when identifying the presence of such microvascular vocal fold lesions is whether the lesion occurs in isolation or in combination with other laryngeal problems. The implications for the contribution of the microvascular lesion to the presenting laryngeal symptoms and the implications for subsequent treatment choices may differ between these two groups.

Only one investigation has addressed the distinction between individuals with isolated microvascular lesions versus those identified with microvascular lesions in combination with other laryngeal problems. Postma et al. (1998) conducted a retrospective study of 800 patients (47% were men, 53% were women) with a diagnosis of benign laryngeal problems who were seen at the Vanderbilt Voice Center between 1992 and 1995. Approximately 29% of the total group consisted of individuals described as professional voice users, with equal numbers of men and women represented. Only 25 individuals exhibited true vocal fold microvascular lesions in isolation. Eleven of these individuals exhibited bilateral microvascular lesions. On average, the isolated true vocal fold microvascular lesion group were 39 years of age (ranging between 24 and 70 years of age) and consisted primarily of women (76%). In addition, 88% of this group were described as professional voice users. The occupations represented by the latter consisted of professional singers, teachers, public speakers, and auctioneers. An overall microvascular lesion incidence of 3.1% was reported for the total group. Within the latter group, the incidence was 1.6% for men and 4.5% for women. Within the total professional voice user group (n = 232), an overall microvascular lesion incidence was determined to be 5% for men and 14% for women. Female professional voice users thus were more likely to present with a microvascular vocal fold lesion than were male professional voice users, regardless of whether the lesion occurred alone or in concert with other laryngeal problems. In addition, professional voice users were generally more likely to exhibit a microvascular lesion than were nonprofessional voice users.

Symptoms associated with microvascular lesions may vary tremendously. Patients may not report any symptoms at the time of diagnosis, or they may complain of severe symptoms, such as throat pain and vocal quality changes. Sataloff and colleagues reported symptoms consisting of pain and vocal fatigue among patients presenting with abnormal varicosities (Sataloff, Hawkshaw, & Spiegel, 1998; Sataloff, Heuer, & Hawkshaw, 1994). Postma et al. (1998) identified "hoarseness" as the primary complaint in 72% of the individuals in the isolated vocal fold varices group. The latter group also listed vocal fatigue, pain, and reduced range as secondary symptoms. The report of vocal quality and range changes may relate to altered vocal fold vibratory patterns, depending upon the severity of the microvascular lesion. With greater disruption of the microvasculature, vocal fold mass changes can occur, resulting in swelling and pooling of fluids. In addition, increased swelling in the superficial layer of the lamina propria may increase the viscosity of the vocal fold "cover," resulting in increased stiffness. Subsequently, pitch range and the amplitude of mucosal excursion will be reduced.

Microvascular lesions related to phonotrauma tend to be located at the midpoint of the vocal folds, where the greatest impact force occurs (Hochman et al., 1999). They may also develop within the vocal folds subsequent to repeated bouts of vocal fold inflammation (Hochman et al., 1999; Postma et al., 1998). The preponderance of female professional singers diagnosed with microvascular lesions and vocal fold hemorrhage suggests that the role of cyclic hormonal fluctuations associated with altered blood vessel permeability also should be considered (Abitbol, Abitbol, & Abitbol, 1999; Postma et al., 1998).

When microvascular lesions occur, management depends upon the severity and chronicity of the problem. Initially, individuals with microvascular lesions may be put on a strict vocal hygiene regime that includes a period of voice rest. In some cases, intramuscular Decadron (dexamethasone) may be used in conjunction with voice rest to help reduce inflammation within the vocal fold(s) (Postma et al., 1998). Once vocal fold swelling reduces, voice therapy may be necessary to address chronic voice use patterns associated with phonotrauma or inefficient voice production patterns.

In cases where the preceding treatment approach does not adequately resolve the microvascular lesion, more aggressive medical intervention becomes necessary. This may occur, for example, when an individual chronically exhibits an enlarged blood vessel associated with recurrent vocal fold hemorrhage. In such cases, surgery may be necessary to successfully resolve the lesion. The most successful surgical approach to address such microvascular lesions involves cauterizing the lesion (Hochman et al., 1999; Postma et al., 1998). For women, however, the decision to perform surgery needs to take into consideration hormonal influences on the vocal fold vasculature. Microvascular lesions increase in size during the premenstrual and early menstrual period phases associated with reduced permeability of capillaries subsequent to increased levels of progesterone (Abitbol et al., 1999; Postma et al., 1998). Surgery performed during these phases may increase the risk of postoperative hemorrhaging and possible scarring.

The outcome of surgical treatment for microvascular lesions has been reported to be highly successful. In the study by Postma et al. (1998), surgical intervention was necessary in 36% of the persons with isolated vocal fold microvascular lesions. All but one of the individuals who underwent surgery were female professional voice users. Based on the surgeon's report, normal vocal function occurred following surgery in eight of the nine patients. For those persons with a successful outcome, full recovery was reported to occur after an average of 3.5 months (range = 1 mo–11 mos). Long-term follow-up performed from 1 year to 4.5 years postsurgery indicated that the individuals with an initial successful surgical outcome eventually returned to unrestricted vocal use without further problems.

Vocal Fold Hemorrhage

A vocal fold hemorrhage is a large rupture of a vocal fold blood vessel along the superior surface of the vocal folds. This can occur as a result of laryngeal trauma subsequent to a blunt external laryngeal impact or from phonotrauma, such as occurs during excessive coughing, sneezing, screaming, or prolonged and strained voice use. Women may be more predisposed to a vocal fold hemorrhage during the premenstrual and early menstrual phases, as discussed earlier (Abitbol et al., 1999; Hochman et al., 1999). In addition, high blood pressure or medications that alter blood clot formation may increase the risk of a vocal fold hemorrhage.

This type of hemorrhage may affect a portion, or the entire superior surface, of the vocal fold, depending upon its severity. In addition, this hemorrhaging may occur in one fold or both folds. Once a major rupture of a blood vessel occurs, blood is released into the surrounding tissues, causing vocal fold mass and mucosal stiffness to increase. Subsequently, the amplitude of vocal fold vibrational excursion, as well as efficiency of approximation during voicing, will be reduced. The symptoms of vocal fold hemorrhage can be described as a sudden change in voice quality characterized by a lowered pitch, reduced pitch and volume ranges, and onset of hoarseness.

Treatment for vocal fold hemorrhage primarily entails complete voice rest for 1 week to 2 weeks. Complete voice rest dramatically reduces vocal fold contact time and movement, which allows the vocal fold tissues to recover and repair damage suffered from the hemorrhage. Beyond complete voice rest, limited and noneffortful talking may be introduced. Low-effort speaking techniques utilize increased breathiness and reduced volume, thereby reducing the force of impact between the vocal folds during voicing. Instruction in this modified voice rest combines voice therapy methods such the yawn–sigh and easy voice onset with a generalized breathy and relaxed voice quality while speaking, referred to as *confidential voice use* (Colton & Casper, 1990). Amplification can also be used to facilitate low-effort speaking while adequately projecting the voice.

In addition to modified speaking techniques, other behaviors associated with phonotrauma, such as throat clearing, coughing, excessive talking, and excessively loud talking, are monitored and reduced. As the individual recovers more fully from the hemorrhage, vocal retraining may be necessary to address voicing behaviors that can lead to reinjury or strain. Professional voice users will need to refrain from their typical vocal routines for 6 to 8 weeks, until the hemorrhage heals fully and they recover their vocal range and strength. Once vocal rehabilitation approaches completion, vocal coaching can be incorporated into the retraining program to facilitate a gradual return to performance. In the majority of cases, vocal fold hemorrhage can be successfully treated without surgical intervention.

In some cases, individuals may recover from their initial vocal fold hemorrhage only to suffer repeated recurrences. In these individuals, chronic microvascular lesions may be visualized on the vocal fold(s) between hemorrhagic recurrences (Hochman et al., 1999). In such cases, surgical treatment of the chronic microvascular lesions, as described in the previous section, will reduce the likelihood of hemorrhagic recurrence (Hochman et al., 1999; Postma et al., 1998).

One of the most common benign lesions of the larynx are polyps (Kleinsasser, 1982). Polyps can take on various forms, such as those attached to the mucosa by a stalk, giving a pedunculated appearance, versus those that form along the mucosa and that appear similar to ones seen in nodules. The latter are referred to as *sessile polyps.* In a study reported by Kleinsasser (1982), of 900 individuals treated at the University of Marburg for vocal fold polyps, 76% were men and 24% were women, with an average age between 30 and 50 years. None of these patients were below 20 years of age. The majority (80% to 90%) reported that they smoked. In addition, many of the 900 individuals treated for laryngeal polyps reported vocal and laryngeal behaviors associated with phonotrauma. It was not reported whether onset of polyp symptoms began after a specific vocal event, such as is typically associated with the onset of laryngeal polyps (McFarlane & Von Berg, 1998).

Polyps associated with severe phonotrauma tend to form subsequent to hemorrhaging at the midpoint of the vocal folds, where maximum impact force occurs (Kleinsasser, 1982; McFarlane & Von Berg, 1998; Sataloff et al., 1994). Kleinsasser described the progression of polyp formation as originating from ruptured or dilated blood vessels that form grape-like clusters and become gradually more pedunculated (Kleinsasser, 1982). Most commonly, microvascular lesions become engulfed in a transparent gelatin that is enclosed within the overlying mucosal epithelium (Kleinsasser, 1982). Depending upon the extent of tissue damage preceding polyp formation, increasing vascularization within the pedunculated polyp gives it the appearance of being filled with blood. Permeability of the blood vessels forming within the polyp leads to gradual accumulation of additional fluids, in turn leading to growth in polyp size over time.

Treatment of hemorrhagic polyps is the same as for other forms of polyps. Initially, either complete or modified voice rest is implemented to reduce the amount of vocal fold contact force related to voice production. In some cases, steroids are administered in low doses to help reduce inflammation (Sataloff, 1998). Vocal hygiene promotes reduction of voicing and laryngeal behaviors associated with phonotrauma. Finally, vocal retraining may be necessary to address voicing patterns that may be associated with the formation of the polyp.

In most cases, polyps will not fully resolve without surgical intervention (Kleinsasser, 1982; Sataloff, 1998). If a vocal fold polyp does not resolve and is not surgically removed, tissue changes may occur where the polyp hits the opposing vocal fold. Although surgeons try to preserve as much of the vocal fold edge as possible when removing the polyp, scarring may occur as a consequence of polyp removal. Because scar formation leads to stiffer mucosa, the vocal fold mucosal wave will be reduced in areas of scarring.

References

Abitbol, J., Abitbol, P., & Abitbol, B. (1999). Sex hormones and the female voice. *Journal of Voice, 13,* 424–446.

Amenta, F., & Mione, M. C. (1988). Age-related changes in the noradrenergic innervation of the coronary arteries in old rats: A fluorescent histochemical study. *Journal of the Autonomic Nervous System, 22,* 247–251.

Amerini, S., Mantelli, L., Filippi, S., & Ledda, F. (1994). Effects of aging and hypertension on vasorelaxant activity of calcitonin gene-related peptide—A comparison with other vasodilator agents. *Journal of Cardiovascular Pharmacology, 23,* 432–437.

Andersen, P., & Saltin, B. (1985). Maximal perfusion of skeletal muscle in man. *Journal of Physiology, 366,* 233–249.

Anderson, K. M., & Faber, J. E. (1991). Differential sensitivity of arteriolar alpha 1- and alpha 2-adrenoceptor constriction to metabolic inhibition during rat skeletal muscle contraction. *Circulation Research, 69,* 174–184.

Andrews, T. J., Li, D., Halliwell, J., & Cowen, T. (1994). The effect of age on dendrites in the rat superior cervical ganglion. *Journal of Anatomy, 184*(1), 111–117.

Anversa, P., Li, P., Sonnenblick, E. H., & Olivetti, G. (1994). Effects of aging on quantitative structural properties of coronary vasculature and microvasculature in rats. *American Journal of Physiology, 267,* H1062–H1073.

Armstrong, W. B., & Netterville, J. L. (1995). Anatomy of the larynx, trachea, and bronchi. *Otolaryngologic Clinics of North America, 28,* 685–699.

Arnstein, D. P., Berke, G. S., Trapp, T. K., & Natividad, M. (1989). Regional blood flow to the canine vocal fold at rest and during phonation. *Annals of Otology, Rhinology & Laryngology, 98,* 796–802.

Balon, T. W., & Nadler, J. L. (1994). Nitric oxide release is present from incubated skeletal muscle preparations. *Journal of Applied Physiology, 77,* 2519–2521.

Bombeli, T., Schwartz, B. R., & Harlan, J. M. (1999). Endothelial cells undergoing apoptosis become proadhesive for nonactivated platelets. *Blood, 93,* 3831–3838.

Bouchayer, M., & Cornut, G. (1988). Microsurgery for benign lesions of the vocal folds. *Ear, Nose and Throat Journal, 67,* 446–466.

Brancatisano, A., Kelly, W. T., Baile, E. M., Pare, P., & Engel, L. A. (1993). Blood flow distribution to upper airway muscles. *Journal of Applied Physiology, 74,* 1928–1933.

Brondbo, K., Dahl, H. A., & Teig, E. (1985). The histochemistry of the posterior cricoarytenoid (PCA) muscle in the dog, compared with the diaphragm, the sternothyroid and the sternomastoid muscle. *Acta Oto-Laryngologica, 100,* 289–298.

Burnstock, G. (1987). Mechanisms of interaction of peptide and nonpeptide vascular neurotransmitter systems. *Journal of Cardiovascular Pharmacology, 10,* s74–s81.

Burnstock, G. (1990). *Overview: Purinergic mechanisms.* In G. R. Dubyak & J. R. Fedan (Eds.), *Biological actions of extracellular ATP* (pp. 1–14). New York: New York Academy of Sciences.

Chen, B. M., & Grinnell, A. D. (1995). Integrins and modulation of transmitter release from motor nerve terminals by stretch. *Science, 269,* 1578–1580.

Christ, G. J., Spray, D. C., el-Sabban, M., Moore, L. K., & Brink, P. R. (1996). Gap junctions in vascular tissues: Evaluating the role of intercellular communication in the modulation of vasomotor tone. *Circulation Research, 79,* 631–646.

Claassen, H., & Klaws, G. R. (1992). Preparation of four-color arterial corrosion casts of the laryngeal arteries. *Surgical and Radiologic Anatomy, 14,* 301–305.

Coggan, A. R., Spina, R. J., King, D. S., Rogers, M. A., Brown, M., Nemeth, P. M., et al. (1992). Histochemical and enzymatic comparison of the gastrocnemius muscle of young and elderly men and women. *Journal of Gerontology, 47*, B71–B76.

Colton, R., & Casper, J. (1990). *Understanding voice problems: A physiological perspective for diagnosis and treatment.* Baltimore: Williams & Wilkins.

Cook, J. J., Wailgum, T. D., Vasthare, U. S., Mayrovitz, H. N., & Tuma, R. F. (1992). Age-related alterations in the arterial microvasculature of skeletal muscle. *Journal of Gerontology, 47*, B83–B88.

Cortes, V., Donoso, M. V., Brown, N., Fanjul, R., Lopez, C., Fournier, A., et al. (1999). Synergism between neuropeptide Y and norepinephrine highlights sympathetic cotransmission: Studies in rat arterial mesenteric bed with neuropeptide Y, analogs, and BIBP 3226. *Journal of Pharmacology and Experimental Therapeutics, 289*, 1313–1322.

Courey, M., & Ossoff, R. (1996). Lesions of the lamina propria. In W. S. Brown, B. P. Vinson, & M. A. Crary (Eds.), *Organic voice disorders: Assessment and treatment* (pp. 245–260). San Diego, CA: Singular.

Cunha, R. A., & Sebastiao, A. M. (1993). Adenosine and adenine nucleotides are independently released from both the nerve terminals and the muscle fibres upon electrical stimulation of the innervated skeletal muscle of the frog. *Pflugers Archives, 424*, 503–510.

Davis, J. R., & Lyon, M. J. (2000, February). *A quantitative stereological and microsphere study of age-related vascular changes in the rat utricular macula.* Paper presented at the Association for Research in Otolaryngology 23rd midwinter meeting, St. Petersburg, FL.

Degens, H. (1998). Age-related changes in the microcirculation of skeletal muscle. *Advances in Experimental Medicine and Biology, 454*, 343–348.

Delp, M. D., & Laughlin, M. H. (1998). Regulation of skeletal muscle perfusion during exercise. *Acta Physiologica Scandinavica, 162*, 411–419.

Desaki, J., Kawakita, S., & Yamagata, T. (1997). Occurrence of capillaries with fenestrae in the intrinsic laryngeal muscles of the guinea pig after unilateral denervation. *Journal of Electron Microscopy, 46,* 491–495.

Desaki, J., Oki, S., Matsuda, Y., & Sakanaka, M. (2000). Morphological changes of capillaries in the rat soleus muscle following experimental tenotomy. *Journal of Electron Microscopy, 49,* 185–193.

Deussen, A., Moser, G., & Schrader, J. (1986). Contribution of coronary endothelial cells to cardiac adenosine production. *Pflugers Archives, 406,* 608–614.

Domeij, S., Dahlqvist, A., & Forsgren, S. (1991). Studies on colocalization of neuropeptide Y, vasoactive intestinal polypeptide, catecholamine-synthesizing enzymes and acetylcholinesterase in the larynx of the rat. *Cell and Tissue Research, 263,* 495–505.

Drenckhahn, D., & Ness, W. (1997). The endothelial contractile cytoskeleton. In G. V. R. Born & C. J. Schwartz (Eds.), *Vascular endothelium: Physiology, pathology and therapeutic opportunities* (pp. 1–15). Stuttgart, Germany: Schattauer.

Folkow, B., Sonnenschein, R. R., & Wright, D. L. (1971). Loci of neurogenic and metabolic effects on precapillary vessels of skeletal muscle. *Acta Physiologica Scandinavica, 81,* 459–471.

Forssmann, W. G., & Said, S. I. (1998). VIP, PACAP, and related peptides. In *Annals of the New York Academy of Sciences: Third international symposium.* New York: New York Academy of Sciences.

Franco-Cereceda, A., Matran, R., Alving, K., & Lundberg, J. M. (1995). Sympathetic vascular control of the laryngeo-tracheal, bronchial and pulmonary circulation in the pig: Evidence for non-adrenergic mechanisms involving neuropeptide Y. *Acta Physiologica Scandinavica, 155,* 193–204.

Franz, P., & Aharinejad, S. (1994). The microvasculature of the larynx: A scanning electron microscopic study. *Scanning Microscopy, 8,* 125–130.

Freeland, A. P. (1975). Microfil angiography: A demonstration of the microvasculature of the larynx with reference to tumor spread. *Canadian Journal of Otolaryngology, 4,* 111–127.

Frenzel, H., & Kleinsasser, O. (1982). Ultrastructural study on the small blood vessels of human vocal cords. *Archives of Otorhinolaryngologica, 236,* 147–160.

Granger, D. N., Perry, M. A., & Kvietys, P. R. (1983). The microcirculation and fluid transport in digestive organs. *Federation Procedures, 42,* 1667–1672.

Habler, H. J., Wasner, G., & Janig, W. (1997). Attenuation of neurogenic vasoconstriction by nitric oxide in hindlimb microvascular beds of the rat in vivo. *Hypertension, 30,* 957–961.

Hellsten, Y., & Frandsen, U. (1997). Adenosine formation in contracting primary rat skeletal muscle cells and endothelial cells in culture. *Journal of Physiology, 504*(3), 695–704.

Hirano, M. (1975). Phonosurgery: Basic and clinical investigation. *Otolagia, 21*(Suppl. 1), 254–260.

Hisa, Y., Koike, S., Tadaki, N., Bamba, H., Shogaki, K., & Uno, T. (1999). Neurotransmitters and neuromodulators involved in laryngeal innervation. *Annals of Otology, Rhinology & Laryngology, 108,* 3–14.

Hochman, I., Hillman, R. E., Sataloff, R. T., & Zeitels, S. M. (1999). Ectasias and varices of the vocal fold: Clearing the striking zone. *Annals of Otology, Rhinology & Laryngology, 108,* 10–16.

Hokfelt, T., Broberger, C., Zhang, X., Diez, M., Kopp, J., Xu, Z., et al. (1998). Neuropeptide Y: Some viewpoints on a multifaceted peptide in the normal and diseased nervous system. *Brain Research Reviews, 26,* 154–166.

Ichev, K. (1968). Functional examination of the laryngeal blood circulation in rabbit. *Nauchni Trudove Na Visshiia Meditsinski Institut, Sofiia, 47,* 29–33.

Janicki, J. S., Sheriff, D. D., Robotham, J. L., & Wise, R. A. (1996). Cardiac output during exercise: Contributions of the cardiac, circulatory, and respiratory systems. In L. G. Rowell (Ed.), *Exercise: Regulation and integration of multiple systems* (pp. 649–704). New York: Oxford University Press.

Joris, I., Cuenoud, H. F., Doern, G. V., Underwood, J. M., & Majno, G. (1990). Capillary leakage in inflammation: A study by vascular labeling. *American Journal of Pathology, 137,* 1353–1363.

Kahane, J. C. (1983). Boundaries of the cricothyroid, thyroarytenoid and lateral cricoarytenoid muscles formed by arterial pedicles from the superior and inferior laryngeal arteries. In I. Titze & R. C. Scherer (Eds.), *Vocal fold physiology: Biomechanics, acoustics and phonatory control* (pp. 15–25). Denver, CO: Denver Center for the Performing Arts.

Kleinsasser, O. (1982). Pathogenesis of vocal cord polyps. *Annals of Otology, Rhinology & Laryngology, 91,* 378–381.

Kobzik, L., Reid, M. B., Bredt, D. S., & Stamler, J. S. (1994). Nitric oxide in skeletal muscle. *Nature, 372,* 546–548.

Korneliussen, H. (1975). Fenestrated blood capillaries and lymphatic capillaries in rat skeletal muscle. *Cell and Tissue Research, 163,* 169–174.

Krogh, A., Harrop, G. A., & Rehberg, P. B. (1922). Studies on the physiology of capillaries: III. The innervation of the blood vessels in the hind legs of the frog. *Journal of Physiology, 56,* 179–189.

Kurjiaka, D. T., & Segal, S. S. (1995). Conducted vasodilation elevates flow in arteriole networks of hamster striated muscle. *American Journal of Physiology, 269,* H1723–H1728.

Lartaud, I., Bray, D. B., Chillon, J. M., Atkinson, J., & Capdeville-Atkinson, C. (1993). In vivo cerebrovascular reactivity in Wistar and Fischer 344 rat strains during aging. *American Journal of Physiology, 264,* H851–H858.

Lasjaunias, P., Halimi, P., & Choi, I. S. (1983). Clinical and angiographic anatomy of the arteries of the larynx. *Journal of Neuroradiology, 10,* 281–299.

Laughlin, M. H., Korthuis, R. J., Duncker, D. J., & Bache, R. J. (1996). *Control of blood flow to cardiac and skeletal muscle during exercise.* In L. G. Rowell, J. T. Shepherd, J. A. Dempsey, et al. (Eds.), *Exercise: Regulation and integration of multiple systems* (pp. 705–769). New York: Oxford University Press.

Levick, J. R., & Smaje, L. H. (1987). An analysis of the permeability of a fenestra. *Microvascular Research, 33,* 233–256.

Lundberg, J. M., Franco-Cereceda, A., Lacroix, J. S., & Pernow, J. (1990). Neuropeptide Y and sympathetic neurotransmission. *Annals of the New York Academy of Sciences, 611,* 166–174.

Luts, A., Uddman, E., Grunditz, T., & Sundler, F. (1990). Peptide-containing neurons projecting to the vocal cords of the rat: Retrograde tracing and immunocytochemistry. *Journal of the Autonomic Nervous System, 30,* 179–192.

Lyon, M. J. (2000a). [Apoptosis within the aging human thyroarytenoid and posterior cricoarytenoid muscles]. Unpublished observations.

Lyon, M. J. (2000b). Nonadrenergic innervation of the rat laryngeal vasculature. *Anatomical Record, 259,* 180–188.

Lyon, M. J., & Wanamaker, H. H. (1993). Blood flow and assessment of capillaries in the aging rat posterior canal crista. *Hearing Research, 67,* 157–165.

Malmgren, L. T., Fisher, P. J., Bookman, L. M., & Uno, T. (1999). Age-related changes in muscle fiber types in the human thyroarytenoid muscle: An immunohistochemical and stereological study using confocal laser scanning microscopy. *Archives of Otolaryngology—Head & Neck Surgery, 121,* 441–451.

Malmgren, L. T., & Gacek, R. R. (1981). Histochemical characteristics of muscle fiber types in the posterior cricoarytenoid muscle. *Annals of Otology, Rhinology & Laryngology, 90,* 423–429.

Malmgren, L. T., Gacek, R. R., & Etzler, C. A. (1983). Muscle fiber types in the human posterior cricoarytenoid muscle: A correlated histochemical and ultrastructural morphometric study. In I. R. Titze & R. C. Scherer (Eds.), *Vocal fold physiology: Biomechanics, acoustics and phonatory control* (pp. 41–56). Denver, CO: Denver Center for the Performing Arts.

Malmgren, L. T., Lovice, D. B., & Kaufman, M. R. (2000). Age-related changes in muscle fiber regeneration in the human thyroarytenoid muscle. *Archives of Otolaryngology—Head & Neck Surgery, 126,* 851–856.

Malmgren, L. T., & Lyon, M. J. (2000). [Age-related changes in rat laryngeal blood flow]. Unpublished observations.

Mantelli, L., Amerini, S., & Ledda, F. (1995). Bradykinin-induced vasodilation is changed to a vasoconstrictor response in vessels of aged normotensive and hypertensive rats. *Inflammation Research, 44*(2), 70–73.

Marin, J. (1995). Age-related changes in vascular responses: A review. *Mechanisms of Aging and Development, 79*(2–3), 71–114.

Marshall, J. M. (2000). Adenosine and muscle vasodilatation in acute systemic hypoxia. *Acta Physiologica Scandinavica, 168,* 561–573.

Matsuo, K., Oda, M., Tomita, M., Maehara, N., Umezaki, T., & Shin, T. (1987). An experimental study of the circulation of the vocal fold on phonation. *Archives of Otolaryngology—Head & Neck Surgery, 113,* 414–417.

Mayhan, W. G., Faraci, F. M., Baumbach, G. L., & Heistad, D. D. (1990). Effects of aging on responses of cerebral arterioles. *American Journal of Physiology, 258,* H1138–H1143.

McCullough, W. T., Collins, D. M., & Ellsworth, M. L. (1997). Arteriolar responses to extracellular ATP in striated muscle. *American Journal of Physiology, 272,* H1886–H1891.

McFarlane, S. C., & Von Berg, S. (1998). Facilitative techniques in intervention for dysphonia. *Current Opinion in Otolaryngology & Head and Neck Surgery, 6,* 161–165.

McGillivray-Anderson, K. M., & Faber, J. E. (1990). Effect of acidosis on contraction of microvascular smooth muscle by alpha 1- and alpha 2-adrenoceptors: Implications for neural and metabolic regulation. *Circulation Research, 66,* 1643–1657.

McKinney, R. V. J., Singh, B. B., & Brewer, P. D. (1977). Fenestrations in regenerating skeletal muscle capillaries. *American Journal of Anatomy, 150,* 213–218.

Michel, C. C., & Curry, F. E. (1999). Microvascular permeability. *Physiological Reviews, 79,* 703–761.

Nakai, Y., Masutani, H., Moriguchi, M., Matsunaga, K., & Sugita, M. (1991). Microvascular structure of the larynx: A scanning electron microscopic study of microcorrosion casts. *Acta Otolaryngology Supplement, 486,* 254–263.

Nakane, M., Schmidt, H. H., Pollock, J. S., Forstermann, U., & Murad, F. (1993). Cloned human brain nitric oxide synthase is highly expressed in skeletal muscle. *Federation of European Biochemical Studies Letters, 316,* 175–180.

Nielsen, H., Hasenkam, J. M., Pilegaard, H. K., Mortensen, F. V., & Mulvany, M. J. (1991). Alpha-adrenoceptors in human resistance arteries from colon, pericardial fat, and skeletal muscle. *American Journal of Physiology, 261,* H762–H767.

Ohyanagi, M., Nishigaki, K., & Faber, J. E. (1992). Interaction between microvascular alpha 1- and alpha 2-adrenoceptors and endothelium-derived relaxing factor. *Circulation Research, 71,* 188–200.

Oki, S., Desaki, J., Matsuda, Y., Okumura, H., & Shibata, T. (1995). Capillaries with fenestrae in the rat soleus muscle after experimental limb immobilization. *Journal of Electron Microscopy, 44,* 307–310.

Postma, G. N., Courey, M. S., & Ossoff, R. H. (1998). Microvascular lesions of the true vocal fold. *Annals of Otology, Rhinology & Laryngology, 107,* 472–476.

Radegran, G. (1997). Ultrasound Doppler estimates of femoral artery blood flow during dynamic knee extensor exercise in humans. *Journal of Applied Physiology, 83,* 1383–1388.

Radegran, G., & Saltin, B. (1998). Muscle blood flow at onset of dynamic exercise in humans. *American Journal of Physiology, 274,* H314–H322.

Renkin, E. M. (1977). Multiple pathways of capillary permeability. *Circulation Research, 41,* 735–743.

Rowell, L. B., O'Leary, D. S., & Kellogg, D. L. (1996). Integration of cardiovascular control systems in dynamic exercise. In L. G.

Rowell, J. T. Shepherd, J. A. Dempsey, et al. (Eds.), *Exercise: Regulation and integration of multiple systems* (pp. 770–838). New York: Oxford University Press.

Saltin, B., Radegran, G., Koskolou, M. D., & Roach, R. C. (1998). Skeletal muscle blood flow in humans and its regulation during exercise. *Acta Physiologica Scandinavica, 162,* 421–436.

Sataloff, R. T. (1998). Common medical diagnoses and treatments in professional voice users. In R. T. Sataloff (Ed.), *Vocal health and pedagogy* (pp. 107–122). San Diego, CA: Singular.

Sataloff, R. T., Hawkshaw, M., & Spiegel, J. R. (1998). Varicosities, hemorrhages and vocal fold masses. *Ear, Nose and Throat Journal, 77,* 808.

Sataloff, R. T., Heuer, R. J., & Hawkshaw, M. J. (1994). Vocal fold varicosities and pain on phonation. *Ear, Nose and Throat Journal, 73,* 807.

Sato, K., Hirano, M., & Nakashima, T. (1999). Electron microscopic and immunohistochemical investigation of Reinke's edema. *Annals of Otology, Rhinology & Laryngology, 108,* 1068–1072.

Seals, D. R. (1989). Sympathetic neural discharge and vascular resistance during exercise in humans. *Journal of Applied Physiology, 66,* 2472–2478.

Segal, S. S. (1991). Microvascular recruitment in hamster striated muscle: Role for conducted vasodilation. *American Journal of Physiology, 261,* H181–H189.

Segal, S. S., & Duling, B. R. (1986a). Communication between feed arteries and microvessels in hamster striated muscle: Segmental vascular responses are functionally coordinated. *Circulation Research, 59,* 283–290.

Segal, S. S., & Duling, B. R. (1986b). Flow control among microvessels coordinated by intercellular conduction. *Science, 234,* 868–870.

Segal, S. S., Welsh, D. G., & Kurjiaka, D. T. (1999). Spread of vasodilatation and vasoconstriction along feed arteries and arterioles of hamster skeletal muscle. *Journal of Physiology, 516*(1), 283–291.

Shepherd, J. T. (1987). Circulatory response to exercise in health. *Circulation, 76*(6, Pt. 2), 13–10.

Shin, T., Rabuzzi, D. D., & Reed, G. F. (1970). Vasomotor responses to laryngeal nerve stimulation. *Archives of Otolaryngology—Head & Neck Surgery, 91*, 257–261.

Simionescu, M., & Simionescu, N. (1984). Ultrastucture of the microvascular wall: Functional correlations. In E. M. Renkin, C. C. Michel, & S. R. Geiger (Eds.), *Handbook of physiology: Vol. 4. The cardiovascular system—Microcirculation, Part 1* (pp. 41–101). Bethesda, MD: American Physiological Society.

Sokjer, H., & Olofsson, J. (1979). Arterial anatomy in the normal larynx and in laryngeal carcinoma: Radiography of specimens. *Acta Radiologica Supplementum, 20*, 917–927.

Song, H., & Tyml, K. (1993). Evidence for sensing and integration of biological signals by the capillary network. *American Journal of Physiology, 265*, H1235–H1242.

Starling, E. H. (1896). On the absorption of fluids from the connective tissue spaces. *Journal of Physiology, 19*, 312–326.

Tateishi, J., & Faber, J. E. (1995). ATP-sensitive K+ channels mediate alpha 2D-adrenergic receptor contraction of arteriolar smooth muscle and reversal of contraction by hypoxia. *Circulation Research, 76*, 53–63.

Teig, E., Dahl, H. A., & Thorkelsen, H. (1978). Actomyosin ATPase activity of human laryngeal muscles. *Acta Otolaryngology, 85*, 272–281.

Thomas, G. D., Hansen, J., & Victor, R. G. (1994). Inhibition of alpha 2-adrenergic vasoconstriction during contraction of glycolytic, not oxidative, rat hindlimb muscle. *American Journal of Physiology, 266*, H920–H929.

Thurston, G., Maas, K., LaBarbara, A., McLean, J. W., & McDonald, D. M. (2000). Microvascular remodelling in chronic airway inflammation in mice. *Clinical and Experimental Pharmacology and Physiology, 27*, 836–841.

Tomita, M., Matsuo, K., Maehara, N., Umezaki, T., & Shin, T. (1988). Measurements of oxygen pressure in the vocal fold during laryngeal nerve stimulation. *Archives of Otolaryngology—Head and Neck Surgery, 114,* 308–312.

Tsuda, K., Shin, T., & Masuko, S. (1992). Immunohistochemical study of intralaryngeal ganglia in the cat. *Otolaryngology—Head & Neck Surgery, 106,* 42–46.

van Brummelen, P., Jie, K., Timmermans, P. B., & van Zwieten, P. A. (1985). Postjunctional alpha-adrenoceptors and the regulation of arteriolar tone in humans. *Journal of Cardiovascular Pharmacology, 7*(Suppl. 6), S149–S152.

van Brummelen, P., Jie, K., & van Zwieten, P. A. (1986). Alpha-adrenergic receptors in human blood vessels. *British Journal of Clinical Pharmacology, 21*(Suppl. 1), 33S–39S.

Weibel, E. R. (1980). Basic stereological principles and finite section thickness. In E. R. Weibel (Ed.), *Stereological methods* (pp. 105–139). London: Academic Press.

Welsh, D. G., & Segal, S. S. (1996). Muscle length directs sympathetic nerve activity and vasomotor tone in resistance vessels of hamster retractor. *Circulation Research, 79,* 551–559.

Welsh, D. G., & Segal, S. S. (1997). Coactivation of resistance vessels and muscle fibers with acetylcholine release from motor nerves. *American Journal of Physiology, 273,* H156–H163.

Welsh, D. G., & Segal, S. S. (1998). Endothelial and smooth muscle cell conduction in arterioles controlling blood flow. *American Journal of Physiology: Heart and Circulatory Physiology, 274,* H178–H186.

Chapter 5

Intervention for Vocal Fold Atrophy, Vocal Fold Bowing, and Immobility

Leslie T. Malmgren and Leslie Glaze

Malmgren and Glaze emphasize that the vocal folds have a complex histological makeup that is prone to the effects of aging. They point out that aging effects are most often acquainted with vocal fold bowing or vocal fold atrophy and with a condition that has been termed presbylaryngeus. *The authors explain the mechanisms underlying atrophy and bowing and the clinical manifestations and symptoms of these two vocal fold conditions.*

1. *List at least three laryngeal physical changes that accompany the normal aging process.*

2. *What is the relationship between exercise and muscle disuse/use? How could this information be incorporated into a treatment program for conditions such as vocal fold atrophy or bowing?*

3. *Why has current theory invalidated the use of the push–pull technique for improving vocal fold adduction?*

The vocal folds have a layered structure that consists of the epithelium, the lamina propria, and the thyroarytenoid (TA) muscle (Hirano, 1977). Studies concerning the basic cellular and molecular mechanisms underlying vocal fold atrophy and bowing have been carried out primarily in relation to the aging process. The mechanisms underlying vocal fold aging differ between layers and involve not only atrophy and cell death but also a complex, age-related remodeling of the tissue in the lamina propria, as well as in the TA muscle.

Remodeling of the Vocal Fold Mucosa

A number of studies have suggested that age-related remodeling of the layered structure of the lamina propria may contribute to an age-related change in the voice. According to the cover-body theory of phonation, the epithelium, the superficial layer of the lamina propria, and much of the intermediate layer of the lamina propria vibrate as a "cover" on a relatively stationary "body," which consists of the remainder of the intermediate layer, the deep layer, and the TA muscle (Hirano, 1977). Hirano, Kurita, and Sakaguchi (1989) reported that there is an age-related decrease in the depth of the superficial and intermediate layers of the lamina propria of the vocal fold, and Tanaka, Hirano, and Chijiwa (1994) suggested that this may result in vocal fold bowing. Because elastin likely plays a key role in the biomechanics of the lamina propria (Gray, Titze, Alipour, & Hammond, 2000), age-related changes in the density of elastin staining have also been examined. These studies are in disagreement. In a qualitative study, Sato and Hirano (1997) reported an age-related loss of elastin. However, a more recent quantitative study demonstrated an 879% increase in the density of elastin staining in geriatric participants, with no significant gender-related difference (Hammond, Gray, Butler, Zhou, & Hammond, 1998). In addition, Hammond et al. found an age-related increase in the thickness of the intermediate layer, and a decrease in the superficial layer, of the lamina propria. They noted that the decrease in the relative thickness of the superficial layer indicated an age-related change in the cover-to-body ratio, and Gray et al. (2000) suggested that this remodeling process contributes to the formation of sulci or to bowed vocal folds. In contrast to the results obtained for age-related changes in vocal fold elastin, Hammond, Gray, and Butler (2000) found no significant age-related difference in the density of collagen staining in the lamina propria. However, both female adult and geriatric vocal folds had substantially less (59%) collagen staining than male vocal folds.

Remodeling of the TA Muscle

Age-Related Fiber Loss and Atrophy

Because laryngeal motor units differ from those of limb muscles with respect to their pattern of innervation, ultrastructure, and contractile proteins (Bendiksen, Dahl, & Teig, 1981; Briggs & Schachat, 2000; Lucas, Rughani, & Hoh, 1995; Malmgren & Gacek, 1981; Malmgren, Gacek, & Etzler, 1983; Merati et al., 1996; Perie, St. Guily, Callard, & Sebille, 1997), it cannot be assumed that the aging process in the TA is identical to that in the limb muscles. Recent studies concerning age-related changes in the muscle-fiber-type content of the TA muscle (see color Figure 5.1, located at the back of the book) have demonstrated a complex remodeling process that includes a pattern of muscle fiber loss and atrophy that differs from that of most other aging skeletal muscles (Malmgren, Fisher, Bookman, & Uno, 1999; Malmgren, Fisher, Jones, Bookman, & Uno, 2000; Malmgren, Jones, & Bookman, 1999).

It is well known that age-related losses of motor neurons and muscle fibers, as well as muscle fiber atrophy, contribute to decreased contraction speed, strength, and endurance in limb muscles in the elderly (W. F. Brown, Strong, & Snow, 1988; Doherty, Vandervoort, Taylor, & Brown, 1993; Grimby, 1995; Jennekens, Tomlinson, & Walton, 1971; Larsson, 1978; Lexell, Henriksson-Larson, Winblad, & Sjostrom, 1983; Tomonaga, 1977; Wang, dePasqua, & Delwaide, 1999). In limb muscles, this process is characterized by a selective loss and atrophy of Type 2 (fast twitch) muscle fibers (Grimby, 1995; Larsson & Edstrom, 1986; Lexell, 1995). Stereological studies on the human TA muscle have demonstrated a preferential 27% loss in the length density (Lv fiber-type muscle) of Type 1 (slow twitch) muscle fibers, however, which indicates an age-related loss in the number of Type 1 fibers (Malmgren, Fisher, et al.,

1999). In contrast, there is no significant age-related decrease in the length density of Type 2 fibers in the TA or an overall decrease in the mean diameters of Type 2 fibers. There is a significant age-related decrease in the surface density of Type 2 fibers, as well as an increase in the atrophy factor, which is an index of the content of very small, atrophic fibers (Malmgren, Fisher, et al., 1999). These findings indicate that although there is no significant age-related overall atrophy of Type 2 fibers in the TA muscle, as in the limb muscles, there is selective atrophy of a small part of the Type 2 fiber population.

Age-Related Changes in Muscle Fiber Regeneration

An age-related change in the balance between the frequency of cell death or injury and the rate and viability of nerve fiber and muscle fiber regeneration contributes to the loss and atrophy of muscle fibers in the TA muscle. Studies conducted on limb muscles have suggested that a reduced capacity for muscle fiber regeneration may contribute to age-related losses in fiber numbers and muscle mass and to a decline in strength (Brooks & Faulkner, 1994; Carlson, 1995). In spite of the importance of muscle fiber regeneration to the maintenance of muscle mass and strength, the technical challenge of obtaining quantitative estimates of this infrequent process has discouraged relevant studies. Quantitative estimates of the content of regenerating muscle fibers in entire volume of the human TA muscle have recently been obtained using stereological techniques (Malmgren, Fisher, et al., 2000). Because the developmental myosin heavy chain isoform is expressed only in regenerating muscle fibers in adults (d'Albis, Couteaux, Janmot, Roulet, & Mira, 1988), these studies detected regenerating fibers using immunocytochemical techniques to image this contractile protein (see color Figure 5.2, located at the back of the book).

It was demonstrated that muscle fiber regeneration plays an important role in compensating for muscle fiber injury and cell death in the TA muscle (Malmgren, Fisher, et al., 2000). Although regenerating muscle fibers make up only a very small proportion of the total fiber population at any one time, by the age of 70, regeneration has replaced almost twice the original muscle fiber population in the human TA muscle (Malmgren, Lovice, & Kaufman, 2000). Muscle fiber regeneration may involve either the entire muscle fiber or an injured segment (Hall-Craggs, 1974); therefore, the contribution of regeneration to the maintenance of muscle mass and strength is most clearly indicated by the total regenerated muscle fiber length rather than the number of regenerated fibers. These stereological studies demonstrated a 610% age-related increase in the ratio of the length of regenerating muscle fibers to the total muscle fiber length in the entire volume of the human TA muscle (Malmgren, Lovice, & Kaufman, 2000). This increase in the relative length of regenerating fibers likely represents a compensatory response to an age-related increase in muscle fiber cell death and injury, rather than an increase in regenerative capacity, because there is an age-related decrease in Type 1 fibers (Malmgren, Fisher, et al., 1999; Malmgren, Lovice, & Kaufman, 2000), as well as an age-related increase in the frequency of programmed cell death (*apoptosis*) in Type 1 fibers (Malmgren, Jones, & Bookman, 1999). The demonstrated age-related increase in muscle fiber death and regeneration in the human TA muscle is paralleled by an age-related increase in cycles of denervation and reinnervation in laryngeal motor neurons (Malmgren, 1989; Malmgren, Fisher, & Brandes, 1997; Malmgren & Ringwood, 1988; Takeda, Thomas, & Ludlow, 2000). Age-related changes in the interaction of these processes probably contribute to the observed age-related loss of muscle fibers in the TA muscle, as well as to an age-related increase in the remodeling of TA motor units. With advancing age, there is a loss of motor neurons (W. F. Brown et al., 1988; Doherty et al., 1993; Wang et al., 1999), and the capacity for both nerve (Choi, Harii, Lee, Furuya, & Ueda, 1995; Kawabuchi, Chongjian, Islam, Hirata, & Nada, 1998; Verdú, Butí, & Navarro, 1995) and muscle fiber (Cannon, 1998; Carlson & Faulkner, 1998; Marsh, Criswell, Hamilton, & Booth, 1997; Sadeh, 1988) regeneration is diminished. Each cycle of muscle fiber death and regeneration requires successful reinnervation for functional recovery. Consequently, the demonstrated age-related increase in cycles of muscle fiber injury and regeneration increase the demand for reinnervation of regenerated muscle fibers. Because the capacity for reinnervation decreases with age, this increase in the frequency of muscle fiber regeneration contributes to an age-related increase in muscle fiber denervation and atrophy (Carlson & Faulkner, 1996, 1998).

Myonuclei and Muscle Fiber Diameter

The prevention and treatment of age-related muscle fiber loss and atrophy in the TA muscle requires an understanding of the underlying cellular and molecular mechanisms. A recent study suggested that muscle fiber atrophy is generally the result of a decrease in the number of nuclei in the muscle fiber and, conversely, that fiber hypertrophy is the result of an increase in the number of myonuclei (Allen, Roy, & Edgerton, 1999). Most cells have a single nucleus, with a volume of cytoplasm that is relatively constant and specific to the cell type, which suggests that some unknown mechanism regulates the amount of cytoplasm that can be supported by a nucleus in a particular cell type (Hughes & Schiaffino, 1999). Muscle fibers differ from other cell types in that they generate force over a long distance, which requires a relatively high cellular volume. Because the transcriptional capacity of a single nucleus is spatially limited, muscle fibers have evolved specialized regulatory mechanisms that are based on a syncytium (multiple nuclei in a single cell) in which the cytoplasmic volume maintained by an individual myonucleus can be regulated by changes in the number of myonuclei in the muscle fiber (see color Figure 5.3, located at the back of the book).

This makes it possible for a single muscle fiber to be very long and to vary in diameter but to maintain a constant amount of cytoplasm controlled by each myonucleus (nuclear domain). The diameter of the muscle fiber thus is a function of the nuclear domain and the number of myonuclei. These relationships have recently been examined in the human TA muscle through stereological estimates of the numerical densities of myonuclei in muscle fiber types that were identified using immunocytochemical techniques (Malmgren, Fisher, et al., 2000). The numerical density of myonuclei was demonstrated to be relatively high for both Type 1 ($71,303/mm^3$ of fiber volume) and Type 2 fibers ($66,072/mm^3$ of fiber volume) in the TA muscle, with no significant difference between the fiber types. Tseng, Kasper, and Edgerton (1994) found that such high numerical densities of myonuclei occur in fatigue-resistant muscle fiber types that are specialized for oxidative metabolism by having a small diameter and a high mitochondrial content. According to Tseng et al., a high numerical density of myonuclei is thought to provide an increased transcriptional capacity to support a relatively high requirement for mitochondrial gene expression, which compensates for the very limited coding capacity of the mitochondrial genome (Scarpulla, 1997). The human TA muscle is composed almost entirely of Type 1 and Type 2a fibers (Claassen & Werner, 1992; Guida & Zorzetto, 2000), both of which have a high mitochondrial content (Rivero, Talmadge, & Edgerton, 1998) consistent with this relationship. Furthermore, muscle fiber diameters in the TA muscle are substantially smaller than in most other human muscles (Malmgren, Fisher, et al., 1999). This is an adaptation for a high capacity for oxidative metabolism because smaller fiber diameters facilitate the diffusion of oxygen and nutrients from the capillaries (Sieck, Zhan, Prakash, Daood, & Watchko, 1995). In addition, Malmgren, Fisher, et al. (2000) demonstrated that the numerical density of myonuclei increased with decreasing fiber diameter in the human TA muscle in both Types 1 and 2 fibers, which also is likely an adaptation to support an increase in mitochondrial transcriptional requirements with decreasing fiber diameter (Sieck et al., 1995; Tseng et al., 1994).

Relationship of Satellite Cells to Injury and Myonuclei

Because the mass and strength of a muscle is largely a function of the number of myonuclei, muscle atrophy and hypertrophy result from changes in the relative rates of loss and replacement of myonuclei (Allen et al., 1999). Muscle fibers are postmitotic; therefore, the number of myonuclei is determined by the numerical density and proliferative capacity of satellite cells (see Figure 5.3), which are the source of myonuclei (Bischoff, 1999). Stereological studies have demonstrated relatively high numerical densities of satellite cells in the human TA muscle (Malmgren, Fisher, et al., 2000). This is consistent with reports indicating that satellite cells are more numerous in oxidative, fatigue-resistant muscles (e.g., Bischoff, 1999). In addition, the numerical density of satellite cells has been shown to be significantly higher for Type 1 fibers than for Type 2 fibers, and this difference increases with increasing total satellite numerical density (Malmgren, Fisher, et al., 2000). Because the number of satellite cells increases in response to challenges such as injury, overwork, denervation, exercise, or stretch (Allen et al., 1999; Bischoff, 1999), the relatively high numerical density demonstrated for Type 1 fiber satellite cells may be a response to some form of cellular injury or to some change in trophic interactions. This would be consistent with a hypothesis that the Type 1 fibers in the TA muscle are more frequently exposed to injury and that the number of satellite cells on this fiber type increases selectively as the extent of the challenge increases.

Age-Related Change in Satellite Cell Numbers

It has been suggested that decreases in satellite cell numerical densities or in their proliferative capacity may contribute to age-related limb muscle atrophy (Mezzogiorno, Coletta, Zani, Cossu, & Molinaro, 1993). Design-based stereological techniques have been used to assess age-related changes in the numerical densities of satellite cells and myonuclei in the human TA muscle. An overall significant age-related decrease occurs in the ratio of satellite cells to myonuclei in the TA muscle (Malmgren, Fisher, et al., 2000). This decrease must be considered in relation to (a) an age-related increase in the demand for satellite cell proliferation as evidenced by an increase in muscle fiber regeneration (Malmgren, Lovice, & Kaufman, 2000) and (b) an age-related increase in muscle fiber programmed cell death in the TA muscle (Malmgren, Jones, & Bookman, 1999). This suggests an age-related decrease in the response of satellite cell proliferation to the demonstrated age-related increase in muscle fiber injury and cell death in the human TA muscle.

Age-Related Changes in Apoptosis

Programmed cell death, or apoptosis, appears to play a major role in the mechanisms underlying the demonstrated age-related increase in muscle fiber injury and cell death in the human TA muscle. Apoptosis is a complex program of cell suicide that can be influenced by a variety of regulatory stimuli (Thompson, 1995). This process is characterized by DNA fragmentation, which can be detected in tissue sections using in situ labeling of fragmented nuclear DNA (Gavrieli, Sherman, & Ben-Sasson, 1992; Tidball, Albrecht, Lokensgard, & Spencer, 1995). In studies using these techniques on nonlaryngeal skeletal muscles, apoptosis of myonuclei and satellite cells contributed to a wide variety of pathological conditions. These conditions included hind-limb unloading-induced muscle atrophy (Allen et al., 1997), exercise-induced muscle fiber damage (Pod-horska-Okolov et al., 1999; Sandri et al., 1995; Sandri et al., 1997), and denervation atrophy (Tews et al., 1997; Yoshimura & Harii, 1999). Mampuru, Chen, Kalenik, Bradley, & Lee (1996) demonstrated that diminished supplies of trophic factors and oxidative stress (Stangel et al., 1996) also result in apoptosis of myonuclei and satellite cell nuclei. Qualitative studies have shown that myonuclei apoptosis accounts for an age-related loss of muscle fibers in the rhabdosphincter (Strasser, Tiefenthaler, Steinlechner, Bartsch, & Konwalinka, 1999). Recent stereological studies have found a significant age-related increase in the numerical density of apoptotic myonuclei and apoptotic satellite cell nuclei in Type 1 fibers—but not in Type 2 fibers—in the entire volume of the human TA muscle (Malmgren, Jones, & Bookman, 1999, 2001). This suggests that an increased frequency of some form of cellular injury contributes to the demonstrated selective loss of Type 1 fibers in the human TA muscle. However, as indicated, apoptosis has been shown to play a role in a variety of pathological conditions, and the cellular and molecular mechanisms underlying this increase in apoptosis are presently unknown.

Remodeling of Motor Units

In addition to the demonstrated loss and atrophy of muscle fibers, an age-related increase in the remodeling of the motor units in the TA muscle occurs. A number of studies have indicated that this is due to an ongoing cycle of denervation and reinnervation. Consistent with this mechanism, there is an age-related increase in the numbers of degenerating and regenerating myelinated nerve fibers in the recurrent laryngeal nerve (Malmgren & Ringwood, 1988). In addition, the number of extremely small, atrophic Type 2 fibers in the human TA muscle also increases, with no significant loss in the total number of Type 2 fibers (Malmgren, Fisher, et al., 1999). An age-related increase also occurs in the content of muscle fibers in the human TA muscle that have a coexistence of both slow and fast myosin heavy chain isoforms (Malmgren, Fisher, et al., 1999), which is consistent with results obtained in aging limb muscles (Klitgaard et al., 1990). Changes in myosin heavy chain isoform expression have been found with altered motor unit activity patterns and a number of other factors (Pette & Staron, 1997). These transitions between muscle fiber types may also result, however, from age-related remodeling of motor units caused by cycles of denervation and reinnervation that accompany age-related loss of motor neurons (Larsson, 1995). In this process, denervated muscle fibers are reinnervated by local sprouting of axons, and muscle-fiber-type conversions occur consistent with the type of the new motor unit. Because this process is local, the normally random topographical distribution of muscle fiber types can progress to clusters of fibers of the same type (muscle fiber "type grouping"; Ansved, Wallner, Larsson, 1991). This process probably contributes to the observed increase of transitional fiber types in the aging human TA muscle. More direct evidence for this mechanism is the finding by Malmgren et al. (1997) that muscle fiber "type grouping" in the human TA muscle increases. Muscle-fiber-type grouping is a well-established indicator of partial denervation followed by reinnervation. The process of motor unit remodeling that results in muscle-fiber-type grouping can also be detected using electromyography. Consistent with these findings is a recent report that demonstrates a significant age-related increase in motor unit duration in the human TA muscle (Takeda et al., 2000).

Effect of Muscle Use and Misuse

A better understanding of the relationship of muscle use and misuse to age-related changes in the laryngeal muscles may provide a basis for improved forms of intervention. It is well known that age-related muscle atrophy and loss of strength in limb muscles can be slowed or even reversed through exercise (Frischknecht, 1998; Singh et al., 1999). Changes in muscle use, such as exercise, stretch, or immobilization, cause changes in the mitotic activity and numerical density of satellite cells (Darr & Schultz, 1989; Delp & Pette, 1994; Kadi, Eriksson, Holmner, Butler-Browne, & Thornell, 1999; Snow, 1990). The resulting change in the number of myonuclei leads to a corresponding increase or decrease in the muscle fiber diameter and in the mass and strength of the muscle (Allen et al., 1996). Although it has been demonstrated that intensive voice and respiration training can improve vocal fold adduction in patients with Parkinson's disease (Ramig, Countryman, O'Brien, Hoehn, & Thompson, 1996; Ramig & Drumey, 1996), strength or endurance training techniques have not been systematically studied in relation to the prevention or reversal of age-related changes in the laryngeal muscles.

The relationship between specific types of muscle use and contraction-induced muscle fiber injuries also requires clarification because these injuries may contribute to the observed cycles of muscle and nerve fiber degeneration and regeneration and muscle fiber loss in the aging human TA muscle (Malmgren, Fisher, et al., 1999; Malmgren, Lovice, & Kaufman, 2000; Malmgren, Jones, & Bookman, 1999). In limb muscles, eccentric (lengthening) contractions are common and are particularly damaging in muscles that have not been adequately conditioned (Armstrong, Warren, & Warren, 1991; S. J. Brown, Child, Day, & Donnelly, 1997a, 1997b; Faulkner, Brooks, & Opiteck, 1993; Hunter & Faulkner, 1997; Macpherson, Dennis, & Faulkner, 1997; Mair et al., 1995; McCully & Faulkner, 1986). This type of contraction-induced muscle fiber injury results in an activation of stretch ion channels and prolonged depolarization of muscle fibers (McBride, Stockert, Gorin, & Carlsen, 2000), followed by ultrastructural lesions—including muscle fiber A-band lesions (Ogilvie, Armstrong, Baird, & Bottoms, 1988)—and, ultimately, muscle fiber degeneration. The muscles of old animals are more vulnerable to eccentric contraction-induced injury, and free radicals have been found to contribute to a delayed decrease in maximum isometric tetanic force and morphological fiber damage (Zerba, Komorowski, & Faulkner, 1990). Although these degenerated fibers regenerate completely in young adult animals, regeneration is incomplete in older animals (Brooks & Faulkner, 1990, 1994; Faulkner, Jones, & Round, 1989). Furthermore, because this muscle fiber regeneration process requires reinnervation for recovery of function, contraction-induced fiber injury places an increased demand on a diminished capacity for nerve regeneration in aging muscles (Faulkner, Brooks, & Zerba, 1995).

Gene Therapy

Because apoptosis plays a role in age-related muscle fiber loss and atrophy in the human TA muscle (Malmgren, Fisher, et al., 1999; Malmgren, Lovice, & Kaufman, 2000), it may be possible to use gene therapy to prevent or reverse age-related changes in the mass and strength of the TA muscle by targeting one of the many complex pathways that regulate apoptosis (Thompson, 1995). For example, an age-related decrease in insulin-like growth factor I (IGF-I; Benbassat, Maki, & Unterman, 1997) probably contributes to the demonstrated age-related increase in apoptotic satellite cells in the human TA muscle (Malmgren, Jones, & Bookman, 1999) because withdrawal of IGF-I results in satellite cell apoptosis (Mampuru et al., 1996). Consistent with these findings, gene therapy based on viral-mediated overexpression of IGF-I has been found to prevent an age-related decrease in rat limb muscle mass and strength (Barton-Davis, Shoturma, Musaru, Rosenthal, & Sweeney, 1998), as well as denervation atrophy in the rat TA muscle (Flint, Shiotani, & O'Malley, 1999; Shiotani, O'Malley, Coleman, Alila, & Flint, 1998; Shiotani, O'Malley, Coleman, & Flint, 1999), which probably is due to myonuclear apoptosis (Yoshimura & Harii, 1999). These findings suggest that it may be possible to prevent or reverse the demonstrated age-related increase in satellite cell and myonuclear apoptosis (Malmgren, Jones, & Bookman, 1999, 2001) in the human TA muscle by using gene therapy or pharmacological intervention to block apoptosis. Designing effective therapeutic strategies, however, will require a more complete understanding of the mechanisms underlying myonuclear and satellite cell apoptosis in this highly specialized muscle. Furthermore, it will be necessary to use animal models to clarify the role and interactions of gene therapy with other growth factors (Cannon, 1995; Menetrey et al., 2000) and with variables such as muscle use (Frischknecht, 1998; Singh et al., 1999) and age-related changes in blood flow (Malmgren, 1992).

Vocal Fold Bowing and Atrophy

To this point, this chapter has provided a state-of-the-art overview of the age-related changes in neural mechanisms of skeletal muscles and, specifically, in the known variables responsible for both decline with aging and the self-repair properties of the vocal fold mucosa and the TA muscle. Currently, this information cannot be applied directly to clinical management decisions for individuals with vocal fold bowing or atrophy. Nonetheless, it does provide new evidence of potential mechanisms of physiologic recovery for the TA muscle. This information supports current rationales for collecting treatment efficacy data to improve outcome predictions, especially for aging speakers with complaints due to vocal fold bowing and presumed atrophy.

Efficient vocal fold closure is a mandatory condition for normal voice production. When any form of glottic incompetence threatens bilateral approximation of the vocal folds, regardless of the etiology, voice quality deteriorates dramatically (Omori et al., 1997). Long before voice scientists understood the important contributions of the superficial layers of the vocal fold mucosa, before voice pathologists could rely on essential images of the vibratory waveform, and before physiologic measures of vocal efficiency, glottic resistance, and other aerodynamic parameters were available, otolaryngologists recognized the critical importance of symmetric bilateral vocal fold closure as a fundamental prerequisite to voice quality (Judson & Weaver, 1942; Kirchner, 1986). The deleterious impact of incomplete glottic closure remains one of the most challenging and elusive clinical voice dilemmas, despite our longstanding awareness of its threat to voice quality.

This section examines the clinical process of making assessments, prognoses, and intervention plans for patients who exhibit signs and symptoms of vocal fold bowing or atrophy. We will reconsider the traditional behavioral therapies for these patients, explore contemporary alternatives, and compare that clinical experience to the scientific evidence provided in the first section of this chapter. Our summary will revise the clinical assumptions and directions that can be reasonably inferred from the interdisciplinary cross-mentorship of scientific and clinical data.

Anatomic Information as a Basis for Clinical Approaches

From a clinical perspective, vocal fold bowing is the visual description of vocal folds that fail to meet at the midline due to curving or sagging of the medial edges, resulting in a spindle-shaped midline glottal gap that can be seen on endoscopy during adduction and phonation. The bowing appearance arises most often from idiopathic (unexplained) sources, but the most common etiologies are neuromuscular impairment (e.g., paresis or paralysis), acquired scarring, sulcus vocalis, or atrophy (Koufman, Postma, Cummins, & Blalock, 2000; Stasney, 1996). *Atrophy* is defined here as the wasting or shrinking of a cell or tissue after it has achieved its full size. The presumed sources of atrophy in skeletal muscles are decreased workload, disuse, ischemia, or lack of stimulation (Churchill Livingston, 1989); however, some confirmation of disuse atrophy has been reported in nonoral speakers with permanent tracheostomies (Sasaki, Suzuki, Horiuchi, & Kirchner, 1977).

Vocal fold bowing is the visual characteristic associated with spindle-shaped glottic gaps. Atrophy is the underlying cellular or tissue shrinking that results in midline glottic gaps. Vocal fold bowing thus is the visible effect of presumed vocal fold atrophy, or shrinking. Usually, the exact etiology of the vocal fold bowing is unknown, but it is presumed to arise from degeneration of the superficial vocal fold layer structure (Hammond et al., 1998), the true vocal fold body (the TA muscle), or both. Although vocal fold bowing is easily identified, the disorder has been one of the most poorly understood threats to vocal function because the resulting idiopathic voice disorder has wide variability in symptom severity and in prognosis for improvement through voice therapy.

If clinicians suspect that the source of the unexplained bowing is some form of neurogenic impairment of the TA muscle, the hypothesis can be confirmed through electromyographic testing. Other clinical signs and symptoms include complaints of voice quality decline due to vocal breathiness, lack of vocal endurance, a limited volume range, and intermittent symptoms of vocal fatigue. The suspected presence of atrophy in the TA muscle increases when the patient is in his or her 60s or older, which is when age-related voice changes appear in most individuals (Bless, Glaze, Lowery, Campos, & Peppard, 1993).

The term *presbylaryngeus* is commonly used as a default diagnosis for older individuals who present with bowed vocal folds and symptoms of declining voice efficiency or quality. Age-based change in midline glottic closure is presumed but is difficult to quantify unless longitudinal visual data are available. Nonetheless, it is important to separate the indirect visual appearance of bowed vocal folds from other disorders that may result in spindle-shaped gaps due to midline scarring or sulcus vocalis (Stasney, 1996).

Usually, the latter vocal fold defects will result in stiff vibratory patterns with significantly impaired mucosal wave. Bowing, on the other hand, reveals incomplete glottic closure but functional mucosal wave velocity and amplitude during vibration (Stasney, 1996).

The first section of this chapter provided a comprehensive summary of anatomic data surrounding the age-related changes in the mucosal, neuromuscular, cellular, and genetic components of the TA muscle. In the descriptions of the anatomic processes of muscle fiber loss, decrease in motor neuron pools, and apoptosis in aging TA muscles, we find potential explanations for the clinical observations of apparent deterioration of vocal fold strength, tonicity, and resilience, especially among geriatric speakers. Most important is the anatomic evidence of cellular and neuromuscular regeneration in the TA muscle following injury or due to aging, based on motor neuron and muscle fiber remodeling, increases in muscle fiber diameter, and selective increases in satellite cells to support the myonuclei. All of these processes are important indicators of the potential for recovery.

The challenge for clinicians is to determine whether the anatomic self-restoration and recovery process in the patient with a voice disorder can be enhanced through adjunctive behavioral treatment. At the minimum, these anatomic data suggest that the clinical tasks facing individuals with bowing or atrophy are not limited to preventing further decline; rather, evidence of self-repair of these neuromyal structures strengthens our rationale for targeting significant voice improvement with appropriate therapy. The idea of future gene therapy for denervated or deteriorated cellular structures is speculative at present, but it provides a compelling preview of the potential for future medical interventions for bowed or atrophic folds. In partnership with current interventions using behavioral strategies and phonosurgical techniques, gene therapy could one day hold promise as a first-order rehabilitative approach.

The descriptions in the first half of this chapter provide many critical insights into the anatomic and neuromuscular structures of the TA muscle that advance our understanding of clinical management of voice disorders in aging populations, specifically:

- Age-related changes are multifactorial and exist at every level of neuromotor structure and function.

- The TA muscle is similar to skeletal muscles but has unique structural attributes that protect its integrity to maintain endurance, strength, mass, and contraction speed.
- Evidence of changes in these structures across the age span include evidence of both decline and recovery.

Clinical experience suggests that there are large individual differences in the patterns of vocal fold aging, deterioration, and preservation. Perhaps the individual tissue response to injury and aging processes influences these highly unpredictable outcomes, particularly in the case of individuals with bowing and atrophy. Previous assumptions about the limited potential for voice improvement following diagnosis of vocal fold bowing or atrophy may be fallacious. Although the exact capacity of this tissue and cellular "remodeling" potential is incompletely understood at present, these data allow voice pathologists to reconsider, and tentatively discard, some traditional notions of the clinical efficacy of treating vocal fold bowing and atrophy in the aging speaker, including presumptions that vocal fold decline with aging is inevitable and irreversible, and behavioral therapies are merely compensatory, and will not reverse, but only momentarily arrest, this decline.

Voice Findings

To understand the impact of these new scientific data on the clinical process of assessment and intervention planning, a review of the differential diagnoses of vocal fold bowing or atrophy is in order. The standard components of evaluation include a case history, audio-perceptual judgments, vocal function measures, endoscopic imaging of glottic closure patterns during vibration, and appraisal of the functional impact of the voice disorder on the patient's everyday communication. For patients who experience vocal hypophonia due to bowing or atrophy, the following is a typical synopsis of findings for each of these aspects of the voice evaluation (Stemple, Glaze, & Klaben, 2000a):

- *Case history:* gradual onset of voice deterioration and decline, without any identifiable onset event, illness, or injury

- *Functional impact:* increased dissatisfaction with voice quality; complaints of difficulty being heard over noise, on the telephone, and—particularly in the aging population—by conversational partners who may be hearing impaired
- *Vocal function measures:* vary with symptoms and severity, but generally include increased transglottal airflow and decreased signal-to-noise ratio
- *Audio-perceptual voice quality:* breathiness, voice breaks, diplophonia, mild weakness, symptoms of vocal fatigue and instability; may exhibit strain and effort in maladaptive response to primary glottic incompetence
- *Videostroboscopic examination:* classic spindle-shaped (unilateral or bilateral) glottic gap despite normal vocal fold adduction (posterior closure) and abduction; vibratory waveform displays adequate mucosal wave

Clinicians with experience in voice disorders are familiar with the unpredictable variability of patients who present with vocal fold bowing of unknown etiology. To make these diagnoses, clinicians must rule out other etiologic variables by matching the onset history and symptoms to the characteristics described above (Special Interest Division 3, in press).

Clinical Interventions

Phonosurgical approaches to vocal fold bowing and atrophy include medialization thyroplasty, reinnervation techniques, and vocal fold injections. These procedures include unilateral and bilateral thyroplasty bioimplant medialization (Lu, Casiano, Lundy, & Xue, 1998; Postma, Blalock, & Koufman, 1998), reinnervation techniques, and lipoinjection (Slavit, 1999). Limited outcome data are available for geriatric populations, but Omori, Slavit, Kacker, & Blaugrund (1998) reported less success in the population of speakers with bowing vocal folds than for similar procedures in patients with paralysis. These equivocal phonosurgical outcome data are consistent with behavioral experience with this disorder, where individual results are not consistent as a larger group (Lundy, Silva, Casiano, Lu, & Xue, 1998). There is, however, a growing body of compelling clinical evidence supporting the notion of potential improvement, if not recovery, from vocal fold changes following neuromuscular impairment, especially in idiopathic Parkinson's disease.

The reports of treatment efficacy using the *Lee Silverman Voice Treatment* (LSVT) approach (Ramig et al., 2001) in individuals with idiopathic Parkinson's disease suggest that vocal function improvements can be achieved in adults facing neuromuscular decline and, potentially, concurrent age-related vocal fold changes. Evidence of physiologic improvements in vocal function in this population has been reported for audio-perceptual judgments of voice quality, for videostroboscopic appearance of the vibratory waveform, and for direct electromyographic confirmation of improved muscle activity, all measured in pre- and posttreatment designs (Ramig et al., 2001). Although the hypophonia associated with Parkinson's disease is distinctly separate from the hypophonia common to typical aging speakers with vocal fold bowing, these positive treatment outcomes support the exploration of active behavioral approaches to voice rehabilitation. The LSVT evidence suggests that such treatment paradigms may be successful, even in the context of neuromuscular decline.

To understand the impact of active voice use on voice quality and improvement in individuals with vocal fold bowing or atrophy, data on contrasting effects of age and voice use need to be reviewed. Peppard and Bless (1988) reported preliminary evidence that suggested a potential for individuals to forestall the presumed aging decline in vocal function. They identified improved vocal function measures of acoustic, aerodynamic, stroboscopic and perceptual judgments of voice in a series of geriatric professional singers in comparison to younger nonsinging counterparts. In this study, individuals with a long and active history of healthy voice use appeared to have preserved vocal function and vocal fold appearance. Although this report has no treatment-based conclusions, the authors proposed a "use it or lose it" model of voice preservation and renewal among aging speakers. If, indeed, healthy vocal exercise preserves vocal function capabilities in later years, is there correlative evidence of anatomic longevity of the vocal fold tissues? Perhaps the anatomic evidence of increased satellite cell production and cellular remodeling in response to stretch stimuli may help explain the underlying physiologic processes of deferring age-related changes.

These "active" approaches to voice therapy are somewhat different from older models for treating vocal hypofunction, which used repeated attempts at overadduction by abruptly increasing phonatory effort in pushing and pulling tasks (Aronson, 1990; Prater & Swift, 1984). There is limited evidence of treatment efficacy for these focal hyperadductory tasks, yet common survey textbooks on communication disorders continue to present this option for treating vocal hypophonia (Dalston, 2000; Roth and Worthington, 2001). Colton and Casper (1996) asserted that despite the pervasive claims for improved adduction following pushing and pulling exercise, they have never observed improved midline closure following this technique.

Instead, newer voice rehabilitation tasks that have better documentation of treatment efficacy employ sustained vocal tones that target efficiency and endurance rather than hyperfunctional effort. These contemporary treatments for vocal hypophonia have replaced overadduction gestures with integrated targets of respiration, phonation, and resonance. Using a variety of clinical tasks, the treatments employ sustained tones (Stemple, Lee, D'Amico, & Pickup, 1994) and vowels (Verdolini, 1998), rhythmic tones and words (Kotby, 1995), and novel tasks that demand good breath support and appropriate oral tone focus, for example, trilling, singing, pitch glides, and humming (Lowery, 2000; Rammage, 1996). The distinct characteristic common to all of these treatment approaches is a focus on combining good respiratory support with attention to an open, resonant vocal tract position. This combination of target behaviors in respiration, phonation, and resonance seeks to improve overall systemic improvements in vocal function rather than narrow, focal changes in laryngeal adduction (Stemple, Glaze, & Klaben, 2000b).

Thus, treatment-based approaches to voice rehabilitation in general, and to clinical intervention for bowing and atrophy specifically, have incorporated repeated and consistent voice exercise trials as essential components of successful voice therapy. Voice hygiene and conservation contribute to overall vocal fold health and help to decrease comorbidity factors (e.g., tobacco, alcohol, and caffeine use) in all populations with voice disorders, but symptoms of bowing and atrophy common to hypofunctional voice disorders will not be improved without direct, active voice intervention.

Indeed, case reports for treating vocal fold bowing, presbylaryngeus, and presumed atrophy all incorporate a common theme of active voice exercise involving coordinated targets of the three subsystems of voice: respiration, phonation, and resonance. Stemple (2000), Stemple, Glaze, and Klaben (2000b), and Gorman (2000) reported that a series of vocal function exercises has been used to successfully "close the gap" of vocal fold bowing in idiopathic presbylaryngeus. The authors reported findings of direct improvement in vocal function, voice quality, and functional communication benefits in elderly speakers with symptoms of presbylaryngeus and vocal fold bowing. These exercises have also been used to improve vocal fold closure and voice quality in typical speakers and in singers (Sabol, Lee, & Stemple, 1995; Stemple et al., 1994).

Lowery (2000) applied a vocal exercise singing program to elderly individuals who complained of vocal fatigue, "airiness," and generalized hypophonia due to apparent vocal fold bowing. Benefits in vocal function measures, videostroboscopic appearance, and long-term satisfaction with voice quality improvement occurred. Other clinicians (Verdolini, 1998; Verdolini, Drucker, Palmer, & Samawi, 1998) have supported the concept of a programmed series of voice-building exercises to remediate glottic incompetence in vocal fold bowing or voice hypofunction. These intervention strategies all share a common characteristic of promoting and training healthy, sustained, and repeated trials of active voice exercise to restore and preserve vocal function. It is highly unlikely that the symptoms of vocal fold bowing and atrophy will improve without active voice exercise as a regular and sustained component of the treatment plan.

In our experience, patients with vocal fold bowing are often significantly distressed by this communication limit, perhaps more than for other physical ailments because of the absence of a known etiology. Without an identifiable cause, patients may become disheartened at the lack of concrete information to predict and guide the course of this elusive disorder. The anatomic overview presented here provides beneficial evidence that can be used to educate patients about the nature and pathophysiology of vocal fold atrophy, age-related changes, and the body's potential for remodeling and recovery. Clinicians and patients have reason to encourage motivated clinical trials using appropriate active stimulation of the vocal mechanism in voice-building therapy.

Directions for Future Research

The next important direction for clinical research will be to augment the limited but compelling evidence for treatment outcomes using these therapeutic methods. Ideally, voice pathologists will use single-subject designs to document evidence-based interventions, including their impact on vocal function, physiologic measures, voice quality, vocal fold vibratory patterns, and functional differences in communication potential. If voice pathologists can gather sufficient treatment efficacy data to determine reliable prognoses for improvement with behavioral treatment, we move forward in our quest for understanding the diverse patterns of injury and recovery in aging speakers (Slavit, 1999). In the front half of this chapter, we speculated about the possibility of future genetic interventions addressing vocal fold atrophy and cell deterioration to remediate vocal fold atrophy or bowing. Treatment efficacy data are needed to specify the role of behavioral therapy in preparing, assisting, or maintaining benefits of potential medical and surgical interventions in individuals with these disorders. For voice pathologists and scientists, the research questions remain plentiful:

- Does voice exercise stimulate or augment anatomic reorganization in patients who exhibit vocal fold bowing or atrophy?
- Do behavioral interventions improve the long-term prognosis for individuals with symptoms of presbylaryngeus?
- What lifestyle variables in voice care, conservation, and use influence positive treatment outcome results in this specialized population?

We are certainly far from closing the intellectual gap in our understanding of vocal fold bowing and atrophy, but both the scientific evidence and select treatment outcomes for individuals with these problems reveal progress in our interdisciplinary understanding.

References

Allen, D. L., Linderman, J. K., Roy, R. R., Bigbee, A. J., Grindeland, R. E., Mukku, V., et al. (1997). Apoptosis: A mechanism contributing to remodeling of skeletal muscle in response to hindlimb unweighting. *American Journal of Physiology, 273* (2, Pt. 1), C579–C587.

Allen, D. L., Roy, R. R., & Edgerton, V. R. (1999). Myonuclear domains in muscle adaptation and disease. *Muscle and Nerve, 22,* 1350–1360.

Allen, D. L., Yasui, W., Tanaka, T., Ohira, Y., Nagaoka, S., Sekiguchi, C., et al. (1996). Myonuclear number and myosin heavy chain expression in rat soleus single muscle fibers after spaceflight. *Journal of Applied Physiology, 81,* 145–151.

Ansved, T., Wallner, P., & Larsson, L. (1991). Spatial distribution of motor unit fibres in fast- and slow-twitch rat muscles with special reference to age. *Acta Physiologica Scandinavica, 143,* 345–354.

Armstrong, R. B., Warren, G. L., & Warren, J. A. (1991). Mechanisms of exercise-induced muscle fibre injury. *Sports Medicine, 12,* 184–207.

Aronson, A. E. (1990). *Clinical voice disorders: An interdisciplinary approach* (3rd ed.). New York: Thieme.

Barton-Davis, E. R., Shoturma, D. I., Musaro, A., Rosenthal, N., & Sweeney, H. L. (1998). Viral mediated expression of insulin-like growth factor I blocks the aging-related loss of skeletal muscle function. *Proceedings of the National Academy of Sciences of the United States of America, 95,* 15603–15607.

Benbassat, C. A., Maki, K. C., & Unterman, T. G. (1997). Circulating levels of insulin-like growth factor (IGF) binding protein- 1 and -3 in aging men: Relationships to insulin, glucose, IGF, and dehydroepiandrosterone sulfate levels and anthropometric measures. *Journal of Clinical Endocrinology and Metabolism, 82,* 1484–1491.

Bendiksen, F. S., Dahl, H. A., & Teig, E. (1981). Innervation pattern of different types of muscle fibres in the human thyroarytenoid muscle. *Acta Oto-Laryngologica, 91,* 391–397.

Bischoff, R. (1999). The satellite cell and muscle regeneration. In A. G. Engel & C. Franzini-Armstrong (Eds.), *Myology* (pp. 97–118). New York: McGraw-Hill.

Bless, D. M., Glaze, L. E., Lowery, D. B., Campos, G., & Peppard, R. C. (1993). Stroboscopic, acoustic, aerodynamic, and perceptual analysis of voice production in normal speaking adults. *Status and Progress Report of the National Center for Voice and Speech, 4,* 121–134.

Briggs, M. M., & Schachat, F. (2000). Early specialization of the superfast myosin in extraocular and laryngeal muscles. *Journal of Experimental Biology, 203* (Pt. 16), 2485–2494.

Brooks, S. V., & Faulkner, J. A. (1990). Contraction-induced injury: Recovery of skeletal muscles in young and old mice. *American Journal of Physiology, 258*(3, Pt. 1), C436–C442.

Brooks, S. V., & Faulkner, J. A. (1994). Skeletal muscle weakness in old age: Underlying mechanisms. *Medicine and Science in Sports and Exercise, 26,* 432–439.

Brown, S. J., Child, R. B., Day, S. H., & Donnelly, A. E. (1997a). Exercise-induced skeletal muscle damage and adaptation following repeated bouts of eccentric muscle contractions. *Journal of Sports Science, 15,* 215–222.

Brown, S. J., Child, R. B., Day, S. H., & Donnelly, A. E. (1997b). Indices of skeletal muscle damage and connective tissue breakdown following eccentric muscle contractions. *European Journal of Applied Physiology and Occupational Physiology, 75,* 369–374.

Brown, W. F., Strong, M. J., & Snow, R. (1988). Methods for estimating numbers of motor units in biceps-brachialis muscles and losses of motor units with aging. *Muscle and Nerve, 11,* 423–432.

Cannon, J. G. (1995). Cytokines in aging and muscle homeostasis. *Journal of Gerontology: Series A. Biological Sciences and Medical Sciences, 50,* 120–123.

Cannon, J. G. (1998). Intrinsic and extrinsic factors in muscle aging. *Annals of the New York Academy of Sciences, 854*(20), 72–77.

Carlson, B. M. (1995). Factors influencing the repair and adaptation of muscles in aged individuals: Satellite cells and innervation. *Journal of Gerontology: Series A. Biological Sciences and Medical Sciences, 50*, 96–100.

Carlson, B. M., & Faulkner, J. A. (1996). The regeneration of noninnervated muscle grafts and marcaine-treated muscles in young and old rats. *Journal of Gerontology: Series A. Biological Sciences and Medical Sciences, 51*(1), B43–B49.

Carlson, B. M., & Faulkner, J. A. (1998). Muscle regeneration in young and old rats: Effects of motor nerve transection with and without marcaine treatment. *Journal of Gerontology: Series A. Biological Sciences and Medical Sciences, 53*(1), B52–B57.

Choi, S. J., Harii, K., Lee, M. J., Furuya, F., & Ueda, K. (1995). Electrophysiological, morphological, and morphometric effects of aging on nerve regeneration in rats. *Scandinavian Journal of Plastic and Reconstructive Surgery and Hand Surgery, 29*(2), 133–140.

Churchill Livingstone. *Churchill's illustrated medical dictionary* (2nd ed.). (1989). New York: Author.

Claassen, H., & Werner, J. A. (1992). Fiber differentiation of the human laryngeal muscles using the inhibition reactivation myofibrillar ATPase technique. *Anatomy and Embryology, 186*, 341–346.

Colton, R., & Casper, J. (1996). *Understanding voice problems: A physiological perspective for diagnosis and treatment* (2nd ed.). Baltimore: Williams & Wilkins.

d'Albis, A., Couteaux, R., Janmot, C., Roulet, A., & Mira, J.C. (1988). Regeneration after cardiotoxin injury of innervated and denervated slow and fast muscles of mammals: Myosin isoform analysis. *European Journal of Biochemistry, 174*, 103–110.

Dalston, R. M. (2000). Voice disorders. In R. B. Gillam, T. P. Marquardt, & F. D. Martin (Eds.), *Communication sciences and disorders*. San Diego, CA: Singular.

Darr, K. C., & Schultz, E. (1989). Hindlimb suspension suppresses muscle growth and satellite cell proliferation. *Journal of Applied Physiology, 67*, 1827–1834.

Delp, M. D., & Pette, D. (1994). Morphological changes during fiber type transitions in low-frequency-stimulated rat fast-twitch muscle. *Cell and Tissue Research, 277,* 363–371.

Doherty, T. J., Vandervoort, A. A., Taylor, A. W., & Brown, W. F. (1993). Effects of motor unit losses on strength in older men and women. *Journal of Applied Physiology, 74,* 868–874.

Faulkner, J. A., Brooks, S. V., & Opiteck, J. A. (1993). Injury to skeletal muscle fibers during contractions: Conditions of occurrence and prevention. *Physical Therapy, 73,* 911–921.

Faulkner, J. A., Brooks, S. V., & Zerba, E. (1995). Muscle atrophy and weakness with aging: Contraction-induced injury as an underlying mechanism. *Journal of Gerontology: Series A. Biological Sciences and Medical Sciences, 50,* 124–129.

Faulkner, J. A., Jones, D. A., & Round, J. M. (1989). Injury to skeletal muscles of mice by forced lengthening during contractions. *Quarterly Journal of Experimental Physiology, 74,* 661–670.

Flint, P. W., Shiotani, A., & O'Malley, B. W. J. (1999). IGF-1 gene transfer into denervated rat laryngeal muscle. *Archives of Otolaryngology—Head & Neck Surgery, 125,* 274–279.

Frischknecht, R. (1998). Effect of training on muscle strength and motor function in the elderly. *Reproduction, Nutrition, Development, 38*(2), 167–174.

Gavrieli, Y., Sherman, Y., & Ben-Sasson, S. A. (1992). Identification of programmed cell death in situ via specific labeling of nuclear DNA fragmentation. *Journal of Cell Biology, 119,* 493–501.

Gorman, S. (2000). Management of senile laryngis. In J. Stemple (Ed.), *Voice therapy: Clinical studies* (2nd ed., pp. 182–187). San Diego, CA: Singular.

Gray, S. D., Titze, I. R., Alipour, F., & Hammond, T. H. (2000). Biomechanical and histologic observations of vocal fold fibrous proteins. *Annals of Otology, Rhinology & Laryngology, 109*(1), 77–85.

Grimby, G. (1995). Muscle performance and structure in the elderly as studied cross-sectionally and longitudinally. *Journal of Gerontology: Series A. Biological Sciences and Medical Sciences, 50A,* 17–22.

Guida, H. L., & Zorzetto, N. L. (2000). Morphometric and histochemical study of the human vocal muscle. *Annals of Otology,
Rhinology & Laryngology, 109*(1), 67–71.

Hall-Craggs, E. C. (1974). The regeneration of skeletal muscle fibres
per continuum. *Journal of Anatomy, 117,* 171–178.

Hammond, T. H., Gray, S. D., & Butler, J. E. (2000). Age- and gender-
related collagen distribution in human vocal folds. *Annals of
Otology, Rhinology & Laryngology, 109*(Pt. 1), 913–920.

Hammond, T. H., Gray, S. D., Butler, J., Zhou, R., & Hammond, E.
(1998). Age- and gender-related elastin distribution changes in
human vocal folds. *Archives of Otolaryngology—Head & Neck
Surgery, 119,* 314–322.

Hirano, M. (1977). Structure and vibratory behavior of the vocal
folds. In M. Sawashima & F. S. Cooper (Eds.), *Dynamic aspects of
speech production* (pp. 13–30). Tokyo: University of Tokyo Press.

Hirano, M., Kurita, S., & Sakaguchi, S. (1989). Ageing of the vibratory tissue of human vocal folds. *Acta Otolaryngology, 107,* 428–
433.

Hughes, S. M., & Schiaffino, S. (1999). Control of muscle fibre size:
A crucial factor in ageing. *Acta Physiologica Scandinavica, 167,*
307–312.

Hunter, K. D., & Faulkner, J. A. (1997). Pliometric contraction-
induced injury of mouse skeletal muscle: Effect of initial length.
Journal of Applied Physiology, 82, 278–283.

Jennekens, F. G., Tomlinson, B. E., & Walton, J. N. (1971). Histochemical aspects of five limb muscles in old age: An autopsy
study. *Journal of the Neurological Sciences, 14,* 259–276.

Judson, L. S., & Weaver, A. T. (1942). *Voice science.* New York: F. S.
Crofts.

Kadi, F., Eriksson, A., Holmner, S., Butler-Browne, G. S., & Thornell,
L. E. (1999). Cellular adaptation of the trapezius muscle in
strength-trained athletes. *Histochemistry & Cell Biology, 111*(3),
189–195.

Kawabuchi, M., Chongjian, Z., Islam, A. T. M. S., Hirata, K., & Nada, O. (1998). The effect of aging on the morphological nerve changes during muscle reinnervation after nerve crush. *Restorative Neurology and Neuroscience, 13*(3–4), 117–127.

Kirchner, J. A. (1986). *Pressman and Keleman's physiology of the larynx* (3rd ed.). Rochester, MN: American Academy of Otolaryngology—Head & Neck Surgery Foundation.

Klitgaard, H., Zhou, M., Schiaffino, S., Betto, R., Salviati, G., & Saltin, B. (1990). Ageing alters the myosin heavy chain composition of single fibres from human skeletal muscle. *Acta Physiologica Scandinavica, 140,* 55–62.

Kotby, M. N. (1995). *The accent method of voice therapy.* San Diego, CA: Singular.

Koufman, J. A., Postma, G. N., Cummins, M. M., & Blalock, P. D. (2000). Vocal fold paresis. *Archives of Otolaryngology—Head & Neck Surgery, 122,* 537–541.

Larsson, L. (1978). Morphological and functional characteristics of the ageing skeletal muscle in man: A cross-sectional study. *Acta Physiologica Scandinavica 457,* (Suppl.), 1–36.

Larsson, L. (1995). Motor units: Remodeling in aged animals. *Journal of Gerontology: Series A. Biological Sciences and Medical Sciences, 50A,* 91–95.

Larsson, L., & Edstrom, L. (1986). Effects of age on enzyme-histochemical fibre spectra and contractile properties of fast- and slow-twitch skeletal muscles in the rat. *Journal of the Neurological Sciences, 76,* 69–89.

Lexell, J. (1995). Human aging, muscle mass, and fiber type composition. *Journal of Gerontology: Series A, Biological Sciences and Medical Sciences, 50A,* 11–16.

Lexell, J., Henriksson-Larsen, K., Winblad, B., & Sjostrom, M. (1983). Distribution of different fiber types in human skeletal muscles: Effects of aging studied in whole muscle cross-sections. *Muscle and Nerve, 6,* 588–595.

Lowery, D. (2000). Management of vocal fold bowing. In J. Stemple (Ed.), *Voice therapy: Clinical studies* (2nd ed.; pp. 172–182). San Diego, CA: Singular.

Lu, F. L., Casiano, R. R., Lundy, D. S., & Xue, J. W. (1998). Vocal evaluation of thyroplasty type I in the treatment of nonparalytic glottic incompetence. *Annals of Otology, Rhinology & Laryngology, 107,* 113–119.

Lucas, C. A., Rughani, A., & Hoh, J. F. (1995). Expression of extraocular myosin heavy chain in rabbit laryngeal muscle. *Journal of Muscle Research and Cell Motility, 16,* 368–378.

Lundy, D. S., Silva, C., Casiano, R. R., Lu, F. L., & Xue, J. W. (1998). Cause of hoarseness in elderly patients. *Archives of Otolaryngology—Head & Neck Surgery, 118,* 481–485.

Macpherson, P. C., Dennis, R. G., & Faulkner, J. A. (1997). Sarcomere dynamics and contraction-induced injury to maximally activated single muscle fibres from soleus muscles of rats. *Journal of Physiology, 500*(Pt. 2), 523–533.

Mair, J., Mayr, M., Muller, E., Koller, A., Haid, C., Artner-Dworzak, E., et al. (1995). Rapid adaptation to eccentric exercise-induced muscle damage. *International Journal of Sports Medicine, 16,* 352–356.

Malmgren, L. T. (1989). Aging-related changes in peripheral nerves in the head and neck. In M. A. Goldstein, H. K. Kashima, & C. F. Koopman (Eds.), *Geriatric otorhinolaryngology* (pp. 138–143). Toronto: B. C. Decker.

Malmgren, L. T. (1992). Age-related changes in blood flow rates in the intrinsic laryngeal muscles of young adult and old rats during quiet respiration [Abstract]. *Abstracts of the Fifteenth Midwinter Research Meeting of the Association for Research in Otolaryngology,* p. 31.

Malmgren, L. T., Fisher, P. J., Bookman, L. M., & Uno, T. (1999). Age-related changes in muscle fiber types in the human thyroarytenoid muscle: An immunohistochemical and stereological study using confocal laser scanning microscopy. *Archives of Otolaryngology—Head & Neck Surgery, 121,* 441–451.

Malmgren, L. T., Fisher, P. J., & Brandes, M. (1997, February). Age-related increase in muscle fiber "type grouping" in the human thyroarytenoid muscle. Paper presented at the Association for Research in Otolaryngology 20th midwinter meeting, St. Petersburg, FL.

Malmgren, L. T., Fisher, P. J., Jones, C. E., Bookman, L. M., & Uno, T. (2000). Numerical densities of myonuclei and satellite cells in muscle fiber types in the aging human thyroarytenoid muscle: An immunohistochemical and stereological study using confocal laser scanning microscopy. *Archives of Otolaryngology—Head & Neck Surgery, 123,* 377–384.

Malmgren, L. T., & Gacek, R. R. (1981). Histochemical characteristics of muscle fiber types in the posterior cricoarytenoid muscle. *Annals of Otology, Rhinology & Laryngology, 90*(5, Pt. 1), 423–429.

Malmgren, L. T., Gacek, R. R., & Etzler, C. A. (1983). Muscle fiber types in the human posterior cricoarytenoid muscle: A correlated histochemical and ultrastructural morphometric study. In I. Titze & R. Scherer (Eds.), *Conference on physiology and biophysics of voice* (pp. 41–56). Denver, CO: Denver Center for the Performing Arts.

Malmgren, L. T., Jones, C. E., & Bookman, L. M. (1999, February). *Stereological study of apoptosis in the aging human thyroarytenoid muscle.* Paper presented at the Association for Research in Otolaryngology 22nd midwinter meeting, St. Petersburg, FL.

Malmgren, L. T., Jones, C. E., & Bookman, L. M. (2001). Muscle fiber and satellite cell apoptosis in the aging human thyroarytenoid muscle: A stereologic study with confocal laser scanning microscopy. *Archives of Otolaryngology—Head & Neck Surgery, 125,* 34–39.

Malmgren, L. T., Lovice, D. B., & Kaufman, M. R. (2000). Age-related changes in muscle fiber regeneration in the human thyroarytenoid muscle. *Archives of Otolaryngology—Head & Neck Surgery, 126,* 851–856.

Malmgren, L. T., & Ringwood, M. A. (1988). Aging of the recurrent laryngeal nerve: An ultrastructural morphometric study. In

O. Fujimura (Ed.), *Vocal physiology: Voice production, mechanisms and function* (pp. 159–180). New York: Raven Press.

Mampuru, L. J., Chen, S. J., Kalenik, J. L., Bradley, M. E., & Lee, T. C. (1996). Analysis of events associated with serum deprivation-induced apoptosis in C3H/Sol8 muscle satellite cells. *Experimental Cell Research, 226,* 372–380.

Marsh, D. R., Criswell, D. S., Hamilton, M. T., & Booth, F. W. (1997). Association of insulin-like growth factor mRNA expressions with muscle regeneration in young, adult, and old rats. *American Journal of Physiology, 273*(1, Pt. 2), R353–R358.

McBride, T. A., Stockert, B. W., Gorin, F. A., & Carlsen, R. C. (2000). Stretch-activated ion channels contribute to membrane depolarization after eccentric contractions. *Journal of Applied Physiology, 88*(1), 91–101.

McCully, K. K., & Faulkner, J. A. (1986). Characteristics of lengthening contractions associated with injury to skeletal muscle fibers. *Journal of Applied Physiology, 61*(1), 293–299.

Menetrey, J., Kasemkijwattana, C., Day, C. S., Bosch, P., Vogt, M., Fu, F. H., et al. (2000). Growth factors improve muscle healing in vivo. *Journal of Bone and Joint Surgery, 82*(1), 131–137.

Merati, A. L., Bodine, S. C., Bennett, T., Jung, H. H., Furuta, H., & Ryan, A. F. (1996). Identification of a novel myosin heavy chain gene expressed in the rat larynx. *Biochimica et Biophysica Acta, 1306*(2–3), 153–159.

Mezzogiorno, A., Coletta, M., Zani, B. M., Cossu, G., & Molinaro, M. (1993). Paracrine stimulation of senescent satellite cell proliferation by factors released by muscle or myotubes from young mice. *Mechanisms of Ageing and Development, 70*(1–2), 35–44.

Ogilvie, R. W., Armstrong, R. B., Baird, K. E., & Bottoms, C. L. (1988). Lesions in the rat soleus muscle following eccentrically biased exercise. *American Journal of Anatomy, 182,* 335–346.

Omori, K., Slavit, D. H., Kacker, A., & Blaugrund, S. (1998). Influence of size and etiology of the glottal gap in the glottic incompetence dysphonia. *Laryngoscope, 108,* 514–518.

Omori, K., Slavit, D. H., Matos, C., Kojima, H., Kacker, A., & Blaugrund, S. (1997). Vocal fold atrophy: Quantitative glottic measurement and vocal function. *Annals of Otology, Rhinology & Laryngology, 106,* 544–551.

Peppard, R. C., & Bless, D. M. (1988). Comparison of young adult singers and nonsingers with vocal nodules. *Journal of Voice, 2,* 250–260.

Perie, S., St. Guily, J. L., Callard, P., & Sebille, A. (1997). Innervation of adult human laryngeal muscle fibers. *Journal of the Neurological Sciences, 149*(1), 81–86.

Pette, D., & Staron, R. S. (1997). Mammalian skeletal muscle fiber type transitions. *International Review of Cytology, 170,* 143–223.

Podhorska-Okolov, M., Sandri, M., Zanada, F., Brun, B., Rossini, K., & Carraro, U. (1999). Apoptosis of myofibres and satellite cells: Exercise-induced damage in skeletal muscle of the mouse. *Neuropathology and Applied Neurobiology, 24,* 518–531.

Postma, G., Blalock, P. D., & Koufman, J. A. (1998) Bilateral medialization thyroplasty. *Laryngoscope, 108,* 1429–1434.

Prater, R. J., & Swift, R. W. (1984). *Manual of voice therapy.* Boston: Little, Brown.

Ramig, L. O., Countryman, S., O'Brien, C., Hoehn, M., & Thompson, L. (1996). Intensive speech treatment for patients with Parkinson's disease: Short-and long-term comparison of two techniques. *Neurology, 47,* 1496–1504.

Ramig, L. O., & Dromey, C. (1996). Aerodynamic mechanisms underlying treatment-related changes in vocal intensity in patients with Parkinson disease. *Journal of Speech and Hearing Research, 39,* 798–807.

Ramig, L., Sapir, S., Countryman, S., Pawlas, A., O'Brien, C., Hoehn, M., et al. (2001). Intensive voice treatment (LSVT®) for individuals with Parkinson's disease: A two year follow-up. *Journal of Neurology, Neurosurgery, and Psychiatry, 71,* 493–498.

Rammage, L. A. (1996). *Vocalizing with ease.* Vancouver, CA: Author.

Rivero, J. L., Talmadge, R. J., & Edgerton, V. R. (1998). Fibre size and metabolic properties of myosin heavy chain-based fibre types in rat skeletal muscle. *Journal of Muscle Research and Cell Motility, 19*, 733–742.

Roth, F., & Worthington, C. (2001) *Treatment resource manual for speech-language pathology* (2nd ed.). New York: Delmar.

Sabol, J., Lee, L., & Stemple, J. C. (1995). The value of vocal function exercises in the practice regimen of singers. *Journal of Voice, 9,* 27–36.

Sadeh, M. (1988). Effects of aging on skeletal muscle regeneration. *Journal of the Neurological Sciences, 87,* 67–74.

Sandri, M., Carraro, U., Podhorska-Okolov, M., Rizzi, C., Arslan, P., Monti, D., et al. (1995). Apoptosis, DNA damage and ubiquitin expression in normal and mdx muscle fibers after exercise. *Federation of European Biochemical Studies Letters, 373,* 291–295.

Sandri, M., Podhorska-Okolov, M., Geromel, V., Rizzi, C., Arslan, P., Franceschi, C., et al. (1997). Exercise induces myonuclear ubiquitination and apoptosis in dystrophin-deficient muscle of mice. *Journal of Neuropathology and Experimental Neurology, 56*(1), 45–57.

Sasaki, C. T., Suzuki, M., Horiuchi, M., & Kirchner, J. A. (1977). The effect of tracheostomy on the laryngeal closure reflex. *Laryngoscope, 87,* 1428–1433.

Sato, K., & Hirano, M. (1997). Age-related changes of elastic fibers in the superficial layer of the lamina propria of vocal folds. *Annals of Otology, Rhinology & Laryngology, 106,* 44–48.

Scarpulla, R. C. (1997). Nuclear control of respiratory chain expression in mammalian cells. *Journal of Bioenergetics and Biomembranes, 29,* 109–119.

Shiotani, A., O'Malley, B. W. J., Coleman, M. E., Alila, H. W., & Flint, P. W. (1998). Reinnervation of motor endplates and increased muscle fiber size after human insulin-like growth factor I gene transfer into the paralyzed larynx. *Human Gene Therapy, 9,* 2039–2047.

Shiotani, A., O'Malley, B. W. J., Coleman, M. E., & Flint, P. W. (1999). Human insulinlike growth factor 1 gene transfer into paralyzed rat larynx: Single vs multiple injection. *Archives of Otolaryngology—Head & Neck Surgery, 125,* 555–560.

Sieck, G. C., Zhan, W. Z., Prakash, Y. S., Daood, M. J., & Watchko, J. F. (1995). SDH and actomyosin ATPase activities of different fiber types in rat diaphragm muscle. *Journal of Applied Physiology, 79,* 1629–1639.

Singh, M. A., Ding, W., Manfredi, T. J., Solares, G. S., O'Neill, E. F., Clements, K. M., et al. (1999). Insulin-like growth factor I in skeletal muscle after weight-lifting exercise in frail elders. *American Journal of Physiology, 277*(1, Pt. 1), E135–E143.

Slavit, D. H. (1999). Phonosurgery in the elderly: A review. *Ear, Nose, and Throat Journal, 78,* 505–509, 512.

Snow, M. H. (1990). Satellite cell response in rat soleus muscle undergoing hypertrophy due to surgical ablation of synergists. *Anatomical Record, 227,* 437–446.

Special Interest Division 3. Voice and Voice Disorders. (in press). *Classification manual of voice disorders* (ver. 1.0). San Diego, CA: Singular.

Stangel, M., Zettl, U. K., Mix, E., Zielasek, J., Toyka, K. V., Hartung, H. P., et al. (1996). H_2O_2 and nitric oxide-mediated oxidative stress induced apoptosis in rat skeletal muscle myoblasts. *Journal of Neuropathology and Experimental Neurology, 55*(1), 36–43.

Stasney, C. R. (1996). *Atlas of dynamic laryngeal pathology.* San Diego, CA: Singular.

Stemple, J. (2000). Improvement of vocal fold adduction in a patient with vocal fatigue. In J. Stemple (Ed.), *Voice therapy: Clinical studies* (2nd ed.), pp. 165–171. San Diego, CA: Singular.

Stemple, J., Glaze, L., & Klaben, B. (2000a). Pathologies of the laryngeal mechanism. In *Clinical voice pathology* (pp. 85–148). San Diego, CA: Singular.

Stemple, J., Glaze, L., & Klaben, B. (2000b). Survey of voice management. In *Clinical voice pathology* (pp. 261–396). San Diego, CA: Singular.

Stemple, J. C., Lee, L., D'Amico, B., & Pickup, B. (1994) Efficacy of vocal function exercises as a method of improving voice production. *Journal of Voice, 8*, 271–278.

Strasser, H., Tiefenthaler, M., Steinlechner, M., Bartsch, G., & Konwalinka, G. (1999). Urinary incontinence in the elderly and age-dependent apoptosis of rhabdosphincter cells [letter]. *The Lancet, 354*, 918–919.

Takeda, N., Thomas, G. R., & Ludlow, C. L. (2000). Aging effects on motor units in the human thyroarytenoid muscle. *Laryngoscope, 110*, 1018–1025.

Tanaka, S., Hirano, M., & Chijiwa, K. (1994). Some aspects of vocal fold bowing. *Annals of Otology, Rhinology & Laryngology, 103*(5, Pt. 1), 357–362.

Tews, D. S., Goebel, H. H., Schneider, I., Gunkel, A., Stennert, E., & Neiss, W. F. (1997). DNA-fragmentation and expression of apoptosis-related proteins in experimentally denervated and reinnervated rat facial muscle. *Neuropathology and Applied Neurobiology, 23*(2), 141–149.

Thompson, C. B. (1995). Apoptosis in the pathogenesis and treatment of disease. *Science, 267*, 1456–1462.

Tidball, J. G., Albrecht, D. E., Lokensgard, B. E., & Spencer, M. J. (1995). Apoptosis precedes necrosis of dystrophin-deficient muscle. *Journal of Cell Science, 108*(Pt. 6), 2197–2204.

Tomonaga, M. (1977). Histochemical and ultrastructural changes in senile human skeletal muscle. *Journal of the American Geriatrics Society, 25*, 125–131.

Tseng, B. S., Kasper, C. E., & Edgerton, V. R. (1994). Cytoplasm-to-myonucleus ratios and succinate dehydrogenase activities in adult rat slow and fast muscle fibers. *Cell & Tissue Research, 275*(1), 39–49.

Verdolini, K. (1998). Resonant voice therapy. In K. Verdolini (Ed.), *National Center for Voice and Speech's guide to vocology* (pp. 32–33). Iowa City, Iowa: National Center for Voice and Speech.

Verdolini, K., Drucker, D., Palmer, P., & Samawi, H. (1998) Laryngeal adduction in resonant voice. *Journal of Voice, 12,* 315–327.

Verdú, E., Butí, M., & Navarro, X. (1995). The effect of aging on efferent nerve fibers regeneration in mice. *Brain Research, 696* (1–2), 76–82.

Wang, F. C., dePasqua, V., & Delwaide, P. J. (1999). Age-related changes in fastest and slowest conducting axons of thenar motor units. *Muscle and Nerve, 22,* 1022–1029.

Yoshimura, K., & Harii, K. (1999). A regenerative change during muscle adaptation to denervation in rats. *Journal of Surgical Research, 81,* 139–146.

Zerba, E., Komorowski, T. E., & Faulkner, J. A. (1990). Free radical injury to skeletal muscles of young, adult, and old mice. *American Journal of Physiology, 258*(3, Pt. 1), C429–C435.

Chapter 6

Spasmodic Dysphonia

Medical, Pharmacological, and Behavioral Perspectives

Gayle E. Woodson and Thomas Murry

Woodson and Murry plainly state that spasmodic dysphonia (SD) is a very distinctive voice disorder, yet its etiology and pathophysiologic mechanisms remain obscure. Defining SD as a focal dystonia involving brain stem dysfunction is an important classification, but as the authors suggest, it is possible that SD is not a single disease but rather a symptom complex that may result from a variety of causes. In their overview of SD, the authors suggest two fundamental problems: uncontrolled muscle spasms and the patient's compensatory response. In their discussion of treatments, the authors emphasize that both past and current interventions that treat SD directly with voice therapy have had little success.

1. *Spasmodic dysphonia is a complex focal dystonia affecting the larynx. What are the primary vocal symptoms associated with SD, and how do these symptoms differentially diagnose this disorder from other types of neurological disorders?*

2. *What is the current treatment for relief of the spasms associated with adductor spasmodic dysphonia? How does it work?*

3. *What are three main components of the evaluation process that are crucial for the accurate diagnosis of spasmodic dysphonia?*

Spasmodic dysphonia (SD) is a very distinctive, yet poorly defined, voice disorder. Experienced clinicians can usually identify the disorder easily, but variations of it may make the diagnosis difficult. Patients do not all sound alike, because of irregularities in (a) the pattern and severity of spasms and (b) the compensatory vocal strategies used. There are no truly pathognomonic physical signs or objective tests. The etiology and pathophysiologic mechanisms of the disorder remain obscure. In fact, there is uncertainty as to whether this is a single disease or a group of disorders with similar presenting signs.

Traube first described the signs of spasmodic dysphonia in 1871, calling it *Spastiche Form der nervosen Helserkeit* (spastic form of nervous hoarseness). For many years it was called *spastic dysphonia.* It was regarded as psychosomatic because of a fluctuation in symptoms and the frequent co-occurrence of anxiety and depression. Subsequent reports have documented a high incidence of neuropathology, such as autonomic dysfunction and tremor, in persons with the disorder (Schaefer, 1983). The dramatic response of the disease to recurrent laryngeal nerve section provided strong support for an organic cause (Dedo, 1976). Moreover, there is evidence indicating that anxiety and depression are the result, rather than the cause of the speech problem. In a group of patients who completed psychological questionnaires before and after successful treatment with botulinum toxin, anxiety and depression were common at presentation but normalized after treatment (Murry, Cannito, & Woodson, 1994).

Currently, SD is thought to be a focal dystonia involving brain stem dysfunction. Because the fundamental problem is spasmodic muscle contractions, not muscle spasticity, the correct term is *spasmodic dysphonia,* as opposed to *spastic dysphonia.* Diagnostic criteria for SD are not clearly defined. With clinical experience, the characteristic strained and strangled voice of adductor SD can be easily recognized, particularly if there are audible voice breaks or frequency shifts. Breathy breaks and sustained breathiness, particularly for vowels following a voiceless consonant, suggest abductor SD. It sometimes is difficult to distinguish organic SD from psychogenic voice disorders or muscle tension dysphonia (a voice disorder resulting from chronic hyperadduction of the true or false vocal folds). Voice breaks are an important sign, but they may not be detectable without computerized acoustic analysis. Acoustic analyses of 10 patients with SD, when compared to analyses of 10 patients with muscle tension dysphonia, found phonatory breaks only in the former (Sapienza, Walton, & Murry, 2000). Physical signs that are often observed in SD include observable spasms and intention tremor of the palate, larynx, or pharynx. Asymmetry of laryngeal motion cannot be voluntarily or unconsciously produced; therefore, when it is present, it indicates neuropathology. Differentiation of SD from other neurologic disorders is also important. The dysfunction of SD is limited to voice production. Associated neurological signs, such as dysarthria, dysphagia, or stridor, suggest a different diagnosis (Swenson, Zwirner, Murry, & Woodson, 1992).

Theoretical/Empirical Knowledge

SD is generally regarded to be a focal dystonia of the larynx. Dystonias are defects in motor control that are manifested by forceful, involuntary muscle contractions. A dystonia may be focal, regional, or generalized and may be either primary or secondary to a wide variety of causes, including hereditary syndromes, stroke, trauma, and drug effects. SD not only behaves like a dystonia but also is often associated with other forms of dystonia, such as blepharospasm or writer's cramp. Greene, Kang, and Fahn (1995) found that of 79 patients with focal SD, other muscle groups became involved in 14%. Martinelli et al. (1995) found an enzyme deficiency (lower than normal levels of arylduphatase activity) in patients with adult postural tremor and adult-onset SD. This abnormality had previously been noted only in patients with generalized dystonia.

The pathophysiology of dystonia is not known. Primary dystonia cannot be attributed to any identifiable brain lesions, but secondary dystonias are often associated with lesions in the basal ganglia (Jankovic & Patel, 1983). The blink reflex has been studied in patients with two types of dystonia, blepharospasm and oromandibular dystonia. In these patients, the latency of the blink reflex is normal, but there is evidence of central disinhibition (Tolosa, Montserrat, & Bayes, 1988). The defect does not appear to be at the cortical level, as electroencephalograph (EEG) back averaging studies do not reveal any preceding cortical trigger. This indicates that the defect is either in the pyramidal tract or the basal ganglia (Beradeli, Rothwell, Day, & Marsden, 1985). Some autopsy studies of patients with dystonia have detected altered levels of norepinephrine, serotonin, and dopamine in neurotransmitters in the caudate, putamen, globus pallidus, and dentate nuclei (Hornykiewicz, Kish, Becker, Farley, & Shannak, 1986). Thus, the most likely site of pathology in dystonia is the basal ganglia.

Linkage analysis has located a gene in the 9q region of the gene atlas that causes increased susceptibility to torsion dystonia (Ozelius et al., 1989). SD may also be familial. Blitzer, Brin, and Stewart (1998) found that 23% of 110 patients with SD reported a family history of dystonia. It remains to be seen whether the genetic abnormality responsible for torsion dystonia can be implicated in SD.

Whatever the biochemical or physiologic mechanisms, the spasms and the compensatory reactions to the spasms require the clinician's attention in the remediation process. The spasms, as well as the compensatory activity, tend to be task and situation dependent. Symptoms are usually worse during conversational speech than during recitation or singing, and they increase in severity with stress. Electromyography (EMG) studies conducted in multiple laryngeal muscles have indicated higher levels of EMG activity in SD, regardless of the task (Watson, McIntire, Roark, & Schefer, 1995). This finding suggests nonspecific hyperactivity of the muscles. However, time-frequency analysis of thyroarytenoid (TA) muscle activity during speech showed a high level of discriminability between SD and nondisordered speech. During whispering and nonspeech acts, however, there was little difference between patients with SD and a control group without the disorder (Roark, Dowling, DeGroat, Watson, & Schaefer, 1995). Van Pelt, Ludlow, and Smith (1994) measured laryngeal EMG activity during speech in patients with SD and five individuals without SD. If aphonic intervals were excluded, muscle activation patterns in the patients with SD were normal. In other words, speech mechanism seems to be normal except for the intrusion of spasms. Abductor spasmodic dysphonia (ABSD) seems to be more complex than adductor dysphonia. ABSD is characterized by breathy breaks due to episodically incomplete glottal closure. Some patients have both adductor and abductor symptoms (Cannito & Johnson, 1981). It is often difficult to distinguish between abductor spasms (posterior cricoarytenoid muscle contraction) and hypoadduction (decreased activation of adductor muscles). EMG studies have demonstrated cricothyroid (CT) muscle spasms instead of posterior cricoarytenoid (PCA) muscle spasms in some patients and have documented that in many patients, the fundamental problem is not abductor spasm but failure of adductor activity (Ludlow, Naunton, Terada, & Anderson, 1991). The cause of this decrease in adductor activity is unknown, and the pathophysiology may well vary from patient to patient. It could be due to central inhibition or to voluntary compensation for adductor spasms. It may also be a psychogenic problem or other neurologic problem, such as vocal fold paresis.

Surgical Procedures

Much of what we know about the pathophysiology of spasmodic dysphonia (SD) has come from observing the response of patients to treatment. As mentioned previously, the introduction of surgical transection of the recurrent laryngeal nerve (RLN) was a major turning point in our understanding of SD (Dedo, 1976). Initial results were dramatic in many patients but less satisfactory in others. The voice was often weak and breathy, due to inadequate vocal fold closure. Vocal fold augmentation to increase glottal closure in these patients reduced breathiness, but with too much augmentation, symptoms recurred. To treat such symptoms, relief was given by thinning the vocal fold through use of lasers (Dedo & Izdebski, 1984). The therapeutic benefit thus seemed to depend on a critical reduction of glottal closure—not too much and not too little. A second problem with RLN section is the tendency for symptoms to return over time. One study found that 64% of patients who underwent RLN section developed recurrent symptoms within 3 years (Aronson & DeSanto, 1983). Netterville, Stone, Rainey, Zealear, and Ossof (1991) found regeneration of the nerve to be the mechanism for recurrent symptoms, leading them to propose avulsion, rather than transection, of the nerve to reduce the chances for regeneration. Despite its shortcomings, RLN section remains a viable treatment option for patients with severe SD, particularly for those individuals who require very frequent botulinum toxin injections or who prefer not to have repeated injections.

Medical Treatments

Local injection of botulinum toxin (Botox) is now widely accepted as an effective treatment for spasmodic dysphonia. It does not restore the voice completely, but it reduces voice breaks and decreases the effort required for speaking. One advantage of this treatment over RLN section is that the adductor muscles can be specifically targeted, rather than producing a global paralysis. Moreover, the effects are temporary, so that if results are unsatisfactory, they will wear off with time. The major advantage of botulinum toxin is that the dose can be tritated to produce enough weakness to relieve spasm without causing excess breathiness. Botulinum toxin blocks the release of acetylcholine from motor end plates by disrupting exocytosis. The resulting paresis wears off in several weeks, but the therapeutic effect on SD lasts somewhat longer. There are seven subtypes of botulinum toxin: A through G. Type A is the one used clinically. The toxin molecule is composed of two chains: The heavy chain binds to the cell membrane and therefore confers specificity for the nerve terminal, whereas the light chain, a zinc-dependent endopeptidase, is internalized and impairs exocytosis, so that acetylcholine remains in vesicles within the end plate (Schiavo, Rossetto, & Montecucco, 1994; Simpson, Coffield, & Bakry, 1993). Types A and E cleave Snap-25, a protein in the presynaptic membrane. Recovery requires sprouting of new terminals. Types B, D, F, and G attack synaptobrevin in synaptic vesicles and thus have a shorter duration of action. Type B has been proposed as an alternative treatment for individuals who develop a resistance to Type A; however, its effects appear to be of shorter duration than those of Type A. Type C attacks syntaxin.

The improvement in symptoms correlates with a reduction in voice breaks and increased phonatory airflow (Zwirner, Murry, Swenson, & Woodson, 1991). Study participants primarily reported a decrease in vocal effort. The sound of the voice was noticeably improved but rarely was perceived as normal. Not surprisingly, patients with the most severe symptoms note the most improvement (Cannito, personal communication, June 1, 2003). Older patients usually note more problems with breathiness and vocal weakness, presumably because the vocal muscles are often atrophic in the elderly.

The botulinum toxin mechanism of improvement is more than just a weakening of muscle, with a resultant decrease in the force of contraction. EMG has revealed a significant decrease in the number of spasmodic muscle bursts after injection, and not just in the injected muscles. After unilateral injection, the incidence of spasmodic muscle bursts decreases on both sides (Bielamowicz & Ludlow, 2000).

As with RLN section, results are critically dependent on the precise degree of weakness. It is important to identify the optimal dose and determine whether one or both sides should be treated (Maloney & Morrison, 1994; Woodson, 1998). For adductor SD, the TA muscle is injected. Patients with moderate-to-severe SD generally require bilateral injections from 1.25 to 2.5 units. For mild or intermittent SD, smaller doses are required in order to avoid breathiness and vocal weakness. It is technically difficult to consistently deliver less than 1.25 units; therefore, it is better to switch to a unilateral injection than to reduce the dose. In fact, a unilateral injection requires a larger total dose to produce effects equivalent to that of a bilateral injection. In general, the result of injecting 1.25 units into each vocal fold (2.5 total) is similar to that of 15 units into one side. And a 25-units injection in one side is roughly equivalent to injecting 2.5 units in each side.

Botulinum therapy has been reported to be less effective for patients with abductor SD (Maloney & Morrison, 1994). To reduce spasmodic abduction, toxin is injected into the PCA muscle. A rate-limiting side effect of PCA injection is that significant bilateral abductor weakness leads to unacceptable stridor and reduced exercise tolerance. Abductor SD is characteristically asymmetric, but bilateral injection is required to control the spasm. An effective strategy is to inject a small amount (1.25 units) into the nondominant side and then inject a larger dose into the dominant side, increasing the dose in a stepwise fashion until spasms are controlled, abduction on the dominant side is completely blocked, or there is incipient stridor (Woodson, 1998).

Injection of botulinum toxin into the CT muscle has also been recommended as a treatment for abductor SD, based on the observation of spasms in that muscle in patients. The mechanism of action of such an injection is not clear, because the CT does not abduct the vocal folds. It is conceivable, however, that the breathy breaks could be caused by abductor activation or adductor suppression that is secondary to CT spasm. Medications such as diazepam, baclofen, and propranolol hydrochloride have not proven effective as primary therapy. Some patients do find that baclofen is a useful adjunct to botulinum toxin therapy by reducing vocal tightness in stressful situations. Other patients may find that the use of baclofen prolongs the duration of improvement after botulinum toxin injection.

Behavioral Therapy

Voice therapy used in the treatment of SD is generally inadequate by itself. Success has been demonstrated with intensive therapy, sometimes utilizing inspiratory phonation as a transitional modality of speaking (Cooper, 1990). Most therapists find voice therapy as a primary treatment to be ineffective and frustrating. Because voice therapy emphasizes breath support and easy onset, it has been shown to prolong the duration of benefit from botulinum toxin in patients with adductor spasmodic dysphonia (Murry & Woodson, 1995).

Research

New surgical approaches are being explored as permanent alternatives to botulinum injection. One approach is to resect a portion of the TA muscle via a window in the thyroid cartilage. In experiments on rabbits the muscle did not regenerate, and the vibratory edge was unimpaired (Genack, Woo, Colton, & Goyette, 1993). There are currently no reports in the literature of using this technique in human patients. The major problem with this approach is the identification of just how much muscle tissue to resect. Experiences with RLN section and botulinum toxin treatment indicate that results can be critically dependent on very small differences.

Another approach is to denervate the TA muscle and reinnervate it with another nerve, a branch of the ansa that normally supplies strap muscles (Berke et al., 1999). In theory, this has the advantage of preserving vocal fold volume, and hence glottal closure, because the muscle is eventually reinnervated. The therapeutic effect is attributed to cutting off the spasmodic bursts from the neurons that normally supply the TA muscle.

Initial results are encouraging, but long-term results in large numbers of patients will be required to adequately assess this procedure. Electrical stimulation of the larynx is another therapeutic approach under investigation. An RLN stimulator showed promise, but it has only been used in limited trials in a few patients with adductor SD.

More recently, experimental results indicated that direct stimulation of laryngeal adductor muscles can improve speech in patients with abductor SD (Bidus, Thomas, & Ludlow, 2000). The mechanism of this effect is not known. To date, all SD treatment has worked by using peripheral interventions to reduce symptoms. No treatment has been effective in correcting the underlying disease process in the brain. The most promising avenue at present is characterization of the molecular mechanisms of disease, with the ultimate goal of developing a biochemical or genetic intervention.

Refining the Diagnostic Process

Virtually all patients with SD have tried one or more treatments with inconsistent or nonexistent results prior to botulinum toxin injection. Our current approach includes a comprehensive diagnosis; symptom review consultation with related behavioral and medical specialists, if necessary; botulinum toxin injection; and postinjection voice therapy. The diagnostic process was outlined at the beginning of this chapter. It should be pointed out that flexible endoscopy, coupled with acoustic and perceptual assessment, is absolutely essential in the diagnostic process. The assessment with flexible endoscopy should include sustained phonation and a speech task. The sentence "The puppy bit the tape" can be used to identify the delayed onset of phonation after the voiceless consonant "p" in ABSD. For adductor spasmodic dysphonia (ADSD), a number of measures can be used to identify the hyperadduction and voice breaks common to the disorder. (See Figure 6.1 for a spectrographic example of the ABSD condition.)

Figure 6.2 is a spectrographic example of ADSD. Note the frequency shifts, aperiodic components, and voice break that are common during vowel productions.

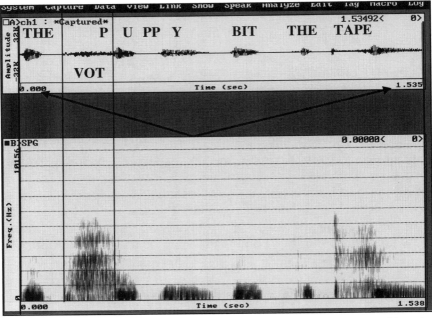

Figure 6.1. Spectrographic example of abductor spasmodic dysphonia. Note the long delay after P.

While vowels and sentences are standard protocol (Woodson, Zwirner, Murry, & Swenson, 1991), the perceptive clinician will sample other sentences as well to help firm up the diagnosis. The sentence "We eat eggs every day" is also very useful, as patients with ADSD have particular difficulty speaking words that begin with vowels. We have found that the voice breaks in ADSD and the delayed voice onset after "s" or "h" in ABSD usually occur at the beginning of a phrase or sentence. The use of sustained vowels during the assessment further helps to distinguish SD from other voice disorders. As stated before, using a reading passage, Sapienza et al. (2000) found phonatory breaks in sustained vowels in patients with ADSD but no phonatory breaks in 10 patients diagnosed with muscular tension dysphonia. This finding suggests that acoustic analysis can be used to help discriminate between two disorders that may have perceptual similarities.

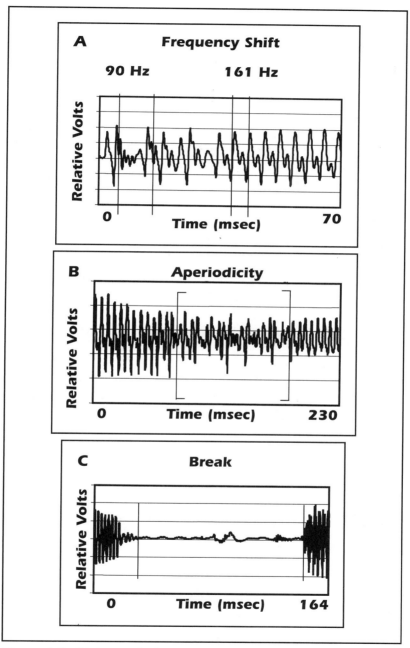

Figure 6.2. Spectrograph showing (A) common frequency shifts, (B) aperiodic components, and (C) voice break during vowel production.

Another part of the evaluation includes sampling the voice during laughter and singing. It has been reported by many researchers that patients with ADSD or ABSD can often produce these two activities without spasmodic episodes. Although this is generally true, it should be pointed out that patients with SD and tremor will retain the tremor in singing. The clinician must be careful not to confuse voice tremor, which occurs in approximately 35% to 50% of patients with SD, with phonatory breaks or voice stoppages. The aerodynamic aspects of ADSD and ABSD also have characteristic signs that provide evidence for the disorders as well as indications for treatment. Airflow rates in ADSD tend to be lower than normal (Zwirner, Murry, Swenson, & Woodson, 1992) and show interruptions or stoppages during speech and sustained phonation. In ABSD, airflow bursts are often seen in conjunction with delayed voice onset after a voiceless consonant. These bursts are associated with high effort levels used by the patient to initiate voicing.

Clearly, the diagnostic workup directs the treatment for SD. Once the diagnosis is made, treatment with botulinum toxin is usually initiated. As Roth, Glaze, Geding, and David (1996) pointed out, however, there are unique cases in which botulinum treatment should be delayed in patients with recent onset of symptoms until a thorough neurological and motor speech examination has been conducted. In our experience, we have seen patients with Parkinson's disease, unilateral vocal fold paralysis, functional dysphonia, and severe gastroesophageal reflux referred for botulinum toxin injection or requesting it based on previous examinations. In all of those cases, a thorough medical and functional assessment indicated the need for other treatments. Examination by a consulting neurologist is an integral part of the diagnosis and treatment planning, and it is standard practice when a patient is seen at the initial visit, as pointed out previously (Swenson et al., 1992).

Treatments

Numerous early researchers (e.g., Blitzer et al., 1988) reported the use of psychotherapy, hypnosis, and traditional voice therapy as nonsurgical methods for treating SD. Crevier-Buchman, Laccourreye, Papon, Nuri, and Brasnu (1997) reported one case in which acupuncture following one injection of botulinum toxin was successful at a 1-year follow-up. Although anecdotal reports occasionally surface, indicating improvement or remission with some single modality behavioral treatment, none of these methods has ever been documented as having long-term success.

In the past, patients diagnosed with SD were referred for voice therapy. Various exercises to reduce laryngeal tension, alter breathing patterns, or change pitch and intonation patterns met with little success outside of the treatment room. Initially, Izdebski (1984) reported on indicators that might be useful markers on which to focus behavioral changes. He found that excess glottic pressure and increased breathlessness accompanied SD. Ludlow, Naunton, Sedory, Schulz, and Hallett (1988), Zwirner et al. (1991), and Zwirner, Murry, and Woodson (1993) found other acoustic parameters (primarily in patients with ADSD) that indicated a possible benefit to combining behavioral therapies with botulinum toxin therapy. In a more recent series, Sapienza, Murry, and Brown (1998) and Sapienza et al. (2000) further defined the acoustic characteristics of ADSD that should be addressed to improve treatment outcomes. Many residual voice symptoms have been identified after botulinum toxin therapy for SD (Ludlow et al., 1988; Ludlow et al., 1991; Murry et al., 1994; Zwirner et al., 1993). Based on these reports, and their own clinical observations, Murry and Woodson (1995) studied treatment that combined botulinum toxin and voice therapy. They compared acoustic and aerodynamic measures and the duration of treatment benefits in two treatment groups: patients who underwent only botulinum toxin injection and patients who were also treated with voice therapy. The combined treatment group had a longer duration of benefit, near normal airflow rates, and lower measures of perturbation than the injection-only group. Voice therapy consisted of three distinct focal points carried out over an average of six treatment sessions beginning 7 to 10 days after injection. The first issue addressed was the phonatory balancing of break flow and breath pressure (subglottic pressure). Exercises included the use of short phrases beginning with voiced consonant–vowel syllables. By prolonging the consonant at the onset, the patient focused on stabilizing the flow of air into the open vowel (see Table 6.1). Eventually,

Table 6.1

Beginning Exercises to Balance and Maintain Airflow After Voice Onset

---

Stimulus Treatment

Prolong the consonant until airflow is stable.
Prolong the consonant /w/.

Stimulus: One

- Shorten the initial consonant.

Stimulus: One

- Keep the air flowing throughout the word and slowly shorten the /w/.

Stimulus: One and One

- Maintain voicing over the entire phrase, after prolongation of the initial /w/. Eventually reduce the prolongation of /w/.

Stimulus: One and One

- Spoken with no breaks between the words.

Stimulus: Why Not Now?

- Focus on airflow maintenance over the entire phrase. Maintain continuous phonation. Vary the intonation once flow can be maintained.

Stimulus: Where Is Our Yard?

- Increase phonetic makeup to include other classes of voiced phonemes. "Where is our yard?"—continuous flow of air.
- Ultimately, add voiceless consonants.

---

voiceless consonants were introduced, and the prolongation time was reduced. This technique is a variation of the flow phonation technique recently designed by Casper and Murry (2000).

The second focus of therapy was voice placement. Exercises were introduced to increase onset pitch and flexibility and to avoid extreme onset pitches (either too low or too high). This technique focused on the classic resonant voice therapy model of Lessac (1973), which has more recently been espoused by Verdolini-Marston, Burke, Lessac, Glaze, and Caldwell (1995).

The third parameter of therapy may be interpreted as vocal hygiene/voice management. This includes education about monitoring laryngeal tension, monitoring voice use in noisy areas, and understanding the basis for the disorder (you do not have to have a psychiatric problem; treatments will probably not return your voice to normal; tremor is a neurological condition that may improve but not be eliminated with injections; you will usually experience difficulty with loudness; etc.).

Vocal hygiene intervention focuses on phonatory-related factors that may predispose the voice to (or prevent the voice from) injury due to internal factors (i.e., hard glottal onset, attempts to shout, or extensive throat clearing) or external factors (i.e., exposure to noxious chemicals, odors, drugs, or dehydration). Using this program, Murry and Woodson (1995) demonstrated prolonged duration between injections, maintenance of near normal airflow rates between injections, and the ability of the patients to time injections to occur at "down times" (e.g., during school-year breaks for teachers, after holidays for clergy, and not during winter months, which was important to elderly individuals or persons who depended on others for transportation). Although this is the only documented report of behavioral treatment combined with botulinum toxin for a group of patients with ADSD, other behavioral techniques may also be appropriate. It remains to be seen if one therapeutic approach is superior to another when combined with the botulinum toxin. Moreover, combined treatment of ABSD using botulinum toxin and voice therapy has yet to be investigated.

Other Factors in Management

Patient satisfaction in the treatment of SD relies on many factors, of which two main ones are botulinum toxin injection and voice therapy. Other aspects, such as emotional stability, reduction of symptoms, return to a more social lifestyle, exploration of other treatments (surgical and nonsurgical), and participation in self-help groups, also have some likely positive contribution to the management of this disorder.

Successful treatment, but no cure, as can be seen from the recent literature, is possible. Treatment is based on accurate diagnosis, combined management, and realistic expectations. The speech–language pathologist plays an integral role in all phases (diagnosis, treatment, and long-term management). Until experimental surgical approaches, medications, biological interventions, and other behavioral techniques can be identified to improve management or cure SD, the current regimen of botulinum toxin injection and voice therapy offers patients symptom reduction, increased communication, and some level of satisfaction.

References

Aronson, A. E., & DeSanto, L. W. (1983). Adductor spastic dysphonia, three years after recurrent laryngeal nerve resection. *Laryngoscope, 93*, 1–8.

Berardelli, A., Rothwell, J. C., Day, B. L., & Marsden, C. D. (1985). Pathophysiology of blepharospasm and oromandibular dystonia. *Brain: A Journal of Neurology, 108*, 593–608.

Berke, G. S., Blackwell, K. E., Gerratt, B. R., Verneil, A., Jackson, K. S., & Sercarz, J. A. (1999). Selective laryngeal adductor denervation-reinnervation: A new surgical treatment for adductor spasmodic dysphonia. *Annals of Otology, Rhinology & Laryngology, 108*, 227–231.

Bidus, K. A., Thomas, G. R., & Ludlow, C. L. (2000). Effects of adductor muscle stimulation on speech in abductor spasmodic dysphonia. *Laryngoscope, 110*, 1943–1949.

Bielamowicz, S., & Ludlow, C. L. (2000). Effects of botulinu toxin on pathophysiology in spasmodic dysphonia. *Annals of Otology, Rhinology & Laryngology, 109*, 194–203.

Blitzer, A., Brin, M. F., & Stewart, C. F. (1998). Botulinum toxin management of spasmodic dysphonia (laryngeal dystonia): A 12-year experience in more than 900 patients. *Laryngoscope, 108*, 1435–1441.

Cannito, M. P., & Johnson, J. P. (1981). Spastic dysphonia: A continuum disorder. *Journal of Communicative Disorders, 14*, 215–233.

Casper, J. K., & Murry, T. (2000). Voice therapy methods in dysphonia. In C. A. Rosen and T. Murry (Eds.), *The Otolaryngologic clinics of North America: Voice disorders and phonosurgery, 2*, 983–1002.

Cooper, M. (1990). Spastic dysphonia simplified. *Asha, 32,* 3.

Crevier-Buchman, L., Laccourreye, O., Papon, J. F., Nuri, T. D., & Brasnu, D. (1997). Adductor spasmodic dysphonia: Case report with acoustic analysis following botulinum toxin injection and accupuncture. *Journal of Voice, 11,* 232–237.

Dedo, H. H. (1976). Recurrent laryngeal nerve section for spastic dysphonia. *Annals of Otology, Rhinology & Laryngology, 85,* 451–459.

Dedo, H. H., & Izdebski, K. (1984). Evaluation and treatment of recurrent spasticity after recurrent laryngeal nerve section. A preliminary report. *Annals of Otology, Rhinology & Laryngology, 93*(4, Pt. 1), 343–345.

Genack, S. H., Woo, P., Colton, R. H., & Goyette, D. (1993). Partial thyroarytenoid myectomy: An animal study investigating a proposed new treatment for adductor spasmodic dysphonia. *Archives of Otolaryngology—Head & Neck Surgery, 108,* 256–264.

Greene P., Kang, U. J., & Fahn, S. (1995). Spread of symptoms in idiopathic torsion dystonia. *Movement Disorders: Official Journal of the Movement Disorder Society, 10,* 143–152.

Hornykiewicz, O., Kish, S. J., Becker, L. E., Farley, I., & Shannak, K. (1986). Brain neurotransmitters in dystonia musculorum deformans. *New England Journal of Medicine, 315,* 347–353.

Izdebski, K. (1984). Overpressure and breathiness in spastic dysphonia: An (LTAS) and perceptual study. *Acta Otolaryngology, 97,* 373–378.

Jankovic, J., & Patel, S.C. (1983). Blepharospasm associated with brain stem lesions. *Neurology, 33,* 1237–1240.

Lessac, A. (1973). *The use and training of the human voice.* New York: Drama.

Ludlow, C. L., Naunton, R. F., Sedory, S. E., Schulz, G. M., & Hallett, M. (1988). Effects of botulinum toxin injections on speech in adductor spasmodic dysphonia. *Neurology, 38,* 1220–1223.

Ludlow, C. L., Naunton, R. F., Terada, S., & Anderson, B. J. (1991). Successful treatment of selected cases of abductor spasmodic dysphonia using botulinum toxin injection. *Archives of Oto-laryngology—Head & Neck Surgery, 104,* 849–855.

Maloney, A. P., & Morrison, M. D. (1994). A comparison of the efficacy of unilateral versus bilateral botulinum toxin injections in the treatment of adductor spasmodic dysphonia. *Journal of Oto-laryngology, 23,* 160–164.

Martinelli, P., Montanari, M., Ippoliti, M., Mochi, M., Sangiorgi, S., & Capocasa, M. (1995). Familial spasmodic dysphonia with low arysulphatase A (ASA) level. *Acta Neurologica Scandinavica, 91,* 196–199.

Murry, T., Cannito, M. P., & Woodson, G. E. (1994). Spasmodic dysphonia: Emotional status and botulinum toxin treatment. *Archives of Otolaryngology—Head & Neck Surgery, 120,* 310–316.

Murry, T., & Woodson, G. E. (1995). Combined modality treatment of adductor spasmodic dysphonia with botulinum toxin and voice therapy. *Journal of Voice, 9,* 460–465.

Netterville, J. L., Stone, R. E., Rainey, C., Zealear, D. L., & Ossoff, R. H. (1991). Recurrent laryngeal nerve avulsion for treatment of spastic dysphonia. *Annals of Otology, Rhinology & Laryngology, 100,* 10–14.

Ozelius, L., Kramer, P. L., Moskowitz, C. B., Kwiatkowski, D. J., Brin, M. J., Bressman, S. B., et al. (1989). Human gene for torsion dystonia located on chromosome 9q32-q34. *Neuron, 2,* 1427–1434.

Roark, R. M., Dowling, E. M., DeGroat, R. D., Watson, B. C., & Schaefer, S. D. (1995). Time-frequency analyses of thyroarytenoid myoelectric activity in normal and spasmodic dysphonia subjects. *Journal of Speech and Hearing Research, 38,* 289–303.

Roth, C. R., Glaze, L. E., Geding, G. S., & David, W. S. (1996). Spasmodic dysphonia symptoms as initial presentation of amyotrophic lateral sclerosis. *Journal of Voice, 10,* 362–367.

Sapienza, C. M., Murry, T., & Brown, W. S. (1998). Variations in adductor spasmodic dysphonia: Acoustic evidence. *Journal of Voice, 2,* 214–222.

Sapienza, C. M., Walton, S., & Murry, T. (2000). Adductor spasmodic dysphonia and muscular tension dysphonia: Acoustic analysis of sustained phonation and reading. *Journal of Voice, 14,* 502–520.

Schaefer, S. D. (1983). Neuropathology of spasmodic dysphonia. *Laryngoscope, 9,* 1183–1204.

Schiavo, G., Rossetto, O., & Montecucco, C. (1994). Clostridial neurotoxins as tools to investigate the molecular events of neurotransmitter release. *Seminars in Cell Biology, 5,* 221–229.

Simpson, L. L., Coffield, J. A., & Bakry, N. (1993). Chelation of zinc antagonizes the neuromuscular blocking properties of the seven serotypes of botulinum neurotoxin as well as tetanus toxin. *Journal of Pharmacological and Experimental Therapeutics, 272,* 720–727.

Swenson, M. M., Zwirner, P., Murry, T., & Woodson, G. E. (1992). A medical evaluation of patients with spasmodic dysphonia. *Journal of Voice, 6,* 320–324.

Tolosa, E., Montserrat, L., & Bayes, A. (1988). *Blink reflex studies in patients with focal dystonias.* In S. Fahn (Ed.). *Advances in neurology: Vol. 50. Dystonia II* (pp. 517–524). New York: Raven Press.

Traube, L. (1871). Spastische from der Nervosen Heiserkeit [Spastic form of nervous hoarseness]. *Gesammelte Beitrage Zur Pathologic and Physiologic, 2,* 677.

Van Pelt, F., Ludlow, C. L., & Smith, P. J. (1994). Comparison of muscle activation patterns in adductor and abductor spasmodic dysphonia. *Annals of Otology, Rhinology & Laryngology, 103,* 192–200.

Verdolini-Marston, K., Burke, M. K., Lessac, A., Glaze, L. E., & Caldwell, E. A. (1995). Preliminary study on two methods of treatment for laryngeal nodules. *Journal of Voice, 9,* 74–85.

Watson, B. C., McIntire, D., Roark, R. M., & Schefer, S.D. (1995). Statistical analyses of electromyographic activity in spasmodic dysphonia and normal control subjects. *Journal of Voice, 9,* 3–15.

Woodson, G. E. (1998). *Spasmodic dysphonia.* In G. A. Gates (Ed.), *Current therapy in otolaryngology: Head and neck surgery* (pp. 436–439). St. Louis, MO: Mosby.

Woodson, G. E., Zwirner, P., Murry, T., & Swenson, M. D. (1991). Use of flexible fiberoptic laryngoscopy to assess patients with spasmodic dysphonia. *Journal of Voice, 5,* 85–91.

Zwirner, P., Murry, T., Swenson, M., & Woodson, G. E. (1991). Acoustic changes in spasmodic dysphonia after botulinum toxin injection. *Journal of Voice, 5,* 78–84.

Zwirner, P., Murry, T., Swenson, M. M., & Woodson, G. E. (1992). Effects of botulinum toxin therapy in patients with adductor spasmodic dysphonia: Acoustic, aerodynamic, and videoendoscopic findings. *Laryngoscope, 102,* 400–406.

Zwirner, P., Murry, T., & Woodson, G. E. (1993). Perceptual acoustic relationships in spasmodic dysphonia. *Journal of Voice, 7,* 165–171.

Chapter 7

Dysphonia Due to Paradoxical Vocal Fold Movement/Episodic Paroxysmal Laryngospasm

Medical and Pharmacological Perspectives

Gregory Gallivan and Mary Andrianopoulos

Gallivan and Andrianopoulos emphasize that paradoxical vocal fold movement (PVFM) is a complex disorder in which adduction of the vocal folds occurs on inspiration. According to the authors, this condition, formerly considered to be rare, mimics other common types of disorders. Gallivan believes that it is essential for physicians, including laryngologists, pulmonologists, thoracic surgeons, internists, general practitioners, and emergency room physicians; speech–language pathologists; singing teachers; and other professionals who care for patients with voice, airway, or breathing problems to become informed about the concept of episodic paroxysmal laryngospasm (EPL). The authors present information delineating the basic history, examination, testing, and treatments of the condition, in an orderly series of steps.

1. *Numerous terms have been used to describe the nature of PVFM. The current label is EPL. Why is this label more acceptable than labels used in the past? Should speech–language pathologists be concerned with the current use of disease descriptors?*

2. *EPL may be difficult to differentially diagnose from other similar conditions, such as asthma. What types of objective or subjective information can be gathered to assist in differentially diagnosing this condition from others?*

3. *What is the central premise behind reframing a patient's behavior when dealing with EPL?*

Auseful synonymous descriptor for paradoxical vocal fold movement (PVFM) with dysphonia is episodic paroxysmal laryngospasm (EPL). Whereas PVFM describes the intrinsic laryngeal abnormal activity, EPL describes the laryngeal dysfunction. EPL is an event, or a reversible series of events, complete in itself but forming part of a larger and uncommon but increasingly frequently recognized, recurring, and disturbing clinical condition. It is paroxysmal in that it is a sudden attack or intensification of symptoms, recurring periodically. Once the episode of EPL has commenced during inspiration, the forceful vocal fold adduction/spasm, sometimes likened to a "cramp of the larynx," may carry over transiently into the expiratory phase of breathing in some patients. PVFM/EPL can masquerade as asthma, vocal fold paralysis, laryngeal edema, voice disorders with diminished phonatory intensity during a sudden attack, and anatomic airway obstruction (such as stenosing lesions of the upper airways). The intermittent inspiratory and respiratory distress of EPL may precipitate emergency clinical maneuvers, resulting in unnecessary endotracheal intubation, cardiopulmonary resuscitation (CPR), or tracheostomy (Gallivan, Hoffman, & Gallivan, 1996).

There is a lack of consensus regarding terminology and nomenclature in the medical, neurological, otolaryngological, psychiatric, pulmonary, and surgical literature. The terms *paradoxical vocal fold movement* or *motion, paradoxical vocal cord movement* or *motion, paradoxical vocal cord dysfunction, vocal cord dysfunction,* and *episodic paroxysmal laryngospasm* are interchangeable, representing the same condition. All of these terms may be a subdivision of, or related to, irritable larynx syndrome (ILS). PVFM and EPL seem to be the most descriptive of what happens and how it happens, although why it happens and how it is best treated continue to evoke controversy.

To understand the plethora of terms historically used to describe this syndrome or symptom complex, it is useful to view the terminology from a historical perspective. The list of terms used to describe this disorder, in approximate historical chronology, includes the following, running from the earliest to the most current:

- motor neurosis spasmodic closure of glottis, orifice of the larynx, or both
- functional dysphonia and aphonia

- psychogenic stridor or emotional laryngospasm
- Münchausen's stridor
- paradoxical vocal fold movement in dysphonia
- hysterical aphonia
- factitious asthma
- paradoxical vocal cord motion causing stridor
- vocal cord dysfunction presenting as asthma
- laryngeal spasm mimicking bronchial asthma
- functional upper airway obstruction as a somatization disorder
- stridor caused by vocal cord malfunction associated with emotional factors
- episodic laryngeal dyskinesia
- laryngeal dysfunction and pulmonary disorder
- variable vocal cord dysfunction presenting as wheezing
- exercise-induced asthma
- paradoxic vocal cord motion in presumed asthmatics
- psychogenic vocal cord dysfunction masquerading as asthma
- stridor in childhood asthma
- psychogenic stridor
- masqueraders in clinical allergy
- dyspnea caused by laryngeal dysfunction
- functional laryngeal obstruction as a somatization disorder
- functional upper airway obstruction with inspiratory vocal fold adduction
- hysterical laryngeal spasm
- episodic psychogenic pharyngeal constriction
- simultaneous functional laryngeal stridor and functional dysphonia
- respiratory dystonia
- adductor laryngeal breathing dystonia
- episodic paroxysmal laryngospasm
- paradoxical vocal fold movement with stridor
- vocal cord dysfunction with exertional dyspnea
- irritable larynx syndrome
- paradoxical vocal cord motion with dystonia
- PVFM–PVCD–EPL—ILS

Jackson and Jackson (1942) appear to have been the first to describe a motor neurosis spasmodic closure of the glottis, orifice of the larynx, or both. They surmised that it was a reflex reaction to a local irritation, such as would be caused by instrumentation, gases, foreign particles or agents, secretions, impaired esophageal drainage, or an elongated uvula. They cited a central or peripheral neurological lesion as a possible etiology and believed the condition occasionally was seen as a result of hysteria. Jackson and Jackson described a patient typically awakening at night, gasping for air, springing from bed, frantically grasping hold of any object, hastening to a window, and opening it because of air hunger. Inspiration was associated with a loud stridor, and expiration was unobstructed. They described a closing cellar-door mechanism—the tight closure of the glottic chink by the inspiratory blast—comparing it to the mechanical principle of a check valve: the greater the respiratory effort exerted, the tighter the glottic closure. The patient's only chance of getting in enough air to survive was to breathe very gently and slowly, allowing the spasm to relax and breathing to come more freely. A brassy cough and hoarse voice resulted from some attacks. Those bouts that occurred in the daytime as a sudden seizure could cause the patient to fall in the street and would continue until the patient became unconscious. In other cases, relaxation came just before unconsciousness supervened. Prophetically, they stated that if an opportunity were afforded for a laryngoscopic examination during a spasm, the diagnosis would be promptly and conclusively made. Jackson and Jackson believed that the best treatment was a proper psychic preparation for the patient, who must be made to feel there was no danger and be informed that the greater the effort to breathe in, the less air would get in.

A. E. Aronson, Peterson, and Litin (1966) described psychiatric symptoms in functional dysphonia and aphonia. Patterson, Schatz, and Horton (1974) described Münchausen's stridor as a nonorganic laryngeal obstruction. Rogers and Stell (1978) recognized paradoxical vocal cord movement in episodes of dysphonia known to be associated with functional conditions and initiated by mild infections. On indirect laryngoscopy, their two patients presented with stridor caused by approximation of the vocal folds during inspiration. A 36-year-old divorced woman with neuroses and a childhood history of asthma and edematous vocal folds had hoarseness, noisy breathing, and throat tightness. A 19-year-old student nurse who was considered to be immature and emotional and was unable to cope with working in an operating theater developed a bovine cough with noisy breathing and bilateral vocal fold edema after an upper respiratory infection. A speech therapist helped her to become free of symptoms within 2 days. Rogers and Stell stated that the diagnosis of PVFM merited consideration when stridor was found in an otherwise healthy patient and noted that the condition could easily be misdiagnosed as bronchospasm.

Appelblatt and Baker (1981) discussed a new syndrome of cases of hysterical aphonia with tightly adducted vocal folds during spasms, yet without signs of respiratory tract obstruction. They stated that functional upper airway obstruction might be difficult to diagnose initially in the presence of severe respiratory tract disease. They believed that tracheostomy early in the course of the disorder seemed justified, if it were indicated on clinical grounds. The cases they reported occurred before the era of videolaryngoscopy. Downing, Braman, Fox, and Corrao (1982) called the disorder *factitious asthma* and described a physiological approach to diagnosis. Kellman and Leopold (1982) reported three cases of paradoxical vocal cord motion causing stridor. One patient had two separate tracheostomies performed before the correct diagnosis was made. Two patients were young women with recent upper respiratory infections, weak phonation, an inability to cough, noisy inspirations, stridor, and what was felt to be, at the time, critical upper airway obstruction requiring tracheostomy. Kellman and Leopold's pivotal contribution was the recognition that indirect laryngoscopy while the patient was awake, rather than direct laryngoscopy under general anesthesia, allowed a normal anatomical examination for assessment of vocal fold function. They considered possible underlying brain stem abnormalities or cortical dysfunction. Also, they postulated that the etiology may be functional and that once medical personnel paid attention to the problem, its seriousness became more exaggerated by the patient. Although they recognized that indirect laryngoscopy may reveal a normal larynx with normal vocal fold motion, they did not correlate this with the episodic nature of the paroxysmal laryngospasm. They even mused about the potential of laryngeal electromyographic evaluation to contribute to the clinical documentation of the disorder. Kellman and Leopold believed that awareness of the problem would encourage use of endotracheal intubation rather than an unnecessary tracheostomy, particularly after meticulous exclusion of bilateral vocal fold paralysis, subglottic stenosis, and tumor.

Christopher et al. (1983) presented their landmark work on vocal cord dysfunction presenting as asthma. They introduced two important technological advances by using either a flexible fiberoptic rhinolaryngoscope or a Hopkins-rod right-angle telescopic laryngoscope and performing the laryngoscopies during an episode of wheezing and dyspnea and during a symptom-free period. They added photography with a 16-mm motion picture running at 16 frames per second. Christopher et al. used a motion analysis projector to select representative frames for still reproduction. In addition, they introduced the concept of pulmonary function assessment. To assess upper airway obstruction, the maximum expiratory and inspiratory flow-volume loop relationships were determined during an episode of wheezing and dyspnea and during a symptom-free period. During the wheezing and dyspnea episodes, they observed marked limitation of maximal inspiratory flow rates in all five of their patients. The expiratory/inspiratory ratios were uniformly greater than 2. Their pulmonary function data suggested the presence of a variable extrathoracic upper airway obstruction. When their study participants were tested while asymptomatic, the flow–volume relationships in expiratory/inspiratory ratios were approximately normal. Christopher et al. stressed obtaining a careful history of the episodic nature of the symptoms and used auscultation to identify wheezing and stridor of variable quality, suggesting upper airway origin. During a typical episode of wheezing or stridor, they documented almost complete adduction of the vocal folds—with a small, posterior, and diamond-shaped glottic chink—in each patient. The arytenoids maintained a lateral position, and they did not adduct. Ventricular (vestibular) fold adduction was variable. The patients were unable to voluntarily reproduce wheezing sounds or to achieve the characteristic cinelaryngoscopic glottic and still-frame motion-analysis pattern. Arterial blood gases and alveolar–arterial oxygen tension gradients were normal, and provocative tests for bronchial asthma were negative. Christopher et al. were the first to expand analysis beyond laryngological and physiological evaluations to include psychiatric and speech–pathology considerations. They noted that all five patients had difficulty directly expressing anger, sadness, or fear and had various degrees of secondary gain from respiratory symptoms. Among the variety of psychiatric diagnoses was stress-related exacerbation of symptoms. A speech–language pathologist evaluated all their cases of laryngeal dysfunction.

Chawla, Upadhyay, and MacDonnell (1983) also described laryngeal spasm mimicking bronchial asthma. Starkman and Appelblatt (1984) described functional upper airway obstruction as a possible somatization disorder. Kattan and Ben-Zvi (1985) reported on stridor caused by vocal cord malfunction associated with emotional factors in a pediatric population. Ramirez, Leion, and Rivera (1986) introduced the term *episodic laryngeal dyskinesia* and gave it a clinical and psychiatric characterization. Wood, Jafek, and Cherniak (1986) coined the terms *laryngeal dysfunction* and *pulmonary disorder.* Kivity et al. (1986) described variable vocal cord dysfunction presenting as wheezing and exercise-induced asthma. Martin, Blager, Gay, and Wood (1987), in work emanating from the National Jewish Center for Immunology and Respiratory Medicine in Denver, Colorado, made a landmark entrance into the modern era with their description of paradoxic vocal cord motion in presumed asthmatics (their contributions are detailed later in this chapter). Brown, Merritt, and Evans (1988) described psychogenic vocal cord dysfunction masquerading as asthma. Storr, Tranter, and Lenney (1988) described stridor in childhood asthma. Skinner and Bradley (1989) described psychogenic stridor. O'Halloran (1990) described masqueraders in clinical allergy, wherein laryngeal dysfunction caused dyspnea. Documentation showed that when the vocal folds approximated during inspiration, severe subjective dyspnea occurred without evidence of hypoxia or abnormality in the alveolar–arterial oxygen gradient. Provocative methacholine asthma tests were negative in O'Halloran's group of predominantly female patients with paradoxical vocal fold motion, many of whom had medical professional affiliations and psychological difficulties. Sim, McLean, Lee, Naranjo, and Grant (1990) described functional laryngeal obstruction as a somatization disorder. Ophir, Katz, Tavori, and Aladjem (1990) found functional upper airway obstruction in adolescents by studying flow-volume loops in girls and boys in their early teens who had inspiratory paradoxical vocal fold adduction during symptomatic periods and normal vocal fold movement during asymptomatic periods. The sudden onset of symptoms and the absence of organic disease suggested to Ophir et al. that hysterical laryngeal spasm was induced by emotional stress as an unconscious somatic expression of emotional conflict. They stated that the stridor was not factitious; therefore, the use of the term *Münchausen's stridor* was inappropriate because this appeared to be a true conversion neurosis.

Magnenat and Junod (1991) coined the term *episodic laryngeal dyskinesia* in five cases wherein they excluded organic pathology by visualizing the laryngeal spasm and inspecting flow-volume loops. They differentiated this recurrent and reversible entity from bronchial asthma, laryngeal edema, and upper airway stenosis. Magnenat and Junod emphasized that the use of differential diagnostic criteria avoided taking a too aggressive approach with these patients.

Nagai, Yamaguchi, Sakamoto, and Takahashi (1992) described functional upper airway obstruction that they called *psychogenic pharyngeal constriction,* again with markedly decreased inspiratory flow-volume loops but normal expiratory flows, indicating extrathoracic airway obstruction. However, Nagai et al. did not use videolaryngoscopy to visualize the glottis. Smith, Perez-Darby, Kirchner, and Blager (1993) presented an adolescent with simultaneous functional laryngeal stridor and functional dysphonia.

Grillone, Blitzer, Brin, Annino, and Saint-Hilaire (1994) described adductor laryngeal breathing dystonia (ALBD) as a rare disorder characterized by inspiratory stridor; normal voice; cough; dysphagia; and paradoxical, involuntary, and action-induced adduction spasms of the vocal folds on inspiration. They stated that although the diagnosis might be confused with other disorders characterized by airway noise or cough, such as psychogenic stridor, asthma, or gastroesophageal reflux disease (GERD), their diagnosis of ALBD was further supported by the finding of dystonias involving other segments of the body in an associated respiratory and diaphragmatic dysrhythmia. In the case of a precise diagnosis of ALBD, they found that bilateral injections of botulinum toxin Type A to the thyroarytenoid (TA) muscle were successful in a small number of patients.

Gallivan et al. (1996) contrasted 10 cases of EPL with a case of exercise-induced asthma and a case of laryngeal dystonia of the adductor spasmodic dysphonia type. They presented voice and pulmonary function assessments and management, historical background, diagnostic developments, modern diagnostic techniques, medical therapy, speech–language pathology therapy, psychiatric therapy, relationships with asthma, GERD, psychosomatic/somatization disorders, and thoughts on electromyography and laryngeal dystonias. They stated that EPL was a laryngeal dysfunction, often without specific organic etiology, which might occasionally be a conversion phenomenon masquerading as asthma, vocal fold paralysis, upper airway obstruction, or a voice disorder.

McFadden and Zawadski (1996) described cases of seven elite athletes with vocal cord dysfunction who had received a diagnosis of exercise-induced asthma. Multiple bronchoprovocation tests, including cold-air isocapnic hyperventilation and methacholine, did not provoke symptoms, but exercise challenge did elicit vocal cord dysfunction in six of the seven patients, who were referred for evaluation of dyspnea and a "choking" sensation during competitive physical activity.

Pinho, Tsuji, Sennes, and Menezes (1997) gave a case report of PVFM in one patient with respiratory stridor that was resolved through speech therapy, which they documented by flexible fiberoptic videolaryngoscopy. The patient, a 36-year-old man, had repeated episodes of noisy inspiratory stridor, cyanosis, hypoxia, and nocturnal awakening with paroxysmal dyspnea, as well as dyspnea associated with stressful work conditions, brassy cough, and hoarse voice. The patient had a severe coordination disorder of the glottis and supraglottis, with paradoxical inspiratory adduction of the vocal folds and atypical movements of the arytenoid cartilages. These cartilages folded anteriorly over the vocal folds, either simultaneously or alternating one with the other asystematically. Pinho et al. likened these movements to a cramp crisis of the larynx and actually taught the patient to learn control through means of a modified seven-step speech therapy program (Martin et al., 1987), which is briefly outlined later in this chapter.

Morris, Deal, Bean, Grbach, and Morgan (1999) described vocal cord dysfunction in patients with exertional dyspnea. These patients underwent direct visualization of vocal cords with flexible laryngoscopy before and after exercise to determine the presence of inspiratory vocal cord adduction. Their work is detailed later in this chapter.

Morrison, Rammage, and Emami (1999) described irritable larynx syndrome, which they defined as a hyperkinetic laryngeal dysfunction resulting from an assorted collection of causes in response to a definitive triggering stimulus. They described hyperkinetic laryngeal dysfunction in several forms: muscular tension dysphonia, EPL, chronic cough, throat clearing, and globus pharyngeus (the sensation of a lump in the throat). Their work is also described later in this chapter.

Altman, Mirza, Ruiz, and Sataloff (2000) described 10 patients with PVFM. They offered a detailed description of presentation and treatment options, including flexible nasolaryngoscopic biofeedback and the use of botulinum toxin (Botox) for dystonia in half the cases.

Andrianopoulos, Gallivan, and Gallivan (1999, 2000) presented *paradoxical vocal cord movement, paradoxical vocal cord dysfunction, episodic paroxysmal laryngospasm,* and *irritable larynx syndrome* as essentially interchangeable terms used to describe laryngeal dysfunction masquerading as asthma, upper airway obstruction, or functional and organic voice disorders. Over a period of 10 years, they conducted a retrospective analysis of 27 individuals, ages 15 to 79 years, of which 20 (74%) were women, with a mean age of 48.8 years. These individuals were identified to have paroxysms of inspiratory stridor, acute respiratory distress, and associated aphonia and dysphonia that often resulted, prior to referral to the authors, in misdiagnosis and unnecessary emergency treatments, including massive pharmacotherapy, endotracheal intubation, CPR, and tracheostomy.

All of these described syndromes share episodic laryngospasm or random, intermittent hyperadduction of the vocal folds during the inspiratory phase of the respiratory cycle, with the result being temporary upper airway obstruction or a sense of such obstruction. As noted earlier in this chapter, the terminology presently and most widely used to refer to this symptom complex includes PVFM, paradoxical vocal cord movement, paradoxical vocal cord dysfunction, vocal cord dysfunction, episodic paroxysmal laryngospasm, and ILS. We believe the two most appropriate, definitive terms in the current voice-care lexicon are PVFM, which describes the inspiratory adduction of the vocal folds with associated dysphonia or aphonia, and EPL, which delineates graphically the random, sudden appearance of spasmodic, forceful, and abnormal closure of the vocal folds during inhalation, resulting in intermittent respiratory obstruction and stridor. If one appreciates the viewpoint of Morrison et al. (1999), the PVFM/EPL syndromes may be viewed as a subset of the inclusion criteria for diagnosis of ILS.

Basic Diagnostic Steps

History and Subjective Factors

A valid clinical caveat is "Listen to your patients; they are telling you their diagnosis." In taking a patient's history, the clinician should allow the patient to describe the problem without interruption for 3 minutes. The history may then be amplified by asking specific questions. One such question would be "Is the trouble breathing in, or breathing out?" The key subjective factor in EPL is the inability to breathe in during the inspiratory phase of the respiratory cycle. Choking, stridor, and wheezing usually occur primarily on inhalation rather than on exhalation. In some cases, once the tonic spasm of the laryngeal muscles has commenced during inspiration, the forceful vocal fold adduction may carry over transiently into the expiratory phase of breathing.

A second important subjective criterion is aphonia. If aphonia occurs, as during an episode or attack, it is highly suggestive of the disorder. Dysphonia or hoarseness may occur during, prior to, or following an episode or the feeling of inspiratory upper airway obstruction with transitory aphonia.

All persons with a history of asthma should be asked an open-ended question about where they believe the voice or airway limitation occurs. Many individuals will indicate the area of the larynx, but if the indication is toward the chest, a directed question specifically related to the site of the larynx should be asked. An additional group of patients may acknowledge a sensation of vocal or airway difficulties at the level of the larynx. The result of vocal folds going into spasm during inspiration may cause asthma-like wheezing and breathlessness that has no relation to true asthma or reactive airways disease. Pulmonologists have increasingly recognized that PVFM/EPL is the biggest asthma mimic currently encountered (Bensimhon & Weiland, 2000). During the 1990s, there appeared in the medical literature an increasing number of articles describing paradoxical vocal fold adduction, either on inspiration or throughout the respiratory cycle, that presented or masqueraded as true asthma, particularly in adolescents and in stressful settings (Caraon & O'Toole, 1991; Corren & Newman, 1992; Craig, Sitz, Squire, Smith, & Carpenter, 1991; Fields, Roy, & Ossorio, 1992; Lim, 1991; M. Schmidt, 1993; Sokol, 1993).

Patients with this dysfunction often display GERD symptoms, including, but not limited to, dysphagia (trouble swallowing) and pyrosis (heartburn). Koufman (1993, 1994) suggested that a psychosomatic response to stress may be associated with an increased incidence of GERD. It is known that GERD can cause aerodigestive, particularly asthmatic and laryngopharyngeal, symptoms and signs in patients who do not have a history of pyrosis or regurgitation and who may have dysphonia, hoarseness, cervical dysphagia, globus pharyngeus, asthma, chronic throat clearing, and chronic cough. Koufman postulated that the persistence and degree of inappropriate paradoxical glottic closure determines the degree of apparent airway obstruction; hence, it determines the severity of vocal and respiratory symptoms experienced by the patient. Little, Koufman, Kohut, and Marshall (1985) studied the effects of gastric acid on the pathogenesis of subglottic stenosis. A significant increase in the degree of subglottic stenosis in canines following chronic application of gastric contents to subglottic mucosal tissues was noted. They established a definitive diagnosis of GERD during 24-hour double-probe pH monitoring. Some researchers have suggested that gastroesophageal respiratory disease and respiratory sequelae—and inflammation of the pharynx and upper esophagus—are due to GERD sensitivities of mucosal chemoreceptors, afferent superior laryngeal nerve branches, and vagally mediated neural networks (Allen & Newhouse, 1984). Loughlin, Koufman, and Averill (1996), who studied acid-induced laryngospasm in a canine model, demonstrated that vagally mediated chemoreceptors consistently induced laryngospasm in the larynx when it was exposed to acidic levels of 2.5 pH or lower.

Definitive, Objective Diagnostic Criteria

Evaluation of voice production and the presence or absence of airway obstruction begins with asking the patient several specific questions:

- Is the trouble breathing in or wheezing on inhalation?
- Does the breathing or wheezing problem involve the entire inspiratory/expiratory respiratory cycle?
- Is the sensation of breathing difficulty or choking at the level of the larynx or elsewhere?

Any examination should include the following:

- thorough physical examination, with emphasis on the larynx, trachea, and thorax;
- auscultatory differentiation of inspiratory from expiratory stridor during an attack;
- anatomic assessment of the airway by means of routine anteroposterior and lateral soft tissue films of the neck (preferably computer assisted) and posteroanterior and lateral chest X rays to help rule out anatomical airway obstruction;
- videolaryngoscopy, with or without stroboscopy;
- pulmonary function testing, with particular attention to the inspiratory portion of the flow-volume loops;
- fiber-optic endoscopic evaluation of swallowing (FEES) and videoesophagography; and
- bronchoscopy.

Indirect mirror laryngoscopy, flexible fiberoptic transnasal laryngoscopy, and rigid transoral telescopic laryngoscopy all share the problem of requiring real-time assessment of laryngeal dynamics during the patient examination. Martin et al. (1987) used videolaryngoscopy to document inspiratory paradoxical vocal fold closure as a laryngeal dysfunction masquerading as asthma. A team of otolaryngologists, pulmonologists, psychiatrists, and speech–language pathologists found that many individuals pointed to the area of the larynx. The study participants were mainly women between the ages of 20 and 40 years, many with education above the high school level and medical backgrounds. In severe cases, Martin et al. documented inspiratory stridor during paradoxical vocal fold adduction. During symptomatic episodes, they found attenuation of the inspiratory portion of the flow-volume loop. When videolaryngoscopy and flow-volume loops could not be accomplished during an acute episode, the authors attempted to stimulate reproduction of the paroxysms with repetitive, rapid, and deep inspirations; panting; various phonatory tasks; and physical stimulation of the supraglottic larynx below the epiglottis. They documented the now classic pattern of inspiratory adduction of the anterior two thirds of the vocal folds with a posterior, diamond-shaped glottic chink or gap, whereas during quiescent periods, the only sign suggesting vocal fold abuse was mucus bridging or stranding between the posterior vocal folds.

The definitive examination is videolaryngoscopy, with or without stroboscopy. It is essential to recognize a pathognomonic pattern of paradoxical inspiratory adduction of the anterior two thirds of the vocal folds with a posterior, diamond-shaped glottic chink or gap (see Figure 7.1).

Another definitive test is attenuation of the inspiratory component of the flow-volume loop (discussed previously), indicating partial extrathoracic airway obstruction. Because this examination and other testing criteria must be done during a PVFM/EPL attack of stridor or wheezing, it may prove challenging to both the patient and examiners. It is especially necessary to ensure that both the patient and the pulmonary laboratory technician understand that it is essential to perform the flow-volume loop analysis of the pulmonary function testing while the patient is experiencing an occurrence of respiratory and phonatory distress. (See Figures 7.2 and 7.3 for comparisons of a normal flow-volume loop and one where there is PVFM/ELP.)

Although a posterior glottic chink or gap is pathognomonic in the presence of paradoxical inspiratory adduction of the anterior two thirds of the vocal folds, this chink or gap may not always be found. Its absence, however, does not rule out the diagnosis. If intermittent paradoxical vocal fold movement, that is, adduction, is not visualized on videolaryngoscopy, maneuvers to elicit the behavior may be utilized. Touching the supraglottis or glottis with a rigid transoral or flexible transnasal examining scope or requesting

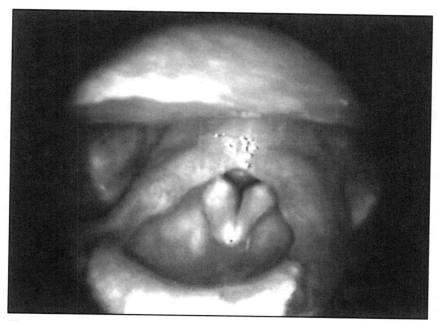

Figure 7.1. Endoscopic picture showing the anterior two thirds of the vocal folds with a posterior diamond-shaped glottic chink.

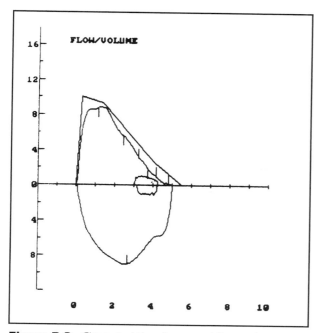

Figure 7.2. Characteristics of a normal flow-volume loop.

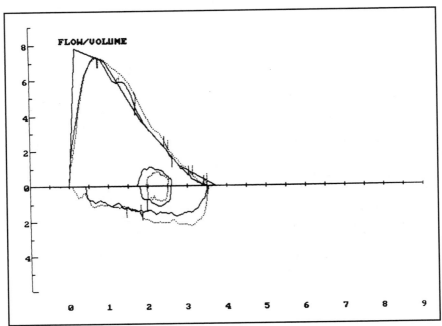

Figure 7.3. Characteristics of a flow-volume loop of a person with paradoxical vocal fold movement/episodic paroxysmal laryngospasm.

voice misuse techniques such as throat clearing, loud coughing, and rapid and loud speaking may precipitate an episode. Conversely, panting, sniffing, and breath holding may result in release of laryngospasm in some cases and may be effective emergency measures for relief of an EPL episode during a diagnostic video-laryngoscopic examination or flow-volume loop testing (Gallivan et al., 1996).

Videoesophagography and FEES may be helpful particularly for those patients with symptoms or signs of GERD. Gallivan et al. (1996) utilized FEES techniques, including 30-frames-per-second slow motion and forward-and-reverse freeze-frame stop motion, with evaluation of laryngeal excursion on deglutition (swallowing) to diagnose occult GERD through visualization of erythema of the arytenoids, mucosal hypertrophic changes of the posterior inter-arytenoid area, and other signs of glottic and supraglottic irritation/

inflammation. The counted freeze-frame and slow-motion video-recording capabilities intrinsic to FEES, as well as contrast radiographic videoesophagography, have also helped implicate occult GERD in selected cases (Andrianopoulos et al., 2000; Gallivan et al., 1996).

Bronchoscopy provides objective confirmation of the absence of laryngotracheal anatomical obstruction in highly selected cases. In the first author's office setting, using only a generic, topical local anesthetic ointment for transnasal passage of the 3.2-mm-diameter flexible fiberscope, the first author has routinely achieved trans-glottic passage of the scope into the trachea and upper bronchial tree while the patient is seated in an examination room chair. Alternatively, in the hospital operating room setting, rigid and flexible fiber-optic bronchoscopy can be performed under topical anesthesia, with or without intravenous sedation, or under general anesthesia in highly selected cases.

If the clinician finds trouble or wheezing on breathing in, aphonia, inspiratory adduction of the anterior two thirds of the vocal folds with a posterior glottal gap, and attenuation of the inspiratory arm of a flow-volume loop during an episode of stridor or wheezing, in all likelihood he or she has unmasked a case of PVFM/EPL.

Differential Diagnosis

The differential diagnosis of PVFM/EPL/ILS is critical to successful medical and behavioral management of the patient, because this laryngeal dysfunction frequently masquerades as asthma with wheezing, pulmonary disease with dyspnea, an allergic reaction, acute respiratory distress, upper airway obstruction with stridor, laryngeal dyskinesia due to neurologic involvement, muscular tension dysphonia or other dysphonias, vocal fold paralysis, globus pharyngeus, esophagospasm, as well as psychogenic, functional, Münchausen's, hysterical, factitious, emotional, somatization, or organic voice/airway disorders. Differentiating this disorder from true asthma or anatomic airway obstruction is very challenging. Aphonia during the paroxysmal attack and subsequent dysphonia from voice misuse/abuse are accompanied by the reality that almost no one with this condition actually has anatomic airway obstruction. Furthermore, categorization into the large group of individuals with psychogenic issues and, much more uncommon, persons with a true dystonia or dyskinesia is important to the selection of appropriate therapeutic strategies.

Andrianopoulos et al. (2000) used the following subjective data during the patient history and examination process to assist in determining or confirming presenting behaviors and symptoms, which aids in differential diagnosis:

- description of obstructive laryngeal symptoms
- location of airway obstruction/limitation (laryngeal vs. chest region)
- nature of respiratory difficulties (inspiratory tridor/wheezing vs. expiratory stridor/wheezing)
- choking episodes
- muscle tightness (neck, chest, generalized)
- intermittent or chronic cough
- phonatory manifestations (aphonia, dysphonia, hoarseness, strained–strangled voice, breathy voice, diplophonia)
- GERD symptoms (dysphagia, pyrosis/heartburn, dyspnea, globus pharyngeus, esophagospasm)
- allergies/allergic reaction
- triggering or exacerbating stimuli
- psychological, emotional, and stress factors

At their pulmonary disease clinic in a U.S. Army tertiary care center, Morris et al. (1999) evaluated for vocal cord dysfunction patients presenting with symptoms of exertional dyspnea. The patients were evaluated through direct visualization of the glottis with flexible fiberoptic videolaryngoscopy, utilizing only a local anesthetic to the right naris and specifically not anesthetizing the vocal folds, before and after exercise, for the presence of inspiratory vocal fold adduction. Morris et al. also avoided stimulation of the glottis. In addition, they did full pulmonary function tests, including spirometry with flow-volume loops, lung volume, diffusing capacity, maximum voluntary ventilation at rest, chest radiographs, methacholine bronchoprovocation and testing, and maximal cardiopulmonary exercise testing with expiratory gas analysis. Ten of 40 patients were found to have evidence of inspiratory vocal cord adduction. Five had evidence of vocal cord dysfunction only after exercise, 3 had GERD, and 6 developed abnormal flow-volume loops after a methacholine challenge. Morris et al. postulated that many patients who had previously been diagnosed with asthma by methacholine challenge might in fact have vocal cord dysfunction (i.e., PVFM/EPL), and they emphasized direct videolaryngoscopic observation of the paradoxical inspiratory vocal fold closure while the patient was in the midst of an acute attack. Although 20% of their patients with the disorder exhibited inspiratory limb trunca-tion of the flow-volume loops during routine spirometry, which was consistent with a variable extrathoracic obstruction to inspiratory flow, had Morris et al. proceeded with flow-volume loop testing while the patient was having an acute attack, or had they precipi-tated an attack, they might have increased their yield of confirma-tory flow-volume loop findings. None of the control group showed evidence of abnormal flow-volume loops on either baseline spirometry or after methacholine challenge. Morris et al. postulated that their patients might have had a combination of reactive airways disease and PVFM/EPL/vocal cord dysfunction. They concluded that paradoxical inspiratory vocal cord closure is a frequent occur-rence in patients with symptoms of exertional dyspnea and should be strongly considered during an evaluation, particularly for indi-viduals who present with exertional dyspnea and for whom other pulmonary, cardiac, and anatomical laryngeal abnormalities have been excluded.

Shao et al. (1995) and Nastasi, Howard, Raby, Lew, and Blaiss (1997) used airway fluoroscopic diagnostic evaluation in the para-doxical vocal fold dysfunction syndrome, utilizing the ability to confirm diaphragmatic dyssynergism with that of the vocal folds. Elshami and Tino (1996) used observation of the usual flattening of the inspiratory limb of the flow-volume loop, to demonstrate ex-trathoracic airway obstruction, in association with a methacholine challenge or bronchodilator medications to evaluate coexistent asthma in patients with paradoxical vocal fold dysfunction.

Etiology of PVFM/EPL

PVFM often occurs without specific organic etiology, and EPL is not an uncommon conversion phenomenon. The etiology of these synonymous entities is controversial. To date, investigators have concurred that psychogenic disturbances (i.e., functional, idiopathic, and nonorganic etiologies, such as anxiety, depression, conversion reactions, panic disorders, borderline personality disorders, and other pervasive psychiatric disturbances) account for the largest category. Emphasis has also been placed on identifying possible precipitating or exacerbating organic etiological factors associated with this symptom complex, such as allergic phenomena, GERD, laryngeal dystonia, and other neurologic/pathophysiologic mechanisms. A small, but important, category is true laryngeal or respiratory dystonia (Koufman, 1994). Stridor, wheezing, laryngeal muscle tension patterns, aphonia, and dysphonia have been associated with all categories.

Psychogenic Factors. Starkman and Appelblatt (1984) explored the temporal association of stressful environmental stimuli and the initiation of symptoms, as well as the evidence of serious underlying psychiatric disturbances. They found features similar to those of asthmatic patients in whom conflicts often stemmed from exaggerated dependency needs and fear of separation. Patients were resistant to psychologic exploration and guarded about descriptions of ongoing family difficulties. PVFM/EPL occurred not necessarily as an isolated, purely conversion reaction but rather in the context of more pervasive psychiatric disturbances, including panic disorder and borderline personality disorder. Upon learning that laryngoscopy did not uncover organic disease, study participants displayed anger, agitation, and resistive behaviors. Starkman and Appelblatt (1984) viewed the behavioral response as possibly warding off dysphoria.

Sim et al. (1990) employed the usual documentation criteria of pulmonary function tests, which suggested the presence of a variable extrathoracic airway obstruction, and laryngoscopy, which showed paradoxical vocal fold adduction during inspiration. Sim et al. found that dependent behavior and high levels of anxiety were the triggers of the functional laryngeal obstruction in their study participant, a 30-year-old woman. Paroxysms with stridor or wheezing could be induced by bizarre triggers and led to multiple pharmacotherapies, including high doses of steroids. Sim et al. emphasized that the episodes occurred suddenly rather than developing over an extending period of time. They postulated that the laryngeal dysfunction might have symbolized a subconscious somatic expression of the woman's dysphoric feelings, with features characteristic of a conversion disorder. Sim et al. used a psychological intervention directed at controlling anxiety, assisted by biofeedback, and then externalizing emotional fear or anger rather than succumbing to a "choking off" internalization mechanism, which may be identified with psychosomatic upper airway dysfunction.

In their prospective study, Morris et al. (1999) supported the concept that PVFM/EPL may be associated with a wide variety of psychological disorders. They pointed out that their patients—young army recruits—were undergoing advanced individual training, which was considered to be a time of great emotional, psychological, and physical stress wherein individual recruits were encouraged by their superiors to achieve high scores in the classroom and during physical training.

PVFM and Laryngeal and Respiratory Dystonias. Altman et al. (2000) postulated that PVFM may be a manifestation of a true respiratory dystonia, as previously described in this chapter. Five of their patients had at least a partial positive response to botulinum toxin injection into the TA muscle, and two of their patients had other dystonias.

The presence of other dystonias and a clinical response to empiric Botox therapy may distinguish those patients with PVFM/EPL who present with a dystonic etiology rather than a psychogenic etiology. Blitzer and Brin (1991, 1992) described laryngeal dystonia as a neurologic disorder of central motor processing that is characterized by action-induced spasm of the vocal folds, producing a clinical voice syndrome termed *spasmodic* or *spastic dysphonia*, with subclassifications of adductor, abductor, and mixed types (see Chapter 6 by Woodson & Murry). Patients with the adductor type had uncontrolled spasms during phonation that were characterized by a strangulated, strained voice pattern with breaks, vocal tremor, harshness, and grunts. The patients with the abductor type had whispery dysphonic breaks and a breathy voice. A third category of patients, who had compensatory abductor dysphonia, voluntarily produced a breathy voice by not contracting their vocal folds in order to prevent the spasms in the broken speech pattern of adductor dysphonia. Blitzer and Brin found an even rarer entity, *compensatory adductor dysphonia,* in which the patient tried to prevent the breathiness of abductor dystonia by tightly contracting the vocal folds.

These four categories of laryngeal dystonias may be successfully treated with Botox Type A injections into the laryngeal musculature. Patients with these dystonias differ from most patients with PVFM/EPL; however, Grillone et al. (1994) described adductor laryngeal breathing dystonia, which was discussed earlier in this chapter. Speech therapy, psychotherapy, and pharmacotherapy all have been used with limited success in treating adductor laryngeal breathing dystonia, but Botox Type A bilateral injections into the TA muscle were successfully used in seven patients in whom the diagnosis needed to be precise before giving the therapy (Grillone et al., 1994).

Irritable Larynx Syndrome. Morrison et al. (1999) used the term *irritable larynx syndrome* to describe a condition in which the larynx is usually normal but there is abnormal laryngeal posturing and palpable muscle tension involving intrinsic and extrinsic laryngeal musculature. Morrison et al. suggested that ILS occurs when brain stem laryngeal–controlling neural networks are held in a perpetual hyperexcitable state and react inappropriately to sensory stimulation. ILS is thought to be due to acquired plastic neural changes to central brain stem nuclei, mainly involving the periaquaductal gray (PAG) area. Morrison et al. referred to this process of altered central neuronal control of the larynx and related structures as "neural plasticity." Their criteria included symptoms attributable to laryngeal tension, such as dysphonia or laryngospasm, with or without a globus pharyngeus or chronic cough. The visible and palpable evidence of tension was noted in laryngoscopic lateral and anteroposterior contraction and palpation of the suprahyoid, thyrohyoid, cricothyroid, and pharyngeal constrictor muscle groups. Suspected sensory triggers included airborne substances, esophageal irritants, and certain odors. Morrison excluded a diagnosis of ILS if there was an apparent organic laryngeal pathology, an identifiable neurologic disease, or an identifiable psychiatric diagnosis. Andrianopoulos et al. (2000) contended that PVFM, EPL, paradoxical vocal cord dysfunction, and paradoxical vocal cord movement are interchangeable terms, and probably a subset of ILS, referring to the same symptom complex or syndrome. These researchers also believed that the disorder may be differentiated from or coexist with identifiable organic laryngeal pathology, such as asthma, laryngeal edema, upper airway stenoses, vocal fold paralysis, laryngeal neurologic disease, and a multiplicity of pervasive psychiatric disturbances.

Multicausal Models. Trudeau (1998) stated that upper airway constriction may arise from at least three different etiologies: psychogenic or conversion reaction, visceral or reflexive laryngeal closure secondary to chronic GERD, and a neurologic form of laryngeal dystonia. Koufman (1994) advocated for a theory that relatively few cases of what he called paradoxical vocal cord motion are psychogenic or functional in origin. In addition to psychogenic stridor, he implicated asthma-associated laryngeal dysfunction, drug-induced laryngeal dystonic reactions, gastroesophageal and laryngopharyngeal reflux disorders, respiratory laryngeal dystonia, and neurologic abnormalities affecting the brain stem. Loughlin and Koufman (1996) identified GERD-induced laryngospasm as causing a sudden, prolonged, and forceful apposition of the vocal folds frequently related to eating or awakening a patient from a sound sleep.

Other Considerations. Kellman and Leopold (1982) reported on a patient with a brain stem abnormality causing PVFM and suggested that the proximity of adductor and abductor neurons to each other in the nucleus ambiguus may permit inappropriate stimulation from the respiratory centers. Maschka et al. (1997) recognized that the Bernoulli effect during inspiration may imitate vocal fold adduction. They also documented two patients with known central neurologic etiologies underlying their laryngeal movement disorders.

Altman et al. (2000) presented a retrospective review of 10 patients, 6 of whom underwent airway intervention and 8 of whom were female, with an age range of 12 years to 53 years and a median age of 36. GERD was present in 8 patients, and psychiatric disorders were present in 7. Six patients had a prior diagnosis of asthma or empiric response to medical treatment of asthma, and of 6 patients who had undergone acute airway intervention, 3 required one or more endotracheal intubations and 3 required tracheotomies. All patients were examined via fiberoptic videolaryngoscopy or video-stroboscopy, which revealed paradoxical vocal fold adduction on inspiration and relaxation on expiration. Altman et al. also observed a pseudoparadoxical adduction in patients with bilateral vocal fold immobility near the midline caused by bilateral vocal fold paralysis, amyotrophic lateral sclerosis, cricoarytenoid joint dysfunction, or Reinke's edema. They postulated that laryngeal electromyography (EMG) may be helpful in confirming or differentiating the diagnosis. Laryngeal EMG may reveal TA muscle activity during inspiration, which may be monitored with contraction of the diaphragm. In 8 of the 10 patients, treating GERD without also addressing the psychiatric and pulmonary conditions was not effective. Altman et al. postulated that increased laryngeal irritability due to GERD laryngitis is a contributor to the multifactorial process.

Management and Treatment of PVFM/EPL with Dysphonia/Aphonia

Medical therapy, speech–language pathology therapy, and psychiatric therapy all appear to be necessary components of an optimal intervention for PVFM/EPL and its associated dysphonia or aphonia.

Medical Therapy

Historically, Christopher et al. (1983) and Martin et al. (1987) found that the wheezing and dyspnea resulting from the airflow turbulence caused by laryngospasm were uniformly relieved by an inhaled gas mixture of 70% to 80% helium and 20% to 30% oxygen. The reason was that the principal factor governing turbulent gas flow is density. Because helium is less dense than nitrogen in air, helium–oxygen mixtures flow with less turbulence across the narrowed glottis.

Although medical treatment of the comorbid conditions, particularly asthma and GERD, should be optimized, Morris et al. (1999) confirmed that treatment with beta agonists and corticosteroids tends to be unsuccessful in patients with PVFM/EPL. On the other hand, Andrianopoulos et al. (2000) stressed that polypharma-cotherapies were counterproductive in the management of upper airway obstructive and episodic paroxysmal laryngospastic symp-toms. Both Andrianopoulos et al. and Altman et al. (2000) empha-sized that any entertained airway intervention must be appropri-ately assessed by a physician, particularly an emergency department physician, who is equipped with and trained in the use of laryn-goscopy, whether by transoral or transnasal approaches. Both groups of researchers also stressed that referral to an appropriate voice-care specialist skilled in videolaryngoscopic and videostro-boscopic techniques may obviate the tragic sequences of multiple endotracheal intubations and even tracheostomies. Altman et al. pointed out the difficulties in decannulating those patients, particu-larly patients with psychiatrically unstable personality disorders, once they have had a tracheostomy.

Pitchenik (1991) utilized a panting maneuver that was largely successful in treating recurrent attacks of functional laryngeal ob-struction. He suggested that panting may be an effective emer-gency measure for relief of PVFM/EPL in those patients for whom a diagnosis has been made through videolaryngoscopy and flow-volume loops. The use of panting has been successful in some of the first author's own patients.

Once medical treatment is directed toward the appropriate use of bronchodilators, steroids, GERD medications, antiallergens, and such, and once triggering or exacerbating stimuli, such as stress, anxiety, food products, environmental factors, air pollutants, perfume products, airborne allergens, airborne chemical agents, ex-ercise, mold, and GERD stimuli, are evaluated and treated, all pa-tients with PVFM/EPL should be referred to a speech–language pathologist.

Speech–Language Pathology Therapy

The seven-step program of Martin et al. (1987) established a speech–language pathology therapeutic standard from which modern therapies, discussed in the next section of this chapter, have learned much. Forceful inspiratory vocal fold adduction results in voice strain, vocal fatigue, hoarseness, voice abuse laryngitis, vocal fold

nodules, polyps, or even ulcers in certain cases. Treatments for reduction of strain on the phonatory mechanism usually involve
pitch change, some type of breathing strategy, and extrinsic muscle-
tension reduction. Patients are taught to utilize these techniques to
maintain airflow at the very first indication of any tightness at the
level of the larynx or any episode of laryngeal stridor or wheezing.
The basic seven-step program of Martin et al. is as follows:

1. Providing the patient with slow direction, acknowledging
   the reality of the stridor, fear, and helplessness.
2. Utilizing behavioral and self-awareness approaches in exercises with good breathing pattern, to allow voluntary control
   when an attack occurs.
3. Teaching "diaphragmatic breathing," similar to the voice
   training utilized by professional singers and professional
   voice users, to direct attention away from the larynx, so that
   refocused body awareness and respiratory effort can be used
   without producing laryngeal, clavicular, or thoracic tension.
   The focus instead is on the abdomen and diaphragm. On exhalation, the patient concentrates on providing support
   through the lower abdominal muscles.
4. Advising use of "wide-open throat" breathing, concentrating
   on having the lips closed, the tongue lying flat on the floor of
   the mouth behind the lower front teeth, with the buccal areas
   of the mouth relaxed, and then releasing the jaw gently and
   using diaphragmatic inhalation/exhalation techniques.
5. Advising patients to focus on exhalation, to interrupt the tendencies of feeling unable to get any more breath and holding
   the breath. The patients are taught to exhale, release the breath,
   and then allow inhalation to follow effortlessly. They are encouraged to develop and maintain an exhalation count and
   avoid gasping for air.
6. Increasing self-awareness of the breathing sequence of inhalation and exhalation and decreasing the feeling of helplessness
   via increased self-awareness of the direct sequence of the
   breathing process.
7. Interrupting effortful breathing by developing the attitude
   that breathing does not have to be actually performed but is

part of a natural body process that can be gradually trusted and practiced.

The first author teaches those patients who have a problem with throat clearing or chronic coughing to use—in addition to hydration therapy—an aphonic cough, followed by swallowing—either a dry swallow or swallowing water—as a substitute for the need to cough or clear the throat. In addition to diet control and GERD protocols for management of acid reflux, vocal hygiene protocols and easy voice-onset techniques are recommended for patients with phonotraumatic symptoms.

Bastian and Nagorsky (1987) introduced laryngeal image biofeedback, which has been shown to be effective for teaching patients to mimic target tasks. It was utilized by Altman et al. (2000), who conducted speech therapy while allowing the patients to view a flexible fiber-optic transnasal videolaryngoscopy display by connecting the flexible laryngoscope to a videocamera and a videomonitor. Biofeedback sessions educated the patients as to the proper position of the vocal folds on inspiration and expiration and allowed them to visualize improper tendencies toward adduction on inspiration. Relaxation maneuvers and breathing control with "sniffing" helped reduce the likelihood of improper vocal fold adduction. Visual laryngoscopic biofeedback may represent an emerging treatment option for selected patients.

Psychiatric Therapy

In a study using a high achievement–oriented group, Martin et al. (1987) noticed that the patients had a feeling they had to "do something" when they were having an attack. The authors emphasized combining speech therapy with short-term psychotherapy as the treatment of choice. The timing of referral for psychotherapy and counseling is necessarily individualized and may be crucial. Christopher et al. (1983) postulated that the abnormal laryngeal function may be learned and may be an unconscious somatization of dysphoric feelings with features characteristic of a conversion disorder, but they found no evidence for malingering. Since the early article by Patterson et al. (1974) on Münchausen's stridor, most researchers have agreed that PVFM is not presently a true malingering situation.

In psychiatric therapy, Martin et al. (1987) utilized the technique of informing patients that they had a problem with paradoxical inspiratory vocal fold motion. They stated that it was helpful to show patients the videotapes of their own and other patients' vocal fold movements. To maximize acceptance of treatment they emphasized that patients should be told that although it is not entirely clear what triggers abnormal vocal fold movements, the condition can be successfully treated with speech therapy and relaxation techniques. Martin et al. made an important point, which the first author has experienced and reinforced to his patients, that people who perceive that they have been told that the problem is "all in their head," whether or not those words have ever specifically been said to them, will actively resist speech therapy or psychotherapy, become angry, and seek another opinion. This experience confirms the principle of allowing the patients to enter into both speech therapy and psychotherapy without having to acknowledge that there may be a psychiatric cause for this condition. The initial aim of the psychotherapy is to allow the patients to retain many of their psychiatric symptoms without needing to utilize PVFM/EPL as a coping syndrome. Alleviation of a patient's fears and fantasies concerning health and dying—and any discussion of changes in health plan, such as for patients misdiagnosed as having asthma—requires gentle and detailed consultation. It is useful to deal with this in a limited paradigm and brief psychotherapy format and to avoid long-term and, most important, insight-oriented dynamic therapy, which may produce paradoxical patient resistance to psychotherapy. The patient resistant to individual psychotherapy may benefit from expansion of that treatment to family therapy, focusing on issues of emancipation from the home and the intensity of the family dynamics that are associated with the illness.

The experience of Martin et al. (1987) and the first author has been that expositional and insight therapy techniques are fraught with failure. Dealing with associated psychiatric conditions—including depression, obsessive–compulsive personality, borderline personality, passive–dependent personality, adjustment reaction, or somatization disorder—and dealing with the common patient factors of difficulty in directly expressing anger, sadness, pleasure, or other emotions are important in speech therapy and psychiatric therapy over the long term. Emphasizing that this syndrome is not a factitious or malingering disorder is also important. One of the reasons that insight therapy is not usually beneficial is that the patient may feel a conscious sense of shame of the disorder and thus have fears in confiding, fears of rejection, and struggles between attachment and interdependence (Vachon, 1990). On the other hand, it may be worthwhile to explain to the patient the role of precipitating psychological factors, muscle tension, and anticipatory anxiety in the production of the disorder. The interaction and effects of organic psychosocial factors may also be reviewed as part of patient preparation. In some cases, hypnosis and hypnotic suggestion may be of value. Proper understanding of the misuse of voluntary musculature in patients with psychological conflicts enables the treating psychiatrist to collaborate more readily with the physician and the speech–language pathologist (Nichol, Morrison, & Rammage, 1993).

As we begin the 21st century, PVFM/EPL may no longer be designated as rare or uncommon but may be more frequently suspected, diagnosed, and successfully treated noninvasively. The differential diagnosis of PVFM/EPL with dysphonia or aphonia is critical to appropriate medical and behavioral management, avoiding unnecessary polypharmacotherapy, emergency room visits, hospitalizations, endotracheal intubations, tracheostomies, and creation of unnecessary comorbidities.

Differential Diagnosis and Management

The differential diagnosis of PVFM is critical to appropriate medical and behavioral management of this condition. An evaluation to establish a differential diagnosis of PVFM and possible etiological factors frequently involves a multidisciplinary team composed of professionals in the following specializations: otolaryngology, pulmonology, speech–language pathology, allergy, neurology, thoracic, and upper airway. The medical and speech–language pathology team should be cognizant of established inclusion criteria consistent with (a) a videolaryngoscopic pattern of paradoxical adduction of the anterior two thirds of the vocal folds during inspiration; (b) a posterior, diamond-shaped glottal gap; and (c) attenuation of the inspiratory component of the flow-volume loop identified during pulmonary function tests (Christopher et al., 1983; Gallivan et al., 1996, Koufman, 1994; Martin et al., 1987). Although it has been described as a pathognomonic pattern, posterior glottal chinking is not uniformly found, and its absence does not rule out the diagnosis (Wood, Jafek, & Cherniak, 1994).

Salient confirmatory signs and symptoms include obtaining key issues through a history; eliciting the patient's inability to inhale; determining the presence or absence of aphonia or dysphonia during or following an episode; and understanding the pattern, frequency, and duration of PVFM symptoms during speech and nonspeech-related activities (Andrianopoulos et al., 1999; Koufman, 1994). Blager (1995) reported that clinical presentations of PVFM include narrow vocal fold opening when symptomatic, twitching laryngeal symptoms, habituated stridor on inspiration and/or expiration, hoarseness, upper chest tightness without lower airway disease or upper chest tightness when lower airway disease is not active, random symptoms, and symptoms with exertion.

During the strobovideolaryngoscopic examination, the mobility, amplitude of the mucosal wave, and symmetry and positioning of the vocal folds should be viewed during speech and nonspeech tasks such as alternatively phonating the [i] sound and sniffing, taking deep breaths, clearing the throat, chuckling or laughing, counting to 50 fast and aloud, reading with a loud voice, and singing. Koufman (1994) reported that patients with probable organic etiologies of PVFM demonstrated consistency of paradoxical vocal fold motion despite the different types of speech and nonspeech tasks performed. Cases due to probable psychogenic causes, however, demonstrated inconsistency of PVFM behaviors during counting and reading tasks.

With respect to the etiology of PVFM, multiple etiologic factors and sequelae have been proposed, ranging from psychogenic and neurologic gastroesophageal reflux to learned-based phenomena (Andrianopoulos et al., 1999; Christopher et al., 1983; Gallivan et al., 1996; Koufman, 1994; Martin et al., 1987; Morrison et al., 1999; Treole & Trudeau, 1996; Trudeau, 1998). Koufman and Trudeau advocated a much broader multicausal model. Trudeau suggested that upper airway constriction or PVFM may arise from at least three distinct etiologies: psychogenic or conversion reaction, visceral or reflexive laryngeal closure secondary to chronic GERD, and a neurologic form of laryngeal dystonia. Koufman suggested that, contrary to popular belief, relatively few cases of PVFM are psychogenic or functional in origin and presented a broader multicausal model consisting of six factors: GERD and laryngopharyngeal reflux, psychogenic stridor, respiratory laryngeal dystonia, drug-induced laryngeal dystonic reactions, asthma-associated laryngeal dysfunction, and neurologic abnormalities affecting the brain stem. The differential and definitive diagnosis of this symptom complex is critical to appropriate medical and behavioral management.

Historical Approaches to Managing PVFM

Historically, managing PVFM has involved a variety of medical and behavioral or symptomatic approaches. These approaches have included behavioral or symptomatic speech therapy (Gallivan et al., 1996; Martin et al., 1987; Pinho et al., 1997), abdominal–diaphragmatic breathing (Koufman, 1994; Martin et al., 1987; Pinho et al., 1997), "wide open throat" breathing (Blager, 1995; Gallivan et al., 1996; Martin et al., 1987; Pinho et al., 1997), focus on exhalation (Blager, 1995; Gallivan et al., 1996; Martin et al., 1987), self-awareness and cessation of effortful breathing (Gallivan et al., 1996; Martin et al., 1987; Pinho et al., 1997), patient–family counseling (Aronson, 1990; Gallivan et al., 1996; Pinho et al., 1997), carryover of breathing strategies to walking activities (Pinho et al., 1997), slow direction (Gallivan et al., 1996; Martin et al., 1987), relaxed throat breathing techniques (Blager, 1995), respiratory–phonatory retraining and relaxation therapy (Blager, 1995; Brugman & Simons, 1998; Treole & Trudeau, 1996), formal or limited psychotherapy (Brugman & Simons, 1998; Fritz, Fritsch, & Hagino, 1997; Martin et al., 1987; Morrison et al., 1999), digital laryngeal musculature manipulation/massage (Aronson, 1990; Roy & Leeper, 1993), and reflux medication and protocols (Koufman, 1994; Morrison et al., 1999; Treole & Trudeau, 1996).

In addition, the following techniques have been used to alleviate PVFM symptoms: the Alexander technique (Austin & Ausubel, 1992), facial-flex mouthpieces for laryngospasm (Spiegel, Creed, & Emerich, 1998), biofeedback techniques (Brugman & Simons, 1998), gas inhalation therapy (Reisner & Borish, 1995), clostridum toxin therapy (Garibaldi, LeBlance, & Hibbett, 1993), the neurolinguistic programming model (Andrianopoulos et al., 1999; Rosen & Sataloff, 1997), and the application of principles of motor learning theory (Andrianopoulos et al., 1999). Although the success of symptomatic–behavioral therapy in managing PVFM has been reported by some authors (e.g., Blager, 1995), the beneficial effects and long-term efficacy of many treatment approaches have not yet been established. The focus of future research should include empirical investigations utilizing scientific methodologies and well-controlled research designs to determine the benefits and efficacy of various medical and behavioral treatment approaches.

Behavioral Management of PVFM

In addition to medical management, an intervention program consisting of three phases of behavioral therapy has been used with PVFM (Andrianopoulos et al., 1999). In Phase 1, a differential diagnosis and inventory of baseline data are established to address etiologic and precipitating factors underlying the PVFM symptoms. Phase 2 emphasizes behavioral management via use of established principles and guidelines of symptomatic–behavioral techniques, motor learning theory, and aspects of the neurolinguistic programming model. Phase 3 consists of carryover of optimal function using "preparatory sets" that were identified in Phases 1 and 2 as achieving the desired change. In Phase 3, self-awareness and independence in controlling exacerbating stimuli and aberrant respiratory and phonatory behaviors are encouraged. The objective is to facilitate sensorimotor changes in the patient by adapting new behaviors that restore optimal function. This differential diagnosis model and baseline data approach is used to establish possible etiological and precipitating factors underlying the PVFM symptoms.

Phase 1: Diagnosis and Inventory of Baseline Data. The objectives of Phase 1 should address establishing a differential diagnosis, advocating for medical management of underlying etiological factors as needed, and determining the need for speech–language therapy and other forms of behavioral interventions. To assist in establishing probable cause-and-effect sequelae, the speech–language pathologist should obtain an inventory of the following variables:

psychological–emotional issues, phonotraumatic behaviors, medical factors, muscle-tension patterns, triggers and exacerbating stimuli, and phonatory and respiratory system involvement. The magnitude of each etiologic variable and the amount it contributes to the presenting problem should be enumerated in hierarchical fashion. Andrianopoulos et al. (1999) recommended that a daily journal be implemented to identify situations in which episodes occur, the duration and frequency of specific symptoms, emotional and medical factors, diet, and triggering stimuli.

Affect and the psychological–behavioral milieu experienced due to PVFM and acute, intermittent upper airway obstruction should be identified. Psychological, emotional, and stress factors may include conversion reaction phenomena; functional disorders resulting from learned, maladaptive physiological compensatory behaviors and psychological–emotional–social sequelae surrounding the aberrant behavior; and natural fears, stress, and anxiety. Moreover, underlying or contributing medical factors, such as chronic coughing, GERD, gastrointestinal problems, sinusitis, rhinitis, organic laryngeal problems, asthma, and other respiratory–pulmonary problems, should be identified and managed by the medical team.

Possible musculoskeletal factors that could exacerbate or coexist with PVFM should be identified. These include laryngospastic episodes, aphonia, muscle-tension dysphonia, and focal and generalized body-tension symptoms. In addition, therapists should list the presence of triggering and exacerbating stimuli, such as emotional and psychological phenomena, food or dietary products, environmental factors, air pollutants, perfumed products, chemical agents, medications, GERD, exercise, allergens, and molds. The speech–language pathologist should determine the degree of involvement of the phonatory and respiratory systems in terms of hyperfunctional vocal and laryngeal behaviors; dysphagia; aberrant respiratory patterns, such as clavicular or diaphragmatic breathing habits; hard glottal behaviors; respiratory insufficiency for phonatory purposes; and phonatory–respiratory incoordination. In addition, any phonotraumatic behaviors, such as throat clearing, chronic coughing, and voice misuse/overuse, should be identified.

Baseline data should be substantiated based on subjective and objective data obtained from the patient's medical history and daily journal, medical reports, laboratory results, and formal/informal batteries administered by the speech–language pathology team. The presence and contribution of each variable and its estimated frequency, duration, and severity constitute the baseline inventory for measuring future change and the beneficial effects of medical and behavioral treatment regimens.

Phase 2: Multidisciplinary Management. Phase 2 utilizes guidelines and general principles for behavioral management involving respiratory–phonatory retraining, motor learning theories, and psychoeducational models in neurolinguistic programming (Andrianopoulos et al., 1999; Duffy, 1995; Rosen & Sataloff, 1997; Rosenbek, 1978; R. A. Schmidt & Bjork, 1992; R. A. Schmidt, 1991). The neurolinguistic programming model is a treatment technique that attempts to facilitate conscious and unconscious behavioral changes in the patient through a multidimensional reframing process (Rosen & Sataloff, 1997). The central premise of reframing involves helping the patient identify the behavior or pattern to be changed and assisting him or her in developing new and more adaptive strategies to replace the maladaptive behavior (Rosen & Sataloff, 1997). Treole and Trudeau (1996) suggested that the patient thus moves from a hyperfunctional state to a more normal level of functioning. For example, a patient needs to gain insight into the nature of his or her respiratory–phonatory problem and physical and nonphysical sequelae resulting in PVFM and acute, intermittent upper airway obstruction. Behavioral treatment goals and objectives should be organized to restore lost function, promote optimal function through purposeful activity, improve performance with instruction, incorporate self-learning techniques, provide essential feedback, and optimize achievement (Andrianopoulos et al., 1999).

To restore sensorimotor function of respiratory and phonatory systems, Rosenbaum (1991) suggested using motor-learning principles, including cognitive, associative, and autonomous/automatic stages. Based on the neurolinguistic programming model, the cognitive stage emphasizes educating the patient in understanding the nature of the problem and the tasks that must be followed to achieve the desired effect. For example, by this point the patient should have implemented the necessary adjustments to eliminate established dietary and medically related factors that precipitated or exacerbated a PVFM episode. The systemic effects of these medical treatments may be monitored by reviewing the patient's daily journal for change from baseline levels in the frequency, duration, and severity of PVFM episodes during nonspeech-related and speech activities. A summary of the involved laryngeal, respiratory, and phonatory systems and projected goals and objectives to rehabilitate these systems, if possible, should be reviewed and addressed. In PVFM cases, behavioral interventions frequently attempt to achieve change through rehabilitation of four systems and related processes:

1. respiratory training utilizing low abdominal breathing, rhythmic inhalatory and exhalatory cycles, and coordinated respiratory timing for speech and nonspeech activities;
2. prevention of focal and generalized muscle-tension patterns for speech and nonspeech activities;
3. phonatory retraining to adapt more optimal laryngeal posturing by monitoring and preventing hyperadduction of the vocal folds and related instrinsic and extrinsic laryngeal musculature; and
4. elimination and prevention of phonotraumatic behaviors.

The associative stage of behavioral intervention consists of helping the patient move from conscious practice to more automatic control of breathing and laryngeal dysfunction through trial-and-error paradigms. Auditory, visual, instrumental, and proprioceptive feedback is essential in this stage. During the autonomous stage, a desired skill can be performed "automatically," and feedback is less crucial (Rosenbaum, 1991). Key ingredients in modifying aberrant respiratory and laryngeal behaviors include early intervention, drills or brief periods of practice distributed over time in lieu of lengthy practices, and daily practice sessions for the patient at home (Andrianopoulos et al., 1999; Singer, 1980; Treole & Trudeau, 1996).

Treatment sessions can be strategically organized to be more frequent in the early stages and in shorter amounts to provide relief to the patient and to remediate the existing problem and its clinical manifestations. Treole and Trudeau (1996) suggested that practice sessions consist of 5-min sessions four times per day, and twice-daily sessions for 10 minutes later in the treatment to decrease the severity and frequency of attacks. Motor-learning behavioral objectives should include consistent and repeated practice on a single task per domain or system that requires modification and variable practice on a range of related tasks across domains and systems (Schmidt & Bjork, 1992; R. A. Schmidt, 1991). Moreover, Rosen and Sataloff (1997) proposed that behavioral and formal psychotherapy interventions employ techniques used in the neurolinguistic programming model, such as guided visualization, enhanced self-awareness, stress-coping repertoires, pacing, modeling, and mirroring.

Similar psychoeducational approaches, such as systematic desensitization, have been successful in remediating fluency disorders. Musculoskeletal relaxation techniques, such as digital and manual laryngeal massage (Aronson, 1990; Roy & Leeper, 1993); head, neck, and shoulder range-of-motion exercises; relaxed whole-body and focal laryngeal and oral posturing; and other relaxation techniques preferred by the patient—such as rest, meditation, body massage, and yoga—are indicated in cases with focal and generalized muscle-tension factors (Duffy, 1995; Treole & Trudeau, 1996;).

Respiratory Retraining Tasks

The focus of respiratory training should be abdominal breathing in which distention of the abdomen during inhalation and maximal use of the abdominal muscles for exhalation are encouraged. Clavicular and diaphragmatic breathing patterns should be eliminated, and the focus of breathing should be away from the larynx. Non-speech tasks to optimize a wide-open airway include panting, blowing, sniffing, pursing the lips during inhalation, and employing nasal inhalation. Initial trials should emphasize abdominal breathing with nasal inhalations and slow and prolonged exhalations, nasal inhalation and exhalation through rounded and pursed lips, inhalation and exhalation through pursed lips, and inhalation and exhalation while prolonging the /s/ sibilant (Blager, 1995).

Moreover, respiratory–phonatory synchronization can be achieved with the following tasks: sibilant prolongation with or without crescendo–diminuendo tasks, upward and downward glides of sibilant sounds, lip trills, humming, nasal sound prolongations with nasal vowel–consonant combinations, counting, reading aloud, singing, and spontaneous speech. Breathing strategies for PVFM have been reported to manage stridor and signs of laryngeal tightness (Blager, 1995).

Stimulus Control

Phonotraumatic behaviors, such as chronic cough and throat clearing, can be eliminated with hydration therapy. It has been suggested that the patient adjust his or her water intake according to current nutrition and dietary standards. In addition, the patient should be encouraged to take a sip of water prophylactically when the need to cough or clear the throat arises. The speech–language pathologist should consult the patient's daily journal to monitor and note change in the frequency of phonotraumatic behaviors in comparison to baseline levels. Vocal hygiene protocols and easy voice–onset techniques are recommended for patients with phonotraumatic speech-related symptoms. Diet control, weight management, and GERD protocols to manage acid reflux should be maintained accordingly (Koufman, 1994).

Phase 3: Carryover. To maximize generalization of desired respiratory and phonatory behaviors, Phase 3 should focus on carryover of tasks using behavioral paradigms noted to facilitate optimal function in Phases 1 and 2. This phase should focus on making the patient more independent in controlling aberrant respiratory and phonatory behaviors due to physiological and emotional triggers or exacerbating stimuli. In Phase 3, carryover strategies composed of preparatory sets to alleviate aberrant symptoms with a high degree of efficiency should be employed.

Conclusion

The patient should be trained to employ effective strategies to manage emotional, physiological, and sensory triggers that exacerbate upper airway obstruction, muscle-tension patterns, and laryngospastic symptoms. Self-awareness, environmental and situational desensitization, relaxed breathing during speech and nonspeech activities, stimulus control, and self-control are emphasized. The beneficial effects and efficacy of medical and behavioral intervention programs for PVFM can be ascertained by consulting medical and behavioral treatment logs as well as the patient's daily journal for empirical changes from baseline levels.

Authors' Note

The invaluable, perceptive, and unflagging computer-structured production, modification, and revision of this chapter, with adherence to formatting and reference structure according to the *Publication Manual of the American Psychological Association*, by Laurie H. Dagesse is deeply and sincerely acknowledged and appreciated.

References

Allen, C. J., & Newhouse, M. T. (1984). Gastroesophageal reflux and chronic respiratory disease. *American Review of Respiratory Disease, 129,* 645–657.

Altman, K. W., Mirza, N., Ruiz, C., & Sataloff, R. T. (2000). Paradoxical vocal fold motion: Presentation and treatment options. *Journal of Voice, 14,* 99–103.

Andrianopoulos, M. V., Gallivan, G. J., & Gallivan, K. H. (1999). PVCM, PVCD, EPL, and irritable larynx syndrome: What are we talking about and How do we treat it? *Journal of Voice, 14,* 607–618.

Andrianopoulos, M. V., Gallivan, G. J., & Gallivan, K. H. (2000). PVCM-PVCD-EPL—Irritable larynx syndrome: What are we talking about and how do we treat it? *Journal of Voice, 14,* 1034–1047.

Appelblatt, N. H., & Baker, S. R. (1981). Functional upper airway obstruction: A new syndrome. *Archives of Otolaryngology—Head & Neck Surgery, 107,* 305–306.

Arnold, G. E. (1973). Disorders of laryngeal function. *Otolaryngology, 3,* 631.

Aronson, A. E., Peterson, H. W., & Litin, E. M. (1966). Psychiatric symptomatology in functional dysphonia and aphonia. *Journal of Speech and Hearing Disorders, 31,* 115–127.

Aronson, A. (1990). *Clinical voice disorders.* New York: Thieme.

Austin, J. H., & Ausubel, P. (1992). Enhanced respiratory muscular function in normal adults after lessons in proprioceptive musculoskeletal education without exercises. *Chest, 102,* 486–490.

Bastian, R. W., & Nagorsky, M. J. (1987). Laryngeal image biofeedback. *Laryngoscope, 97,* 1346–1349.

Bensimhon, M., & Weiland, J. (2000). Asthma and COPD: What's the difference? *Breathe Well, 4*(2), 4–6.

Blager, F. B. (1995). Treatment of paradoxical vocal cord dysfunction. *Voice and Voice Disorders* [SID3 Newsletter], *5,* 8–11.

Blitzer, A., & Brin, M. F. (1991). Laryngeal dystonia: A series with botulinum toxin therapy. *Annals of Otology, Rhinology & Laryngology, 100,* 85–89.

Blitzer, A., & Brin, M. F. (1992). The dystonic larynx. *Journal of Voice, 6,* 294–297.

Blitzer, A., Brin, M. F., Sasaki, C. T., Fahn, S., & Harris, K. S. (1992). *Neurological disorders of the larynx.* New York: Thieme.

Brown, T. M., Merritt, W. D., & Evans, D. L. (1988). Psychogenic vocal cord dysfunction masquerading as asthma. *Journal of Nervous and Mental Disease, 176,* 308–310.

Brugman, S. M., & Simons, S. M. (1998).Vocal cord dysfunction: Don't mistake it for asthma. *The Physician and Sports Medicine, 26,* 1–14.

Caraon, P., & O'Toole, C. (1991). Vocal cord dysfunction presenting as asthma. *Irish Medical Journal, 84,* 98–99.

Chawla, S. S., Upadhyay, B. K., & MacDonnell, K. F. (1983). Laryngeal spasm mimicking bronchial asthma. *Annals of Allergy, 53,* 319–321.

Christopher, K. L., Wood, R. P., Eckert, R. C., Blager, F. B., Raney, R. A., & Souhrada, J. F. (1983). Vocal cord dysfunction presenting as asthma. *New England Journal of Medicine, 308,* 1566–1570.

Corren, J., & Newman, K. B. (1992). Vocal cord dysfunction mimicking bronchial asthma. *Postgraduate Medicine, 92,* 153–156.

Craig, T., Sitz, K., Squire, E., Smith, L., & Carpenter, G. (1991). Vocal cord dysfunction during wartime. *Military Medicine, 157,* 614–616.

Downing, E. T., Braman, S. S., Fox, M. J., & Corrao, W. M. (1982). Factitious asthma: Physiological approach to diagnosis. *Journal of the American Medical Association, 248,* 2878–2881.

Duffy, J. R. (1995) *Motor speech disorders: Substrates, differential diagnosis, and management.* St. Louis, MO: Mosby.

Elshami, A. A., & Tino, G. (1996). Coexistent asthma and functional upper airway obstruction. *Chest, 110,* 1358–1361.

Fields, C. L., Roy, T. M., & Ossorio, M. A. (1992). Variable vocal cord dysfunction: An asthma variant. *Southern Medical Journal, 85,* 422–424.

Fritz, G. K., Fritsch, S., & Hagino, O. (1997). Somatoform disorders in children and adolescents: A review of the past 10 years. *Journal of American Child and Adolescent Psychology, 6,* 1329–1338.

Gallivan, G. J., Hoffman, L., & Gallivan, K. H. (1996). Episodic paroxysmal laryngospasm: Voice and pulmonary assessment and management. *Journal of Voice, 10,* 10, 93–105.

Garibaldi, E., LeBlance, G., & Hibbett, A. (1993). Exercise-induced paradoxical vocal cord dysfunction: Diagnosis with videostroboscopic endoscopy and treatment with clostridium toxin. *Journal of Allergy and Clinical Immunology, 91,* 200.

Grillone, G. A., Blitzer, A., Brin, M. F., Annino, D. J., Jr., & Saint-Hilaire, M. H. (1994). Treatment of adductor laryngeal breathing dystonia with botulinum toxin type A. *Laryngoscope, 104,* 30–32.

Jackson, C., & Jackson, C. L. (1942). *Motor neuroses of the larynx: Disease and injuries of the larynx—A textbook for students and practitioners.* New York: Macmillan.

Kattan, M., & Ben-Zvi, A. (1985). Stridor caused by vocal cord malfunction associated with emotional factors. *Clinical Pediatrics, 24,* 158–160.

Kellman, R. M., & Leopold, D. A. (1982). Paradoxical vocal cord motion: An important cause of stridor. *Laryngoscope, 92,* 58–60.

Kivity, S., Bibi, H., Schwarz, Y., Greif, Y., Topilisky, M., & Tabachnick, E. (1986). Variable vocal cord dysfunction presenting as wheezing and exercise-induced asthma. *Journal of Asthma, 23,* 241–244.

Koufman, J. A. (1993). Aerodigestive manifestations of gastroesophageal reflux: What we don't yet know. *Chest, 104,* 1321–1332.

Koufman, J. A. (1994). The differential diagnosis of paradoxical vocal cord movement. *The Visible Voice, 3,* 3.

Lim, T. K. (1991). Vocal cord dysfunction presenting as bronchial asthma: The association with abnormal thoraco-abdominal wall motion. *Singapore Medical Journal, 32,* 153–156.

Little, F .B., Koufman, J. A., Kohut, R. I., & Marshall, R. B. (1985). Effect of gastric acid on the pathogenesis of subglottic stenosis. *Annals of Otology, Rhinology & Laryngology, 94,* 516–517.

Loughlin, C. J., & Koufman, J. A. (1996). Paroxysmal laryngospasm secondary to gastroesophageal reflux. *Laryngoscope, 106,* 1502–1505.

Loughlin, C. J., Koufman, J. A., & Averill, D. B. (1996). Acid-induced laryngospasm in a canine model. *Laryngoscope, 106,* 1502–1505.

Magnenat, J. L., & Junod, A. F. (1991). Episodic laryngeal dyskinesia: A functional cause of stridor. *Revue des Maladies Respiratoires, 8,*(1), 95–99.

Martin, R. J., Blager, F. B., Gay, M. L., & Wood, R. P. (1987). Paradoxic vocal cord motion in presumed asthmatics. *Seminars in Respiratory Medicine, 8,* 332–338.

Maschka, D. A., Bauman, N. M., McCray, P. B., Jr., Hoffman, H. T., Karnell, M. P., & Smith, R. J. H. (1997). A classification scheme for paradoxical vocal fold motion. *Laryngoscope, 107,* 1429–1435.

McFadden, E. R., Jr., & Zawadski, D. K. (1996). Vocal cord dysfunction masquerading as exercise-induced asthma: A physiologic cause for "choking" during athletic activities. *American Journal of Respiratory and Critical Care Medicine, 153,* 942–947.

Morris, M. J., Deal, L. E., Bean, D. R., Grbach, V. X., & Morgan, J. A. (1999). Vocal cord dysfunction in patients with exertional dyspnea. *Chest, 116,* 1676–1682.

Morrison, M., Rammage, L., & Emami, A. J. (1999). The irritable larynx syndrome. *Journal of Voice, 12*(4), 1–9.

Nagai, A., Yamaguchi, E., Sakamoto, K., & Takahashi, E. (1992). Functional upper airway obstruction: Psychogenic pharyngeal constriction. *Chest, 101,* 1460–1471.

Nastasi, K. J., Howard, D. A., Raby, R. B., Lew, D. B., & Blaiss, M. S. (1997). Airway fluoroscopic diagnosis of vocal dysfunction syndrome. *Annals of Allergy, Asthma, and Immunology, 78,* 586–588.

Nichol, H., Morrison, M. D., & Rammage, L. A. (1993). Interdisciplinary approach to functional voice disorders: The psychiatrist's role. *Archives of Otolaryngology—Head & Neck Surgery, 108,* 643–647.

O'Halloran, M. T. (1990). Masqueraders in clinical allergy: Laryngeal dysfunction causing dyspnea. *Annals of Allergy, 65,* 351–356.

Ophir, D., Katz, Y., Tavori, I., & Aladjem, M. (1990). Functional upper airway obstruction in adolescents. *Archives of Otolaryngology—Head & Neck Surgery, 116,* 1208–1219.

Patterson, R., Schatz, M., & Horton, M. (1974). Münchausen's stridor: Non-organic laryngeal obstruction. *Clinical Allergy, 4,* 307–310.

Pinho, S. M. R., Tsuji, D. H., Sennes, L., & Menezes, M. (1997). Paradoxical vocal fold movement: A case report. *Journal of Voice, 11*(3), 368–372.

Pitchenik, A. E. (1991). Functional laryngeal obstruction relieved by panting. *Chest, 100,* 1465–1477.

Ramirez, J., Leion, I., & Rivera, L. M. (1986). Episodic laryngeal dyskinesia: Clinical and psychiatric characterization. *Chest, 90,* 716–721.

Reisner, C., & Borish, L. (1995). Heliox therapy for acute vocal cord dysfunction. *Chest, 108,* 1477.

Rogers, J. H., & Stell, P. M. (1978). Paradoxical movement of the vocal cords as a cause of stridor. *Journal of Laryngology and Otology, 92,* 157–168.

Rosen, D. C., & Sataloff, R. T. (1997). *Psychology of voice disorders.* San Diego, CA: Singular.

Rosenbaum, D. A. (Ed.). (1991). *Human motor control.* New York: Academic Press.

Rosenbek, J. C. (1978). A treatment for apraxia of speech in adults. *Journal of Speech and Hearing Disorders, 38,* 462–468.

Roy, N., & Leeper, H. A. (1993). Effects of the manual laryngeal musculoskeletal tension reduction technique as a treatment for functional voice disorders: Perceptual and acoustic measures. *Journal of Voice 7,* 242–249.

Schmidt, M. (1993). Not all wheezing is asthma: On functional laryngospasm. *Pneumonologie, 47,* 439–442.

Schmidt, R. A. (1991). Frequent augmented feedback can degrade learning: Evidence and interpretations. In G. E. Stelmach & J. Requin (Eds.), *Tutorials in motor neuroscience* (pp. 59–75). Dordrecht, The Netherlands: Kluwer Academics.

Schmidt, R. A., & Bjork, R. A. (1992). New conceptualizations in practice: Common principles and three paradigms suggest new concepts in training. *Psychological Sciences, 3,* 207.

Shao, W., Chung, T., Berdon, W. E., Mellins, R. B., Griscom, N. T., Ruzal-Shapiro, C., et al. (1995). Fluoroscopic diagnosis of laryngeal asthma (paradoxical vocal cord motion). *American Journal of Radiology, 165,* 1229–1231.

Sim, T. C., McLean, S. P., Lee, J. L., Naranjo, M. S., & Grant A. (1990). Functional laryngeal obstruction: A somatization disorder. *American Journal of Medicine, 88,* 293–295.

Singer, R. N. (1980). *Motor learning and human performance: An application to motor skills and movement behaviors.* New York: Macmillan.

Skinner, D. W., & Bradley, S. R. (1989). Psychogenic stridor. *Journal of Laryngology and Otology, 103,* 383–385.

Smith, M. E., Perez-Darby, K., Kirchner, K., & Blager, F. B. (1993). Simultaneous functional laryngeal stridor and functional dysphonia in an adolescent. *American Journal of Otology, 14,* 366–369.

Sokol, W. (1993). Vocal cord dysfunction presenting as asthma. *Western Journal of Medicine, 158,* 614–615.

Spiegel, J. R., Creed, J. N., & Emerich, K. A. (1998). *The use of facial-flex as an adjunct to speech therapy in treatment of voice disorders.* Retrieved September 17, 2003, from http://www.facialconcepts. com/index.htm

Starkman, M. N., & Appelblatt, N. H. (1984). Functional upper airway obstruction: A possible somatization disorder. *Psychosomatics, 24,* 327–333.

Storr, J., Tranter, R., & Lenney, W. (1988). Stridor in childhood asthma. *British Journal of Diseases of the Chest, 88,* 197–199.

Treole, K., & Trudeau, M. (1996, November). *Paradoxical vocal cord dysfunction.* Paper presented at the annual conference of the American Speech-Language-Hearing Association, Boston, MA.

Trudeau, M. D. (1998). Paradoxical vocal cord dysfunction among juveniles. *Voice and Voice Disorders* [Social Interest Division 3, newsletter], *8*(1), 11–13.

Vachon, L. (1990). Respiratory disorders. In H. J. Kaplan & B. J. Sadock (Eds.), *Comprehensive textbook of psychiatry* (5th ed., pp. 1197–1208). Baltimore: Williams & Wilkins.

Wood, R. P., II, Jafek, B. W., & Cherniak, R. M. (1986). Laryngeal dysfunction and pulmonary disorder. *Archives of Otolaryngology—Head & Neck Surgery, 94,* 374–378.

Chapter 8

Dysphonia Due to Parkinson's Disease

Pharmacological, Surgical, and Behavioral Management Perspectives

Mitchell F. Brin, Miodrag Velickovic,
Lorraine Olson Ramig, and Cynthia Fox

Brin, Velickovic, Ramig, and Fox collectively define Parkinson's disease as a degenerative condition affecting the basal ganglia. It is associated with a myriad of symptoms that involve sensory, musculoskeletal, and autonomic systems, along with emotional effects, such as depression. The symptoms associated with Parkinson's disease vary with the severity of the disease or the stage of the disease process. This chapter provides an overview of the general considerations of Parkinson's disease and a detailed review of the use of pharmocotherapy options, surgical treatments, and behavioral treatments for reducing symptoms.

1. *List at least four of the diagnostic criteria that must exist in order to classify a patient as having idiopathic parkinsonism.*

2. *What is the relationship between degree of voice and articulatory symptoms and stage of the disease?*

3. *What was the justification for using surgical techniques to relieve parkinsonian symptoms? Have they been successful? Why or why not? What are the primary side effects of pallidotomy, if any?*

4. *What are the five essential concepts of the* Lee Silverman Voice Treatment *program?*

Parkinson's disease is a neurological syndrome with the following cardinal features: bradykinesia, postural instability, rigidity, rest tremor, and freezing (motor blocks; Fahn 1986, 1989). At least two of these five cardinal features should be present, with one of them being either tremor or rigidity. Parkinsonism, as a syndrome, can be caused by idiopathic Parkinson's disease (PD), secondary (symptomatic) PD that can be traced to a known and identifiable cause, or parkinsonism plus syndromes (symptoms of parkinsonism are caused by a known gene defect or have a distinctive pathology; see Table 8.1). The specific diagnosis depends on details of the clinical history, the neurological examination, and laboratory tests. No single feature is completely reliable for differentiating among the different causes of parkinsonism.

Idiopathic PD is the most common type of parkinsonism encountered by the neurologist. Pathologically, PD affects many structures in the central nervous system, with preferential involvement of dopaminergic neurons in the substantia nigra pars compacta (SNpc). Lewy bodies, eosinophilic intracytoplasmatic inclusions, can be found in these neurons. Alpha-synuclein is the primary component of lewy body fibrils (Galvin, Lee, & Trojanowski, 2001). However, only about 75% of patients who are clinically diagnosed with PD have pathological central nervous system changes characteristic of PD at autopsy (A. J. Hughes, Daniel, Kilford, & Lees, 1992; Rajput, Rozdilsky, & Rajput, 1991). Several diagnostic criteria have been proposed for the diagnosis of idiopathic PD. In a recent review by Gelb, Oliver, and Gilman (1999), the presence of the following clinical features was noted: resting tremor, bradykinesia, rigidity, and asymmetric onset. The authors also listed criteria that would weigh against such a diagnosis:

1. prominent postural instability, freezing phenomena, and hallucinations in the first 3 years of the disease;
2. dementia preceding motor symptoms or starting in the first year of the disease;
3. supranuclear gaze palsy or slowing of vertical saccades;
4. severe dysautonomia unrelated to medications;
5. a condition known to produce parkinsonism; or
6. neuroleptic use within the past 6 months.

Table 8.1

Classification of Parkinsonism

I. Idiopathic Parkinson's disease

II. Secondary (symptomatic)

  1. Drug-induced

  2. Head trauma

  3. Hemiatrophy–hemiparkinsonism

  4. Hydrocephalus

  5. Hypoxia

  6. Infectious; postencephalitic

  7. Metabolic

  8. Paraneoplastic syndrome

  9. Psychogenic

  10. Syringomesencephalitis

  11. Toxins

  12. Trauma

  13. Tumor

  14. Vascular

III. Parkinsonism plus syndromes

  1. Corticobasalganglionic degeneration (CBGD)

  2. Dementia syndromes

  3. Lytico-Bodig (Guamanian Parkinson's disease, amyotrophic lateral sclerosis)

  4. Motor neuron disease/parkinsonism

  5. Multiple system atrophy

    a) Striatonigral degeneration

    b) Shy-Drager syndrome

    c) Olivopontocerebellar degeneration

  6. Progressive pallidal atrophy

  7. Progressive supranuclear palsy

  8. Other hereditary degenerative disorders

    a) Chorea–acanthocytosis

    b) Familial olivopontocerebellar atrophy

    c) Hallervorden syndrome

    d) Huntington's Chorea

    e) Lubag (X-linked dystonia–parkinsonism)

    f) Mitochondrial disorders

    g) Wilson's disease

Different combinations of these features are required for diagnosis of possible or probable PD. Definite diagnosis, according to this review, requires pathohistological confirmation. Resting tremor and responsiveness of PD symptoms to levodopa, considered by many as highly sensitive for the diagnosis of idiopathic PD, are actually not uncommon in the other types of parkinsonism. For instance, resting tremor was present in 34% of pathologically proven cases of multiple system atrophy (Wenning, Ben Shlomo, Magalhaes, Daniel, & Quinn, 1995) and 17% of progressive supranuclear palsy cases (Collins, Ahlskog, Parisi, & Maraganore, 1995). A response to levodopa was present in 33% to 49% of the patients with pathologically proven parkinsonism plus syndrome (Muller et al., 2001; Wenning et al., 1995). On the other hand, a lack of levodopa responsiveness has been documented in pathologically proven cases of idiopathic PD (Mark, Sage, Dickson, Schwarz, & Duvoisin, 1992). In another clinicopathological study, the presence of at least two of the following four features—autonomic features, early motor fluctuations, poor initial levodopa response, and initial rigidity—were found to have a sensitivity of 87.1% and specificity of 70.5% for the diagnosis of multiple system atrophy (Wenning et al., 2000).

Speech Disorders and Idiopathic PD

The reduced ability to communicate is considered by many patients and their families to be one of the most difficult aspects of PD. Individuals with PD reported significantly less participation in conversations and less confidence in their voice when compared to an age- and gender-matched control group (Fox & Ramig, 1997). Soft voice, monotone, breathy and hoarse voice quality, and imprecise articulation (Darley, Aronson, & Brown, 1975; Logemann, Fisher, Boshes, & Blonsky, 1978; Sapir, Pawlas, Ramig, et al., in press), together with lessened facial expression (masked faces) contribute to limitations in communication in the vast majority of individuals with PD (Pitcairn, Clemie, Gray, & Pentland, 1990a, 1990b). A 1989 study by the Parkinson Study Group indicated that in the early stages of PD, 2% of the patients reported their speech to be the most troublesome aspect of their disease. During the course of the disease, between 45% and 89% of patients will report speech problems (Hartelius & Svensson, 1994; Logemann & Fisher, 1981; Mutch, Strudwick, & Roy, 1986; Sapir, Paulas, Ramig, et al., in press). Hypokinetic dysarthria (Darley et al., 1975), repetitive speech phenomena (Benke, Hohenstein, Poewe, & Butterworth, 2000), and voice tremor (Stewart et al., 1995) can be encountered in individuals with idiopathic PD. Hyperkinetic dysarthria, also reported to occur in idiopathic PD, (Critchley, 1981), is most frequently seen with other motor complications of prolonged levodopa therapy (Critchley, 1976). However, hypokinetic dysarthria, characterized by monotonous and reduced pitch and volume, variable rate, short rushes of speech, imprecise consonants, and a breathy and harsh voice (Darley et al., 1975) is most commonly seen. Logemann et al. (1978) suggested that the speech symptoms they observed in 200 individuals with Parkinson's disease represented a progression in dysfunction, beginning with disordered phonation in recently diagnosed patients and gradually extending to include disordered articulation and other aspects of speech in more advanced patients. Recent findings by Sapir, Pawlas, Seeley, Fox, and Corboy (in press) are consistent with this suggestion. Sapir, Paulas, Seeley, et al. observed primarily voice disorders in individuals with recent onset of PD and low *Unified Parkinson's Disease Rating Scale* (UPDRS; Fahn, Marsden, Colne, & Goldstein, 1987) scores; in individuals with longer duration of disease and higher UPDRS scores, they observed a significantly higher incidence of abnormal articulation and fluency in addition to the disordered voice. In another study of 83 pathologically proven cases of idiopathic PD and parkinsonism plus syndromes, dysarthria was never reported within the first year of the onset of symptoms in idiopathic PD cases (Muller et al., 2001).

Hypokinetic dysarthria of parkinsonism is considered to be a part of basal ganglia damage (Darley et al., 1975); however, no studies have been conducted on pathological changes in hypokinetic dysarthria of idiopathic PD. A significant correlation between neuronal loss and gliosis in SNpc and substantia nigra pars reticulata (SNpr) and severity of hypokinetic dysarthria was found in patients with progressive supranuclear palsy (Kluin et al., 2001). The pathological correlates of repetitive speech phenomena and voice tremor are not known.

Certain aspects of hypokinetic dysarthria in idiopathic PD have been studied extensively. The common report of reduced volume has been supported by the finding that individuals with PD had statistically significantly lower vocal sound pressure levels (2.0–4.0 dB; 30 cm) during speech and voice tasks than an age-matched healthy control group (Fox & Ramig, 1997). Lack of vocal fold closure, including bowing of the vocal cords as well as anterior and posterior chinks (Hanson, Ludlow, & Bassich, 1983; Smith, Ramig, Dromey, Perez, & Samandari, 1995), decreased firing rate and amplitude of muscle fibers of the thyroarytenoid (TA) muscle (Baker, Ramig, Luschei, & Smith, 1998; Luschei, Ramig, Baker, & Smith, 1999), and misperception of voice volume (Ho, Bradshaw, & Iansek, 2000; Ramig, Countryman, Thompson, & Horii, 1995) have been implicated as a cause of reduced volume seen in individuals with idiopathic PD. Videostroboscopic observations have been used to study vocal fold vibration in individuals with idiopathic PD. In individuals with idiopathic PD, altered speech rate and longer and more frequent speech pauses, compared to controls (Hammen & Yorkston, 1996; Solomon & Hixon, 1993), might be due to decreased vital capacity, forced vital capacity, and oral pressure (Solomon & Hixon, 1993; Tamaki, Matsuo, Yanagihara, & Abe, 2000). Speech and voice characteristics may differ in persons with idiopathic PD compared to persons with parkinsonism plus syndromes (e.g., Shy-Drager syndrome, progressive supranuclear palsy, and multiple system atrophy). In addition to the classic hypokinetic symptoms, these patients may have more slurring, strained/strangled voice, palilalia, and hypernasality (Countryman, Ramig, & Pawlas, 1994; Hanson et al., 1983), and the progression of their symptoms may be more rapid.

Medical Treatment

Introduction of a few new dopaminergic agents, catechol-O-methyl transferase inhibitors, and novel surgical techniques have significantly increased the ability to control symptoms of idiopathic PD. Reviews and algorithms of different treatment strategies have been published recently (Olanow & Koller, 1998; Schapira, Obeso, & Olanow, 2000). This chapter will review pharmacotherapy and surgical treatments and their impact on speech and voice disorders. Perspectives regarding behavioral treatment (speech and voice therapy) are also presented.

Pharmacotherapy

In the absence of medications that are undisputedly proven to be neuroprotective, when to start pharmacotherapy remains an unresolved issue. Most movement disorders specialists agree that treatment should be initiated when a patient begins to experience a functional impairment (Olanow & Koller, 1998).

Levodopa. Levodopa is the most effective drug for the treatment of many symptoms of idiopathic PD (Koller & Hubble, 1990). As previously mentioned, patients with pathologically proven idiopathic PD that have a poor response to levodopa are rare (Mark et al., 1992). However, because of concerns of potential neurotoxicity, many choose to postpone treatment (Naudin, Bonnet, & Costentin, 1995; Smith et al., 1995). Potential neurotoxicity has never been proven in animal models or humans, and studies now in progress on the effects of levodopa on disease progression will provide us with more information (Agid et al., 1999).

The pathways of metabolism for levodopa and dopamine provide the framework for current levodopa-related therapy. Levodopa is absorbed in the small intestine via the large neutral amino acid transporter, thus competing with other amino acids for transport (Hardie, Malcolm, Lees, Stern, & Allen, 1986). It is rapidly distributed throughout the tissues and absorbed into the central nervous system via the same transporter (Nutt, Woodward, Hammerstad, Carter, & Anderson, 1984); dietary protein may therefore influence eventual levodopa response at either the gut or central nervous system level (Kempster & Wahlqvist, 1994).

Peripherally, levodopa is rapidly metabolized by aromatic amino acid decarboxylase and catechol-O-methyl transferase, reducing the availability of levodopa to the central nervous system. Levodopa is administered in combination with a decarboxylase inhibitor to prevent a peripheral conversion to dopamine. Insufficient decarboxylase inhibition leads to excessive conversion to dopamine, with resultant nausea, vomiting, and hypotension. In the

United States, the decarboxylase inhibitor carbidopa is combined with levodopa (Sinemet™). In Europe, the decarboxylase inhibitor benserazide is combined with levodopa (Madopar™).

The exact mechanism of action of levodopa is not known. The current hypothesis is that dopaminergic cells in the SNpc take up levodopa, convert it to dopamine, and release it to bind with post-synaptic D1 and D2 receptors. According to this hypothesis, as the number of dopaminergic cells decreases (with the progression of the disease), there should be a continuous loss of levodopa efficacy; however, such a reaction has not been observed. This suggests that there are alternative sites for exogenous levodopa decarboxilation (Koller, 2000).

The effects of levodopa on speech in idiopathic PD have been studied almost since the introduction of levodopa therapy. Improvement in speech production (Bejjani et al., 2000; Fetoni et al., 1997; Nakano, Zubick, & Tyler, 1973; Rigrodsky & Morrison, 1970) and volume (Mawdsley & Gamsu, 1971) in individuals with PD who were taking levodopa has been reported during "on" periods (periods in which the patients responded to levodopa). Levodopa decreases labial bradykinesia (Nakano et al., 1973) and labial and laryngeal rigidity (Jiang, Lin, Wang, & Hanson, 1999; Leanderson, Meyerson, & Persson, 1971) and increases lip pressures during on periods (Cahill et al., 1998). On the other hand, some studies have shown no subjective improvement of speech after taking levodopa (in the on state) in individuals with idiopathic PD compared to their off periods (Klawans, 1986; Quaglieri & Celesia, 1977). This has been supported by findings of unchanged breathing pattern (Solomon & Hixon, 1993), acoustic measures of vowels (Poluha, Teulings, & Brookshire, 1998), and vocal cord movements (K. K. Larson, Ramig, & Scherer, 1994) measured across the levodopa drug cycle.

Dopamine Agonists. Dopamine agonists directly stimulate dopaminergic receptors, but unlike levodopa, they do not require neuronal transformation in order to be effective. They offer the benefit of dopaminergic action without requiring viable dopamine-releasing cells. The half-life of most of the dopamine agonists is longer than for immediate-release levodopa formulations. The individual dose thus can provide more sustained stimulation of dopamine receptors, which potentially can protect against complications of long-term levodopa therapy, such as fluctuations in motor performance or abnormal movements (Olanow, Schapira, & Rascol, 2000; Rascol et al., 2000). By substituting for endogenous or exogenous dopamine sources, dopamine agonists may reduce the generation of free radicals, thereby potentially exerting a neuroprotective effect (Montastruc, Rascol, & Senard, 1993). In contrast to levodopa, they do not compete with circulating amino acids for absorption or transport into the brain. In spite of these putative advantages, the current dopamine agonists have not proved to be as clinically effective as levodopa. Side effects, which are similar for all agonists, include dose-related confusion, hallucinations, nausea, and orthostatic hypotension (Ramaker, van de Beek, Finken, & van Hilten, 2000; Rascol et al., 2000).

In the United States, bromocriptine, pergolide, cabergoline, pramipexole, and ropinirole are available. Lisuride and apomorphine are available in most European countries. Pramipexole, ropinirole, and apomorphine are non-ergot–derived dopamine receptor agonists.

Apomorphine was first described as an antiparkinsonian drug in 1951 (Schwab, Amador, & Lettvin, 1951). Its effects are predominantly through the D_2, D_3, and D_4 receptors and, to a lesser extent, the D_1 and D_5 receptors. After subcutaneous injection, peak plasma concentrations are reached within a few minutes, and the half-life is approximately 30 minutes (Corboy, Wagner, & Sage, 1995). Besides subcutaneous administration, rectal, sublingual, and intranasal routes may be used. Continuous infusion via a minipump is also possible. Coadministration with the antiemetic domperidone is often necessary. In a randomized, double-blind, placebo-controlled study, apomorphine fail to improve articulation and laryngeal function in individuals with idiopathic PD (Kompoliti, Wang, Goetz, Leurgans, & Raman, 2000). However, apomorphine has been shown to have some effect, predominantly on the oral phase of swallowing, in individuals with idiopathic PD and swallowing difficulty (Hunter, Crameri, Austin, Woodward, & Hughes, 1997).

Bromocriptine stimulates the D_2, D_3, D_4, and D_5 receptors and inhibits the D_1 receptors. It has been shown to be effective monotherapy in early idiopathic PD (Ramaker et al., 2000). Like all dopamine agonists, it is less effective than levodopa against parkinsonian symptoms. As a result, only about 30% of patients can be treated with bromocriptine monotherapy for more than 3 years (Ramaker et al., 2000). As monotherapy, bromocriptine is usually dosed at 20 to 40 mg per day; slightly smaller doses are given as an adjunct to levodopa therapy. The effects last from 1 hour to 6 hours. The issue of its effect on chronic nonfluent aphasia remains controversial (Bragoni et al., 2000; Gupta, Mlcoch, Scolaro, & Moritz, 1995; Sabe, Salvarezza, Garcia, Leiguarda, & Starkstein, 1995). There are no studies of its effects on speech impairment in idiopathic PD.

Lisuride is an ergot derivate that stimulates both D_1 and D_2 receptors. It improves parkinsonian symptoms and reduces motor fluctuations when used as an adjunct to levodopa in late-stage PD (Rinne, 1989). Unlike the other dopamine agonists, lisuride is water soluble and may be administered parenterally or even continuously infused via a minipump, although this approach may cause a higher degree of psychosis (Vaamonde, Luquin, & Obeso, 1991). As an oral medication, its duration of action is relatively short (1 hour–3 hours). There are no controlled studies of its effect on speech in individuals with idiopathic PD (Jellinger, 1987).

Pergolide is an ergot-derived dopaminergic agonist that stimulates the D_1, D_2, D_3, D_4, and D_5 receptors. Pergolide has been shown to reduce motor fluctuations by 30% or more and to reduce by 25% the amount of levodopa required for disease management (Langtry & Clissold, 1990; Markham & Benfield, 1997). In a single-blind crossover comparison of pergolide and bromocriptine, pergolide was found to be slightly more effective and better tolerated (Pezzoli et al., 1995). The duration of its effect is 2 to 8 hours. Pergolide may reduce dopamine turnover and have important effects on free radical–scavenging enzymes, thus providing a theoretical basis for early management with this agent (Felten, Felten, Steece-Collier, Date, & Clemens, 1992; Glover, Clow, & Sandler, 1993). There are no studies of its effect on speech in idiopathic PD.

Cabergoline is another ergot-derived dopaminergic agonist. It stimulates the D_2 receptors. Of the dopaminergic agents, it has the longest half-life (approximately 60 hours). Theoretically, this would provide a sustained stimulation of dopamine receptors and protect against motor fluctuations (Olanow et al., 2000). Treatment of early idiopathic PD can reduce the relative risk of motor complications by 50% when compared to treatment with levodopa only (Rinne, Bracco, et al., 1998), and reduce by 18% the amount of levodopa required for disease management in patients that already have developed dyskinesia (Hutton et al., 1996). There are no studies on its effect on speech in individuals with idiopathic PD.

Two non–ergot-derived agents—ropinirole and pramipexole—stimulate the D_2, D_3, and D_4 dopamine receptors. In addition, pramipexole also stimulates alpha$_1$ and alpha$_2$ adrenergic receptors. Recent studies have shown that ropinirole reduces the incidence of dyskinesia (Rascol et al., 2000); in a similar manner, pramipexole reduces the incidence of dyskinesia, wearing-off phenomena, and on-off motor fluctuations (Parkinson Study Group, 2000) in patients with idiopathic PD, compared to the patients treated with levodopa. An initial report by Frucht, Rogers, Greene, Gordon, and Fahn (1999) related these agents to "sleep attacks." However, subsequent reports and studies found that excessive daytime sleepiness occurs with the use of levodopa and other dopaminergic agents (Pal, Bhattacharya, Agapito, & Chaudhuri, 2001; Schapira, 2000) and is usually worse in advanced stages of idiopathic PD (Factor, McAlarney, Sanchez-Ramos, & Weiner, 1990). The effect of these two medications on speech in individuals with idiopathic PD has not been extensively studied.

MAO-B Inhibitors. Dopamine is metabolized to 3,4-dihydroxy-phenylacetic acid by monoamine oxidase B (MAO-B). MAO-B inhibitors, therefore, can enhance the effects of dopamine (and levodopa) by blocking its degradation. The principal MAO-B inhibitor that is important in the treatment of PD is selegiline.

Selegiline is commonly used as early monotherapy or in combination with levodopa. Its mild efficacy in monotherapy was demonstrated in a large, multicenter study known as DATATOP (Parkinson Study Group, 1989). This and other studies have demonstrated the ability of selegiline to postpone levodopa therapy for perhaps 9 months or more (Allain, Pollak, & Neukirch, 1993; Myllyla, Sotaniemi, Vuorinen, & Heinonen, 1993). However, controversy exists regarding the mechanism of this effect. Early researchers hypothesized that selegiline exerted a neuroprotective effect by blocking degradation and subsequent free radical formation, thus prolonging the life of the degenerating nigral cells and postponing the onset of parkinsonian symptoms. Selegiline also has mild, clear symptomatic effects, possibly because of its ability to block dopamine degradation and reuptake (Engberg, Elebring, & Nissbrandt, 1991; Yang & Neff, 1974) or through its metabolism to methamphetamine (Reynolds et al., 1978). Some researchers have interpreted the results of the DATATOP and later studies as indicating symptomatic improvement rather than neuroprotection (Schulzer, Mak, & Calne, 1992), a conclusion supported by follow-up studies showing no statistical difference in therapy needs 3 years after treatment with selegiline versus a placebo (Olanow & Calne, 1992). As a levodopa adjunct in late PD, selegiline has been shown to improve motor fluctuations in one half to two thirds of patients (Birkmayer, Riederer, Youdim, & Linauer, 1975; Golbe et al., 1988; Rinne, Siirtola, & Sonninen, 1978).

The absence of serious side effects in selegiline therapy, combined with its as yet unproven potential as a neuroprotective agent, has led many clinicians to prescribe it at the time of diagnosis (Mytilineou et al., 1998; Mytilineou, Radcliffe, & Olanow, 1997). The standard dose of selegiline is 10 mg per day. Levodopa side effects may be enhanced by selegiline, and its use often requires a decrease in the levodopa dose in patients experiencing peak dose dyskinesias.

The effects of selegiline on speech in individuals with idiopathic PD have not been extensively studied. Combined with levodopa, it has improved certain aspects of articulation and respiration (Shea, Drummond, Metzer, & Krueger, 1993), but it had almost no effect on speech in individuals with idiopathic PD when given alone (Stewart et al., 1995).

Anticholinergics. Anticholinergics are used primarily in de novo patients for whom tremor is the predominant complaint. Anticholinergic therapy may have a mild effect on rigidity and tremor, but it has little effect on akinesia (Quinn, 1984). Because of the propensity to induce confusion (Dubois et al., 1987), use of anticholinergics in elderly patients is not recommended and is contraindicated in patients with dementia. Side effects include constipation, blurred vision, dizziness, and nausea. Another side effect, dry mouth, may actually be welcomed by the patient for whom sialorrhea may be an unpleasant symptom of the disease. Dosing for trihexyphenidyl, the most widely used anticholinergic, is begun at 0.5 to 1.0 mg twice daily and gradually increased to 2 to 3 mg three times daily. Other anticholinergics include benztropine, biperiden, orphenadrine, parsitan, and procyclidine. Their effect on speech in individuals with idiopathic PD has not been studied.

Amantadine. Amantadine is effective against akinesia, rigidity, and to some extent, tremor (Koller, 1986; Mann, Pearce, & Waterbury, 1971; Parkes, Baxter, Marsden, & Rees, 1974). Its mechanism of action is unknown, although it has been shown to have N-methyl-D-aspartate–antagonist properties and anticholinergic properties and to promote the release of stored dopamine in nerve terminals (Kornhuber & Weller, 1993). Because of its NMDA antagonism, amantadine and similar compounds are being explored for their potential neuroprotective effect (Montastruc, Rascol, & Senard, 1997). Amantadine may be started as monotherapy in individuals with PD with mild impairment. Dosage is 100 to 300 mg daily for younger patients. Lower doses, in the form of an elixir, are given to older patients. There are no reports of its effect on speech in individuals with idiopathic PD.

Catechol-O-Methyltransferase (COMT) inhibitors. In the United States, two COMT inhibitors are available for the treatment of idiopathic PD—entacapone (Omtan) and tolcapone (Tasmar). Both of them are reversible inhibitors of the COMT enzyme. They are effective only if given with levodopa. COMT converts levodopa to 3-O-methyldopa (3-OMD), and this is one of the major degradation pathways, particularly after inhibition of Aromatic-L-amino acid decarboxylase by carbidopa or benserazide. 3-OMD cannot be metabolized to dopamine. Entacapone is only a peripheral COMT inhibitor, whereas tolcapone inhibits COMT both peripherally and centrally. However, when given without levodopa, tolcapone—at a dose of 200 mg—had no effects in patients with idiopathic PD (Hauser, Molho, Shale, Pedder, & Dorflinger, 1998). It is conceivable that the central effect of tolcapone is minimal at this dose. Studies have shown an increase in on time by 5% to 15%, a decrease in off time by 10% to 22%, and a decrease in levodopa dose by 12% to 29% when a COMT inhibitor combined with levodopa was compared to a placebo combined with levodopa (Adler et al., 1998; Baas et al.,

1997; Kurth et al., 1997; Parkinson Study Group, 1997; Rinne, Larsen, Siden, & Worm-Petersen, 1998). Three cases of acute liver failure were associated with the use of tolcapone (Olanow, 2000). As a result, special monitoring guidelines were issued in the United States, and tolcapone was withdrawn from the European market. No studies on the effects of COMT inhibitors on speech in idiopathic PD have been published.

Other Medications. Clonazepam, a benzodiazepine, has been shown to improve hypokinetic dysarthria in 10 of 11 individuals with idiopathic PD (Biary, Pimental, & Langenberg, 1988). The effective dose was between 0.25 mg and 0.5 mg per day. In a single case report, both setline and transcranial magnetic stimulation were found to be effective for the treatment of dysarthria in juvenile onset of Parkinson's disease (Sandyk, 1997).

Summary. It seems that pharmacotherapy does not have a major impact on speech impairment in idiopathic PD. Even though there are no studies on the effects of dopamine agonists on speech impairment, it is conceivable that they are not nearly as effective as levodopa, considering their lesser potency to improve motor symptoms. It is possible that nondopaminergic pathways that are affected in idiopathic PD are responsible for speech impairment (Sapir, Pawlas, Ramig, et al., in press). This hypothesis would also explain the fact that the prevalence of dyskinesia affecting the limbs in idiopathic PD is close to 40% with levodopa therapy, whereas there are only a few reports of dyskinetic or hyperkinetic speech as a consequence of levodopa treatment (Critchley, 1981). It may also explain the nearly identical prevalence of voice and articulation abnormalities in medicated (85.7%; Sapir, Pawlas, Ramig, et al., in press) and unmedicated (89%; Logemann et al., 1978) individuals with PD.

Surgical Treatments

Initial surgical techniques for idiopathic PD were aimed at the pyramidal tract, with the belief that induction of paresis would decrease tremor, bradykinesia, and rigidity (Bucy, 1948; Oliver, 1949; Putnam, 1938, 1940; Walker, 1952). The basal ganglia was first tar-

geted in the 1940s by R. Meyers (1940, 1942). Introduction of stereo-
taxic neurosurgery (Spiegel, Wycis, Marks, & Lee, 1946) improved
the accuracy of electrode or probe placement, because the brain
atlas and brain imaging (ventriculography) could be used. Isolated
lesions of either the globus pallidus (pallidotomy; Cooper, 1954;
Cooper & Bravo, 1958) or thalamus (thalamotomy; Stellar & Cooper,
1968) were commonly performed at that time. Because adequate
pharmacotherapy was not available until the late 1960s, surgical
procedures were aimed mostly at relieving one of three symptoms
of idiopathic PD: rigidity, bradykinesia, or tremor. Surgical therapy
reemerged in the late 1980s. This time it was aimed at patients who
were failing medical therapy and who developed motor complications, specifically dyskinesia. Today the targets for surgical intervention are the thalamus, globus pallidus pars interna (GPi), and
subthalamic nucleus. In addition to higher accuracy of the electrode or probe placement (± 1 mm) due to the development of new
imaging techniques (computerized tomography and magnetic
resonance imaging), new forms of surgical treatment were introduced: deep brain stimulation and transplant surgery.

Thalamic Procedures. Thalamic procedures—thalamotomy and deep
brain stimulation of the thalamus—are effective in tremor control
and therefore are indicated mostly in tremor-dominant forms of
idiopathic PD. However, newer procedures, such as deep brain
scan of the subthalamic nucleus, might be as effective as thalamic
procedures in reducing tremor. Nucleus ventralis intermedius
(VIM) is the target area for thalamic procedures. Even though it is
not anatomically clearly delimited, this area can be recognized
through neurophysiological methods (microelectrode recording or
stimulation).

The exact mechanism of action of thalamotomy is not known,
but the assumption is that destruction of "tremorogenic" neurons
(Hayase, Miyashita, Endo, & Narabayashi, 1998; Lenz et al., 1995) is
effective in the treatment of tremor. The other possibility is that by
damaging the nucleus ventralis intermedius, the circuit of globus
pallidus to the VIM, cerebellum to the VIM, and the VIM to the motor cortex is disrupted. Even if tremorogenic neurons were not (or
not entirely) located in the VIM, the destruction of the VIM would

halt the impulse transmission through it to the motor system, and therefore the tremor.

In idiopathic PD, thalamotomy appears to have a long-lasting effect on tremor on the side contralateral to the thalamotomy side (Jankovic, Cardoso, Grossman, & Hamilton, 1995; Nagaseki et al., 1986). However, there are almost no effects on other parkinsonian symptoms on the contralateral side (especially bradykinesia) or to tremor and other parkinsonian symptoms on the ipsilateral side of the thalamotomy (Diederich et al., 1992; Moriyama, Beck, & Miyamoto, 1999; Young et al., 2000). After thalamotomy, both reduction in the dose of levodopa (Moriyama et al., 1999) and no change in its dose (R. C. Hughes, Polgar, Weightman, & Walton, 1971) have been reported.

Dysarthria has been reported after thalamotomy (Matsumoto, Shichijo, & Fukami, 1984; Nagaseki et al., 1986; Quaglieri & Celesia, 1977; Tasker, Siqueira, Hawrylyshyn, & Organ, 1983). Bilateral thalamotomy is even more likely to produce dysarthria (Tasker et al.) or to decrease the fluency and speech volume (45% of patients; Matsumoto et al.).

Thalamic stimulation is a deep brain scan intervention. It uses a deep brain scan lead, which on the intracranial end has four platinum–iridium contacts that are 1.5 mm in length and are separated by 1.5 mm. The other end is connected to an implantable pulse generator that is usually surgically placed under the skin of the chest wall. Any one of the contacts, or any combination of them, can be used for stimulation. Pulse width, amplitude, stimulation frequency, and the number and polarity of active contacts are parameters that can be adjusted. The patient can turn the stimulator on or off by using a handheld magnet. The target is the VIM, the nucleus targeted in thalamotomy. The mechanism of action of stimulation of the thalamus in idiopathic PD is not known, but there are a few theories. First, thalamic neurons could be depolarized by stimulation so that they cannot transfer impulses. Second, the neural circuits may be disrupted by stimulation ("neural jamming"). Third, stimulation might activate inhibitory neurons, with a consequent decrease in thalamic activity (Benazzouz & Hallett, 2000).

Thalamic stimulation has effects on tremor similar to those of thalamotomy and a similar lack of effects on other parkinsonian symptoms. Like thalamotomy, thalamic stimulation can have adverse effects and cause dysarthria (Benabid et al., 1996; Koller et al., 1997; Ondo, Jankovic, Schwartz, Almaguer, & Simpson, 1998; Schuurman et al., 2000). However, these usually can be abolished by changing the stimulation parameters. Recently, a cardioversion causing thalamotomy in a patient with thalamic stimulator was reported (Yamamoto et al., 2000). The advantages of thalamic stimulation over thalamotomy are lack of tissue destruction (reversibility of the effects) and minimization of the side effects through adjustment of the stimulation parameters. The cost of the device, battery replacement (every 3 to 5 years), risk of infection, and equipment failure are disadvantages. A randomized comparison of continuous stimulation and thalamotomy for the suppression of tremor found no statistical differences between these two methods; however, thalamic stimulation had a lower incidence of side effects (Schuurman et al., 2000).

Pallidal Procedures. Pallidal procedures—pallidotomy and deep brain scan of the globus pallidus—are indicated for patients who have idiopathic PD, are responsive to levodopa, and have levodopa-induced dyskinesias. These procedures are not recommended for patients who have cognitive problems or other forms of parkinsonism.

The medial and ventral parts of the internal globus pallidus have been shown to project through the thalamus to the primary motor cortex and premotor areas (Middleton & Strick, 2000). In the primate model of parkinsonism, the internal globus pallidus is overactive (DeLong, 1990), which leads to inhibition of the motor nuclei in the thalamus and brain stem, resulting in hypokinesia (bradykinesia). According to the same model, dyskinesia seen after long-term levodopa therapy might be a consequence of a decreased firing rate of the internal globus pallidus neurons (Hamada & DeLong, 1992). Therefore, destruction of this structure during pallidotomy accounts for improvement of rigidity, bradykinesia, tremor, and dyskinesia contralateral to the site of the surgical procedure (Fine et al., 2000; Herrera et al., 2000; Schrag et al., 1999). Unilateral pallidotomy can improve UPDRS motor scores by approximately 25% in the off state and activities of daily living scores by 20% in both off and on states (Baron et al., 2000; Fine et al., 2000). However, pallidotomy can also cause dysarthria or worsen hypophonia (Herrera et al., 2000; Schrag et al., 1999). Bilateral pallidotomy, even though effective for dyskinesia, can cause even more significant speech difficulty (Favre, Burchiel, Taha, & Hammerstad, 2000). Similar are the effects of staged (not contemporaneous) bilateral pallidotomy (Intemann et al., 2001). Vocal intensity might improve after unilateral pallidotomy in patients who had mild dysarthria preoperatively (Schulz, Greer, & Friedman, 2000).

Unilateral stimulation of the internal globus pallidus produces similar effects on parkinsonian symptoms and activities of daily living as pallidotomy, and these two procedures also had a comparable side effect profile (Merello et al., 1999). Unilateral and bilateral pallidus stimulation improves UPDRS motor scores and activities of daily living scores in both the off and on states (Gross et al., 1997; Krack et al., 1998; Kumar et al., 2000; Pahwa et al., 1997; Volkmann et al., 2001). Reduction of dyskinesia with stimulation, either off or on, has also been significant (Gross et al., 1997; Kumar et al., 2000; Volkmann et al., 2001). Positioning of the electrode might have an impact on the effects of stimulation. Improvement in gait, bradykinesia, and rigidity, but induction of dyskinesia even in an off state, can be seen with stimulation of the dorsal parts of the globus pallidus (Bejjani et al., 1997; Yelnik et al., 2000). Similar to stimulation of the dorsal part, stimulation of the posteroventral part of the globus pallidus worsened gait and bradykinesia but improved rigidity and levodopa-induced dyskinesia (Bejjani et al., 1997, Yelnik et al., 2000). Stimulation of the globus pallidus pars externa improved speech and facial expressions but was more likely to also induce dyskinesia (dystonia/choreoathetosis) in the rest of the body (Yelnik et al., 2000). Some of the side effects of pallidal stimulation, including dysarthria, are probably due to stimulation of the internal capsule, and they disappear with the adjustment of the stimulation parameters (Kumar et al., 2000). There are no studies that have objectively evaluated the effects of pallidal stimulation on speech and voice in individuals with idiopathic PD.

Compared to pallidotomy, pallidal stimulation has a lower incidence of cognitive and speech problems, especially if the procedure is bilateral. There are, however, a few disadvantages, including the cost of the device, battery replacement (every 3 to 5 years), risk of infection, and equipment failure.

Subthalamic Nucleus Procedures. In the primate model of parkinsonism (DeLong, 1990) the subthalamic nucleus is hyperactive. Inhibition of it by the external globus pallidus is lost, and a hyperactive subthalamic nucleus increases the neuronal activity in the internal globus pallidus and the SNpr. The final result is inhibition of thalamic and brain stem nuclei. The subthalamic nucleus was not considered to be a suitable target for treatment of idiopathic PD for many years. Initial experimental data showed hemiballismus as a consequence of subthalamotomy (subthalamic nucleus lesion; Carpenter, Whittier, & Mettler, 1950; Whittier & Mettler, 1949). However, two recent studies have shown that the procedure is safe and usually is not associated with persistent dyskinesia (Alvarez et al., 2001; Barlas et al., 2001). The procedure was associated with significant improvement in both the activity of daily living and motor scores of the UPDRS, but there were no changes in the daily dose of levodopa or the dyskinesia score (Alvarez et al., 2001). No effects of subthalamotomy on speech were reported.

Deep brain scan of the subthalamic nucleus has been successfully employed in many patients with idiopathic PD (Kumar et al., Limousin et al., 1998; Limousin et al., 1995; 1998; Rodriguez-Oroz et al., 2000). This procedure probably decreases the rate of neuronal firing from the subthalamic nucleus. Without stimulation from the subthalamic nucleus, the neuronal firing rate of the internal globus pallidus also decreases. In turn, the firing rate of the ventrolateral and the ventromedial nuclei of the thalamus increases (Benazzouz & Hallett, 2000). Deep brain scan of the subthalamic nucleus reduces off-state motor scores by 50% to 60%, reduces tremor, reduces the dose of levodopa by 40% to 60%, reduces levodopa-induced dyskinesia, and improves activities of daily living scores (Krack et al., 1998; Limousin et al., 1995). Even though no study has compared the effects of deep brain scan of the internal globus pallidus versus the subthalamic nucleus, there is some evidence that the latter could be potentially better. First, the former is not associated with a significant reduction of the daily levodopa dose, and second, the subthalamic nucleus influences not only internal globus pallidus nuclei but also SNpr and other brain stem nuclei (Benabid et al., 2000; Burchiel, Anderson, Favre, & Hammerstad, 1999; Krause et al.,

2001; Volkmann et al., 2001). Deep brain scan of the internal globus pallidus might be better for patients who develop dyskinesia even on a low daily dose of levodopa.

Transient and chronic dysarthria have been reported in deep brain scan of the subthalamic nucleus (Benabid et al., 2000; Hariz et al., 2000; Krause et al., 2001; Volkmann et al., 2001). On the other hand, improvement in sound pressure levels, fundamental frequency variability in response to stimulation in the medication-on condition (Dromey, Kumar, Lang, & Lozano, 2000), and dynamic and static control of the articulatory organ as measured by ramp- and hold-force contractions of the lips and tongue (Gentil, Garcia-Ruiz, Pollak, & Benabid, 2000) have been reported.

Transplant Procedures. Transplant procedures are based on the idea that implantation of dopamine-producing cells into the basal ganglia may compensate for the deficits caused by dopaminergic neuron loss in the substantia nigra pars compacta. Initial studies were done by transplanting adrenal medullary tissue into the striatum of two individuals with parkinsonism (Backlund et al., 1985). Subsequent studies have not shown a major benefit from this procedure (Goetz et al., 1991), and there are no reports concerning effects of this procedure on speech in individuals with idiopathic PD.

Implantation of fetal ventral mesencephalic cells has also been used in treatment of idiopathic PD. The cells are usually obtained from fetuses at 7 to 9 weeks of gestational age. A major limiting factor is that only 3% to 20% of transplanted cells survive (Brundin et al., 2000). Different strategies—including usage of tissue strands but not suspension of cells (Clarkson, Zawada, Adams, Bell, & Freed, 1998) and tropic factors (Espejo, Cutillas, Arenas, & Ambrosio, 2000)—have been suggested. In an open-labeled study, clinical improvement correlated with survival and function of transplanted fetal tissue (Hauser et al., 1999); however, a double-blind, placebo-controlled study failed to show major improvement in PD symptoms (Freed et al., 2001). In the Freed et al. study, however, the surgical technique used during implantation, the technique of recovering and extruding fragments of fetal tissue from the embryos, and the absence of immunosuppression might have contributed to the poor survival rate of the transplanted dopamine neurons seen in two patients from this study who died. The study also did not evaluate the effects of fetal cell transplant on speech production. A study by Baker, Ramig, Johnson, and Freed (1997) revealed no improvement of speech intelligibility in five patients who received fetal cell transplants. All patients, however, had improvement in motor scores on the UPDRS.

Summary. Surgical procedures are not aimed toward the areas of basal ganglia involved in orofacial control. Destructive procedures and deep brain scan of the thalamus, especially if performed bilaterally, are likely to cause or worsen preexisting speech impairment. Deep brain scan of the internal globus pallidus or the subthalamic nucleus can cause a transient worsening of speech that usually improves with adjustment of the stimulation parameters. However, some aspects of speech production might even be improved by deep brain scan of the subthalamic nucleus.

Summary

Available pharmacotherapies and surgical therapies are not nearly as effective for speech as for limb movements. It is possible that non-dopaminergic pathways affected in idiopathic PD are responsible for speech impairment (Sapir, Pawlas, Seeley, et al., in press) and therefore levodopa and dopaminergic medications have little influence on speech production. Similarly, parts of the basal ganglia involved in speech and orofacial control, such as the external globus pallidus (Yelnik et al., 2000), might not be a target of the surgical procedures currently employed. Further studies of the pathophysiology of speech impairment in idiopathic PD are necessary.

Behavioral and Speech and Voice Treatment for Parkinson's Disease

Because neuropharmocological and neurosurgical treatments do not consistently or significantly improve speech and voice disorders in Parkinson's disease, behavioral treatment is needed. Although there is a high incidence of disordered speech and voice in individuals with idiopathic PD, only 3% to 4% of these individuals receive speech treatment (Hartelius & Svensson, 1994; Mutch et al.,

1986). One explanation for this discrepancy is that physicians may not refer these individuals for speech treatment. A common scenario is that "a soft-speaking, monotone" individual with PD (with reduced awareness of his or her speech or voice problem) arrives at the physician's office. The patient expresses no complaint about speech or voice problems, and because the physician is able to understand the patient easily in a quiet examination room, a referral for speech treatment is not made. At each yearly visit, this scenario is repeated. Many years pass, and the patient's communication abilities continue to decline; he or she reduces activities (talks on the phone less, limits social events, may retire from employment or volunteer activities). By the time the speech disorder is obvious in the physician's quiet examination room, the disorder has had a major negative impact on the patient's quality of life. When the referral for speech treatment is finally made, the treatment may be more challenging and the outcome less positive due to the severity of the speech disorder and the likely progression of other PD symptoms, which may make focusing on speech treatment difficult. Another reason for the discrepancy between the number of individuals with PD needing speech treatment and the number actually referred may be that there has been a question about whether speech treatment for individuals with PD is really effective, because carryover and long-term outcomes have been disappointing in the past. In fact, "conventional wisdom" has been that most of the rehabilitation goals that are achieved do not carry over in day-to-day situations (Allan, 1970; Greene, 1980; Sarno, 1968; Weiner & Lang, 1989).

These challenges of carryover and long-term treatment outcomes have been observed consistently over a wide range of speech treatments that have been applied to this population. These treatment approaches have included a combination of training in rate control, prosody, volume, articulation, and respiration (Yorkston, 1996). In addition, some forms of treatment have included devices such as delayed auditory feedback, amplification devices, and pacing boards (Adams, 1997; Downie, Low, & Lindsay, 1981; Helm, 1979; Ludlow & Bassich, 1983). Certain of these approaches probably are valuable for select patients (e.g., pacing board for cases of palilalia and speech augmentation for certain individuals at later stages of PD, when the ability to control the speech mechanism is severely disordered). In general, however, it has been observed that when individuals with idiopathic PD are in the speech treatment room and receiving direct stimulation or feedback from the speech clinician or an instrument (Adams, 1997; Rubow & Swift, 1985; Scott & Caird, 1983), they are able to improve speech and voice production. Maintaining these improvements (training the ability to internally cue outside of the treatment room) has been a long-term challenge, however, and has made speech treatment outcomes disappointing over the years.

These challenges to treatment success provide potential insight into the underlying basis for the speech problems in most individuals with PD. It has been generally assumed that the disordered speech in idiopathic PD can be explained by select motor symptoms (bradykinesia, hypokinesia, and rigidity). It is becoming apparent, however, that additional factors, including the sensory processing, internal cueing, and impaired movement scaling problems frequently experienced in limb systems (Barbeau, Sourkes, & Murphy, 1962; Berardelli, Dick, Rothwell, Day, & Marsden, 1986; Boecker et al., 1999; R. G. Brown & Marsden, 1988; Contreras-Vidal & Stelmach, 1995; Jobst, Melnick, Byl, Dowling, & Aminoff, 1997; Schneider, Diamond, & Markham, 1986), should be considered when determining the origin and treatment of the speech and voice disorders (Fox, Morrison, Ramig, & Sapir, in press; Sapir, Pawlas, Ramig, et al., in press). In addition, decreased cognitive function (e.g., slow thinking, problems shifting set, problems with procedural memory), which may occur in 40% to 60% of individuals with PD (Mahler & Cummings, 1990), may affect the ability to benefit from treatment (Fox et al., in press).

Intensive Voice Treatment for Parkinson's Disease

Recently, Ramig, Pawlas, and Countryman (1995) developed an approach to the treatment of speech in individuals with PD. Unlike approaches that focus on the motor disorders of rate or articulation, the *Lee Silverman Voice Treatment* (LSVT) focuses on disordered voice—the speech problem observed most often in individuals with PD—and sensory processing—the feedback disorder that appears to limit awareness of the individual with PD of his or her speech disorder (e.g., the person says, "My voice is not too soft, but my spouse needs a hearing aid!" or when the person brings the voice to a normal volume, he or she says, "I can't speak this loud, I feel like I am shouting!").

The idea of training volume and the specific techniques of LSVT bring together clinical concepts from literature in the areas of motor speech (Berry & Sanders, 1983; Duffy, 1995; Froeschels, Kastein, & Weiss, 1955; Hardy, 1967; Rosenbek & LaPointe, 1985; Wertz, 1978; Yorkston, Beukelman, & Bell, 1988) and voice (Aronson, 1990; Boone & McFarlane, 1988; Colton & Casper, 1996; Stemple, 1993). LSVT integrates these concepts and techniques in a manner specifically designed for individuals with PD. In addition, LSVT is administered in a manner consistent with principles of exercise science (A. B. Brown, McCartney, & Sale, 1990; Frontera, Meredith, O'Reilly, Knuttgen, & Evans, 1988), skill acquisition (Verdolini, 1997), and motor learning (Schmidt & Lee, 1999; e.g., high effort, multiple repetitions, intensive, simple), with a focus on sensory awareness. These elements have previously not been systematically combined in a speech treatment program for individuals with PD (Yorkston, 1996; Yorkston et al., 1988), and they are consistent with approaches to facilitate learning in individuals who have the profile of cognitive impairments seen in PD (Fox et al., in press).

Ramig and colleagues hypothesized that there are at least three features underlying the voice disorder in individuals with PD. These features are an overall scale-down of amplitude (Albin, Young, & Penny, 1989; Barbeau et al., 1962; Penny & Young, 1983) to the speech mechanism (reduced amplitude of neural drive to the muscles of the speech mechanism), which may result in a "soft voice that is monotone"; problems in sensory perception of effort (Barbeau et al., 1962; Berardelli et al., 1986), which prevents the individual with PD from accurately monitoring his or her vocal output; and difficulty in independently generating (internal cueing/scaling) the right amount of effort (Demirci, Grill, McShane, & Hallet, 1995; Stelmach, 1991) to produce adequate volume. The combination of reduced amplitude of output, problems in sensory perception of effort, and problems scaling adequate output effort may be significant factors that underlie the speech and voice problems in these individuals and make them particularly resistant to successful treatment. The LSVT, which has been designed to address these problems, is based on five essential concepts:

1. increasing the amplitude of phonatory output,
2. improving sensory perception of effort (i.e., "calibration"),
3. administering treatment in a high-effort style,
4. administering treatment intensively (four times a week for 16 sessions in 1 month), and
5. quantifying all speech and voice output.

Every element of treatment that is delivered is consistent with these five concepts. Treatment techniques are designed to scale up amplitude to the respiratory and phonatory systems and train sensory perception of effort and internal cueing and scaling of adequate output. Administration of treatment four times a week for 1 month is consistent with the principles of motor learning and skill acquisition (Schmidt, 1975, 1988) and muscle training (Astrand & Rodahl, 1970). In addition, the LSVT is administered in a manner to maximize patient compliance by assigning treatment activities that make an immediate impact (after first treatment session) on daily functional communication (see also Figure 8.1).

Treatment Efficacy Data for the LSVT

The LSVT was initially developed during the late 1980s, and initial Phase I studies (e.g., case studies, single-subject designs, non-randomized studies) were published based upon that early work (Ramig, 1992; Ramig, Bonitati, Lemke, & Horii, 1994). These studies documented the first evidence of successful treatment outcomes and suggested that intensive treatment focusing on increasing phonatory effort could improve communication in individuals with PD (see Figure 8.2).

Based upon those findings, a number of Phase II experimental studies (e.g., randomized, blind) were carried out. In one study, 45 individuals with idiopathic PD were randomly assigned to one of two forms of treatment: respiratory treatment or respiratory and voice treatment (LSVT). Short- and long-term (Dromey, Ramig, & Johnson, 1995; Ramig, Countryman, O'Brien, Hoehn, & Thompson,

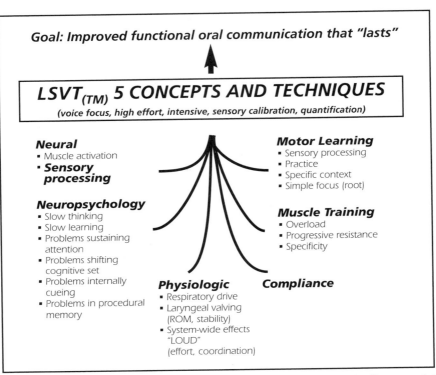

Figure 8.1. Graphical summarization of the rationale underlying the five essential concepts and techniques of the *Lee Silverman Voice Treatment* from neural, speech mechanism physiology, motor learning, muscle training, neuropsychological, and compliance perspectives. *Note.* LSVT = *Lee Silverman Voice Treatment.*

1996; Ramig, Sapir, Countryman, et al., 2001; Ramig, Sapir, Fox, & Countryman, 2001) outcome data have been reported from these studies. Significant pretreatment to posttreatment improvements were observed for more variables and were of greater magnitude for the study participants who received LSVT than for the participants who received the respiratory treatment alone. Only the individuals who received LSVT rated a significant decrease on the impact of PD on their communication posttreatment. Corresponding perceptual ratings by "blind" raters (Baumgartner, Sapir, & Ramig, 2001) revealed that listeners' perception of articulation and hoarseness pretreatment to posttreatment improved for men in both treatment groups; however, only the men who had LSVT im-

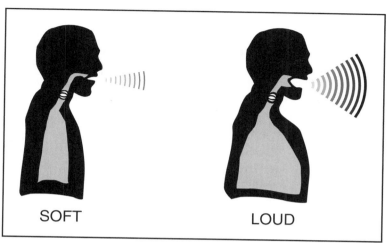

SOFT   LOUD

Figure 8.2. *The Lee Silverman Voice Treatment* is designed to improve the phonatory source and scale up amplitude across the speech mechanism with the global variable "LOUD." Increases in volume can trigger increases in respiratory volumes, vocal fold adduction, articulatory valving, and vocal tract opening. These factors may all contribute to improved speech intelligibility with the cognitively simple target of "LOUD."

proved in ratings of breathiness and intonation. These findings were supported in studies at 1-year (Ramig et al., 1996; Sapir, Pawlas, Seeley, et al., in press) and 2-year follow-up (Ramig, Sapir, Countryman, et al., 2001). Only the LSVT group improved or maintained vocal intensity above pretreatment levels. In addition, perceptual reports by patients and family members supported the positive impact of the treatment on functional daily communication.

In another study (Ramig et al., 2001), 29 individuals with idiopathic PD were studied over 6 months. Half the group received LSVT; the other half served as untreated controls. In addition, an age-matched, nontreated control group of individuals without the disorder was studied over this time period. Only the persons who received LSVT demonstrated significant increases in variables such as sound pressure level (related to volume) and semitone standard deviation (related to intonation) at pretreatment, posttreatment, and 6-month follow-up.

An important aspect of this work was to evaluate the underlying speech mechanism changes accompanying treatment. A study by Smith et al. (1995) documented increases in vocal fold closure following treatment in individuals who received LSVT, but not in individuals who received respiratory treatment only. These data were collected outside of the treatment clinic by clinicians not directly involved in the study and therefore support generalization of treatment effects. Of note, there was no evidence of increased hyperfunction (ventricular hyperadduction or anterior–posterior foreshortening) associated with volume training in these individuals (Smith et al., 1995). It is important to clarify that the goal of LSVT is to maximize phonatory efficiency, not to teach "tight or pressed" voice, but rather to improve vocal fold adduction for optimum, healthy volume and quality. In fact, mild to moderate hyperfunction observed pretreatment in some individuals with PD, which was hypothesized to be a compensation for hypoadduction of true vocal folds, resolved post-LSVT with training of improved true fold adduction (Countryman, Hicks, Ramig, & Smith, 1997; Smith et al., 1995).

Consistent with these findings, Ramig and Dromey (1996) reported increased subglottal air pressure and improved maximum flow declination rate accompanying increased vocal sound pressure level following LSVT. Finally, preliminary data from laryngeal electromyography pre-LSVT to post-LSVT in two individuals with PD have documented positive increases in TA muscle activity accompanying increased vocal volume across a range of speech tasks (Ramig, Sapir, et al., 2000). These findings were interpreted to be consistent with increased respiratory drive and improved vocal fold adduction accompanying successful treatment.

To evaluate application of LSVT to individuals with other neurological disorders or conditions, a number of case studies were carried out during this time as well. In one study, LSVT was applied to an individual with idiopathic PD who had had bilateral thalamotomies (Countryman & Ramig, 1993). In another study, the LSVT was applied to three individuals who had the parkinsonism plus syndromes of multiple system atrophy, Shy-Drager, and progressive supranuclear palsy (Countryman et al., 1994). Although improvements were documented in speech and voice characteristics in these individuals following treatment, the magnitude was not as great as for the persons with idiopathic PD. Countryman et al. recommended that application of LSVT to individuals such as these be done on a case-by-case basis and that the patients be referred for treatment early in the course of the disease.

A finding of interest following LSVT use has been the apparent generalization of phonatory effort from a focus on phonation to additional changes throughout the vocal tract. Not only does increased phonatory effort apparently improve vocal characteristics (volume, pitch variability, vocal quality), it appears to trigger effort and coordination across the speech mechanism. The observation of apparently larger movements in the upper articulatory system following LSVT is consistent with the reports by Schulman (1989) that as a speaker talks "louder" there are accompanying vocal tract and articulatory changes. Ramig, Dromey, Johnson, and Scherer (1994) first reported documentation of this observation in individuals with PD from pretreatment to posttreatment. These generalized effects have since been reported by Dromey et al. (1995) at posttreatment, 6-month follow up, and 12-month follow-up and compared by Johnson, Strand, and Ramig (2003) to the effects on participants who received LSVT and respiratory treatment. In addition, Spielman, Ramig, Story, and Fox (2000) documented increases in vowel space (decreased centralization) associated with positive changes in vowel formant frequencies during the speech of individuals with PD post-LSVT. The increase in vowel space reflected differential changes in formant 1 and formant 2, which raised or lowered, depending on the vowel, despite an overall increase in sound pressure level. This suggests that the formant frequency changes may represent improvements in articulatory range and coordination rather than simply the increase in sound pressure level. These changes in articulatory measures post-LSVT are functionally relevant because it has been well documented that individuals with PD have imprecise articulation, reduced amplitude, and reduced speed of articulatory movements (Ackerman & Zeigler, 1991; Caligiuri, 1989; Connor, Abbs, Cole, & Gracco, 1989; Forrest, Weismer, & Turner, 1989; Leanderson et al., 1971; Netsell, Daniel, & Celesia, 1975). Improvements in articulatory function post-LSVT may be related to an increased neural drive to the orofacial muscles associated with increased vocal effort (Ramig, Sapir, et al., 2000; Wohlert & Hammen, 2000), improved coordination of the orofacial system, or enhanced excursion of the articulators accompanying increased volume (Schulman, 1989).

Posttreatment data have also documented changes in facial expression (Spielman, Ramig, & Borod, 2001). Observations of increased facial expression accompanying improved volume and intonation following voice treatment, but not an alternative treatment, suggest these facial changes may reflect more than just posttreatment feelings of happiness or the results of positive reinforcement from 1 month of treatment (Spielman et al., 2001). Rather, these findings suggest that training loud phonation may also stimulate neural centers considered important in the regulation and conscious experience of affect and emotion (Borod, 2000; Eccles, 1980) and the vocal expression of emotion (Cummings, Benson, Houlihan, & Gosenfeld, 1983; Jurgens & von Cramon, 1982; P. Meyers, 1976; Porges, 1995).

In addition, positive improvements in the nonspeech motor function of swallowing in eight individuals with PD having a mild swallowing disorder have been reported following LSVT (El Sharkawi et al., 2002). El Sharkawi et al. noted a 51% reduction in swallowing motility disorders for these individuals. The combination of greater articulatory excursions and intensive exercise of the speech mechanism associated with volume training may have contributed to the positive changes that were documented. In addition, increased tongue strength, which has been reported following LSVT (Ward, Theodoros, & Murdoch, 2000), may contribute to improvements in oral tongue and tongue base function for swallowing that were reported post-LSVT. Future studies are needed to clarify the simultaneous effects of LSVT on voice and swallowing of individuals with PD.

To examine neural correlates of the speech disorder in PD and neural changes associated with behavioral improvements post-LSVT, a study using positron emission tomography in five individuals with mild PD was conducted. This pilot study revealed a reduction of abnormally increased activation in cortical premotor areas pre-LSVT and a shift to greater activation in the basal ganglia and anterior insula region post-LSVT (Liotti et al., 2003; Liotti et al., 1999). These observations suggest a change from an abnormally effortful volitional control (cortex), to compensate for disordered voice and speech, to more effortless and automatic implementation of speech motor actions (basal ganglia, anterior insula). It is important to note that these effects required training of vocal volume (LSVT), because stimulated increases in loudness pre-LSVT had no effect on the pretreatment abnormalities. These are initial data documenting potential neural changes accompanying LSVT and will be followed up in studies of a similar nature to confirm these findings.

The apparent multisystem spreading of effects of LSVT may be valuable in attempts to improve efficiency and simplify speech treatment for individuals who may have multiple speech mechanism problems as well as cognitive limitations, as is common in PD and other motor speech disorders. It appears that increasing and systematically training vocal volume may offer a single motor organizing theme that stimulates effort and coordination across multiple levels of speech production. By targeting volume in treatment, well-established, centrally stored motor patterns for speech may be triggered. Speech production is a learned, highly practiced motor behavior that becomes relatively automatic; scaling volume is a task we engage in all our lives. For example, it is common to increase volume to improve speech intelligibility when speaking against noise or when the listener is far away. Intensive volume training thus may provide the stimulation needed for individuals with PD to activate and appropriately modulate speech motor programs that are still intact. Volume training may be deceptively simple because the patient focuses only on increasing volume, but an array of positive, system-wide changes contribute to improved speech production.

The goal of LSVT is to improve functional communication for at least 6 to 12 months without additional treatment. After the 16 sessions of individual treatment in 1 month, most patients will be able to maintain speech and voice changes for at least 6 months, and sometimes for up to 2 years (Ramig, Countryman, et al., 1995; Ramig, Sapir, Countryman, et al., 2001), without additional speech treatment. Within the 16 initial treatment sessions, patients are encouraged to establish a daily homework routine that they maintain on their own once treatment is completed. All patients are encouraged to return for a reassessment at 6 months, at which time some patients may benefit from a few "tune-up" sessions. LSVT has been described in detail elsewhere (Ramig, Pawlas, & Countryman, 1995).

Treatment data suggest that individuals with mild to moderate PD have the most positive treatment outcomes following LSVT.

Patients with co-occurring mild to moderate depression and dementia have succeeded in treatment as well (Ramig et al., 1996). Because treatment focuses on voice, all patients must have a laryngeal
examination before treatment to rule out any contraindications (vocal nodules, gastric reflux, laryngeal cancer).

The extent to which the effects of LSVT are specific to hypokinetic dysarthria associated with PD is not clear. Data from using
intensive voice treatment with select individuals with neurological
disorders other than idiopathic PD (e.g., ataxia, multiple sclerosis,
stroke, traumatic brain injury) have indicated increased vocal
sound pressure level following treatment with corroborating perceptual ratings of improved loudness, voice quality, and functional
communication (Fox, Ramig, Countryman, Sapir, & Spielman, 2000;
Ramig, Fox, Countryman, Sapir, & Spielman, 2000; Sapir, Pawlas,
Seeley, et al., in press; Solomon et al., 2000). In addition, articulatory acoustic data of improved formant transitions and increased
vowel space, along with perceptions of improved articulatory precision, have been reported in a woman with ataxic dysarthria
(Countryman et al., 2000; Sapir et al., 1999). Although positive outcomes in perceptual and acoustic measures have been reported,
the physiological mechanism of change associated with improved
speech production in these individuals with varied neurological
disorders has not been established. At this time, we may speculate
that positive outcomes could be related to a combination of improved motor stability and enhanced coordination of respiratory,
laryngeal, and orofacial systems accompanying intensive treatment with a simple focus. Additional studies examining the impact of LSVT on individuals with neurological disorders other
than idiopathic PD are needed.

Although studies of LSVT for individuals with PD are promising, there clearly are limitations to existing knowledge. First, current published clinical efficacy studies fall into Phase I through
Phase III (Robey & Schulz, 1998) and have examined treatment effects in ideal experimental conditions. Reports of real-world clinical
application have been positive, but large-scale, multisite clinical
trials have yet to be conducted. Second, prognostic variables for
predicting treatment success remain to be clearly defined. Although
the Ramig, Countryman, et al. (1995) study examined the magnitude of treatment-related change and participant characteristics

and reported no significant correlations among age, stage of disease, rating on motor UPDRS, time since diagnosis, severity of pretreatment speech disorder, glottal incompetence, cognitive ability, and depression, future studies examining these factors in a greater number of participants may indicate otherwise. Third, studies examining modifications of LSVT at different levels of intensity, with variable versus blocked practice of treatment tasks, treatment in groups, and shorter or longer periods of treatment, will help elucidate the best mode of administration for optimal treatment results. Fourth, studies comparing individuals with idiopathic PD who receive LSVT (with its focus on phonation) with individuals who receive alternative treatment approaches that are administered in a parallel mode and intensity but with a focus on articulation or rate are needed to further delineate the key elements for treatment success (e.g., is it the focus on phonation, the intensity of treatment, or sensory awareness training that contributes most to successful outcomes?). Finally, despite positive, long-term (2-year) treatment outcomes for groups as a whole, successful retraining of sensory awareness for individual patients continues to offer challenges. Efforts to develop feedback and at-home data collection devices to improve this key element of treatment are ongoing.

In summary, data from systematic training of increased volume as part of LSVT provides experimental support for improving the phonatory source and stimulating effort and coordination across the speech mechanism in individuals with idiopathic PD. These changes are most likely related to increased neural drive to respiratory, laryngeal, and orofacial system motor neuron pools that facilitates overcoming hypokinetic and bradykinetic movements of the speech musculature. In addition, these changes observed across the speech mechanism with increased vocal effort and volume may conceivably involve a common central mechanism, such as the fronto-limbic system and its link to the basal ganglia, periaqueductal gray, and reticular formation (Davis, Zhang, Winkworth, & Bandler, 1996; Devinsky, Morrell, & Vogt, 1995; Jurgens & von Cramon, 1982; C. Larson, 1985). LSVT thus may be geared toward both the motor system and an emotive system of speech production that is characterized by the limbic system, basal ganglia, thalamus, and periaqueductal gray. As a result, LSVT does not involve deautomatization of speech production by requiring individuals to slow down or overarticulate; instead, it rescales amplitude or amplifies the emotive system, which has simultaneous effects on respiration, phonation, and articulation. Concurrently, learning is facilitated by the nature of the tasks and the emotional salience of the treatment activities (e.g., the patient self-identifies potent communication situations and contributes to selection of treatment materials and activities that are deemed important and relevant). Future research should continue to examine the nature of motor and neural changes associated with post-LSVT improvements, move outcome data from efficacy studies (ideal treatment conditions) to larger scale effectiveness studies, and enhance understanding of the mechanism of change associated with LSVT.

Summary

Speech and voice problems occur in most individuals with idiopathic PD and may limit quality of life. Although all aspects of speech production may be affected, disordered voice is one of the most common problems. Because neuropharmacological and neurosurgical treatments have limited effects on improving speech and voice production, behavioral treatment is necessary. Previous forms of treatment (rate, articulation) for the disorder of speech and voice in individuals with idiopathic PD have been modestly effective. LSVT, which addresses increased vocal effort and improved sensory perception of effort and is administered in 16 high-effort sessions in 1 month, has been extensively documented to be a successful approach in both the short and long terms. The ability to communicate is essential to quality of life. Management of individuals with PD can be optimized by early referral for speech treatment and follow-up by teams of speech–language pathologists, otolaryngologists, and neurologists.

Authors' Note

This chapter has been supported in part by NIH-NIDCD Grant R01 DC-01150. Select portions of this chapter have been published previously.

References

Ackerman, H., & Ziegler, W. (1991). Articulatory deficits in Parkinsonian dysarthria. *Journal of Neurology, Neurosurgery, and Psychiatry, 54*, 1093–1098.

Adams, S. G. (1997). Hypokinetic dysarthria in Parkinson's disease. In M. R. McNeil (Ed.), *Clinical management of sensorimotor speech disorders* (pp. 261–285). New York: Thieme.

Adler, C. H., Singer, C., O'Brien, C., Hauser, R., Lew, M., Marek, K., et al. (1998). Randomized, placebo-controlled study of tolcapone in patients with fluctuating Parkinson disease treated with levodopa-carbidopa: Tolcapone Fluctuator Study Group III. *Archives of Neurology, 55*, 1089–1095.

Agid, Y., Ahlskog, E., Albanese, A., Calne, D., Chase, T., De Yebenes, J., et al. (1999). Levodopa in the treatment of Parkinson's disease: A consensus meeting. *Movement Disorders, 14*, 911–913.

Albin, R. L., Young, A. B., & Penny, J. B. (1989). The functional anatomy of basal ganglia disorders. *Trends in Neuroscience, 12*, 366–375.

Allain, H., Pollak, P., & Neukirch, H. C. (1993). Symptomatic effect of selegiline in denovo parkinsonian patients. *Movement Disorders, 8*(Suppl. 1), S36–S40.

Allan, C. M. (1970). Treatment of non-fluent speech resulting from neurological disease: Treatment of dysarthria. *British Journal of Disordered Communication, 5*(1), 3–5.

Alvarez, L., Macias, R., Guridi, J., Lopez, G., Alvarez, E., Maragoto, C., et al. (2001). Dorsal subthalamotomy for Parkinson's disease. *Movement Disorders, 16*(1), 72–78.

Aronson, A. E. (1990). *Clinical voice disorders* (3rd ed.). New York: Thieme-Stratton.

Astrand, P. O., & Rodahl, K. (1970). *Textbook of work physiology.* New York: McGraw-Hill.

Baas, H., Beiske, A. G., Ghika, J., Jackson, M., Oertel, W., Poewe, W., et al. (1997). Catechol-O-methyltransferase inhibition with tolcapone reduces the "wearing off" phenomenon and levodopa requirements in fluctuating parkinsonian patients. *Journal of Neurology, Neurosurgery, and Psychiatry, 63*, 421–428.

Backlund, E. O., Granberg, P. O., Hamberger, B., Knutsson, E., Martensson, A., Sedvall, G., et al. (1985). Transplantation of adrenal medullary tissue to striatum in parkinsonism: First clinical trials. *Journal of Neurosurgery, 62*, 169–173.

Baker, K. K., Ramig, L. O., Johnson, A. B., & Freed, C. R. (1997). Preliminary voice and speech analysis following fetal dopamine transplants in 5 individuals with Parkinson disease. *Journal of Speech, Language, and Hearing Research, 40*, 615–626.

Baker, K. K., Ramig, L. O., Luschei, E. S., & Smith, M. E. (1998). Thyroarytenoid muscle activity associated with hypophonia in Parkinson disease and aging. *Neurology, 51*, 1592–1598.

Barbeau, A., Sourkes, T. L., & Murphy, C. F. (1962). Les catecholamines de la maladie de Parkinson's [Catecholamines in Parkinson's disease]. In J. Ajuriaguerra (Ed.), *Monoamines et systeme nerveux central* [Monoamines and the central nervous system]. Geneva, Switzerland: George.

Barlas, O., Hanagbreve, H. A., Imer, R., Sahin, H., Sencer, S., Emre, M., et al. (2001). Do unilateral ablative lesions of the subthalamic nucleus in parkinsonian patients lead to hemiballism? *Movement Disorders, 16*, 306–310.

Baron, M. S., Vitek, J. L., Bakay, R. A., Green, J., McDonald, W., Cole, S., et al. (2000). Treatment of advanced Parkinson's disease by unilateral posterior GPi pallidotomy: 4-year results of a pilot study. *Movement Disorders, 15*, 230–237.

Baumgartner, C., Sapir, S., & Ramig, L. (2001). Voice quality changes following phonatory-respiratory effort treatment (LSVT) versus respiratory effort treatment for individuals with Parkinson disease. *Journal of Voice, 15*(1), 105–114.

Bejjani, B., Damier, P., Arnulf, I., Bonnet, A. M., Vidailhet, M., Dorment, D., et al. (1997). Pallidal stimulation for Parkinson's disease: Two targets? *Neurology, 49*, 1564–1569.

Bejjani, B. P., Gervais, D., Arnulf, I., Papadopoulos, S., Demeret, S., Bonnet, A., et al. (2000). Axial parkinsonian symptoms can be improved: The role of levodopa and bilateral subthalamic stimulation. *Journal of Neurology, Neurosurgery, and Psychiatry, 68,* 595–600.

Benabid, A. L., Krack, P. P., Benazzouz, A., Limousin, P., Koudsie, A., & Pollak, P. (2000). Deep brain stimulation of the subthalamic nucleus for Parkinson's disease: Methodologic aspects and clinical criteria. *Neurology, 55*(12, Suppl. 6), S40–S44.

Benabid, A. L., Pollak, P., Gao, D., Hoffman, D., Limousin, P., Gay, E., et al. (1996). Chronic electrical stimulation of the ventralis intermedius nucleus of the thalamus as a treatment of movement disorders. *Journal of Neurosurgery, 84,* 203–214.

Benazzouz, A., & Hallett, M. (2000). Mechanism of action of deep brain stimulation. *Neurology, 55*(12, Suppl. 6), S13–S16.

Benke, T., Hohenstein, C., Poewe, W., & Butterworth, B. (2000). Repetitive speech phenomena in Parkinson's disease. *Journal of Neurology, Neurosurgery, and Psychiatry, 69,* 319–324.

Berardelli, A., Dick, J. P., Rothwell, J. C., Day, B. L., & Marsden, C. D. (1986). Scaling of the size of the first agonist EMG burst during rapid wrist movements in patients with Parkinson's disease. *Journal of Neurology, Neurosurgery, and Psychiatry, 49,* 1273–1279.

Berry, W. R., & Sanders, S. B. (1983). *Clinical dysarthria.* San Diego, CA: College-Hill Press.

Biary, N., Pimental, P. A., & Langenberg, P. W. (1988). A double-blind trial of clonazepam in the treatment of parkinsonian dysarthria. *Neurology, 38,* 255–258.

Birkmayer, W., Riederer, P., Youdim, M. B., & Linauer, W. (1975). The potentiation of the anti akinetic effect after L-dopa treatment by an inhibitor of MAO-B, Deprenil. *Journal of Neural Transmittors, 36,* 303–326.

Boecker, H., Ceballos-Baumann, A., Bartenstein, P., Weindl, A., Siebner, H., Fassbender, T., et al. (1999). Sensory processing in

Parkinson's and Huntington's disease: Investigations with 3D H(2)(15)O-PET. *Brain, 122,* 1651–1665.

Boone, D., & McFarlane, S. C. (1988). *The voice and voice therapy.* Englewood Cliffs, NJ: Prentice Hall.

Borod, J. (2000). *The neuropsychology of emotion.* New York: Oxford University Press.

Bragoni, M., Altieri, M., Di, P. V., Padovani, A., Mostardini, C., & Lenzi, G. L. (2000). Bromocriptine and speech therapy in non-fluent chronic aphasia after stroke. *Neurological Sciences, 21*(1), 19–22.

Brown, A. B., McCartney, N., & Sale, D. G. (1990). Positive adaptations to weight-lifting training in the elderly. *Journal of Applied Physiology, 69,* 1725–1733.

Brown, R. G., & Marsden, C. D. (1988). An investigation of the phenomenon of "set" in Parkinson's disease. *Movement Disorders, 3,* 152–161.

Brundin, P., Karlsson, J., Emgard, M., Schierle, G., Hansson, O., Peterson, A., et al. (2000). Improving the survival of grafted dopaminergic neurons: A review over current approaches. *Cell Transplant, 9,* 179–195.

Bucy, P. C. (1948). Cortical extirpation in the treatment of the involuntary movements. *American Journal of Surgery, 75,* 257–263.

Burchiel, K. J., Anderson, V. C., Favre, J., & Hammerstad, J. P. (1999). Comparison of pallidal and subthalamic nucleus deep brain stimulation for advanced Parkinson's disease: Results of a randomized, blinded pilot study. *Neurosurgery, 45,* 1375–1382.

Cahill, L. M., Murdoch, B. E., Theodoros, D. G., Triggs, E. J., Charles, B. G., & Yao, A. A. (1998). Effect of oral levodopa treatment on articulatory function in Parkinson's disease: Preliminary results. *Motor Control, 2,* 161–172.

Caliguri, M. P. (1989). The influence of speaking rate on articulatory hypokinesia in Parkinsonian dysarthria. *Brain Language, 36,* 493–502.

Carpenter, M. B., Whittier, J. R., & Mettler, F. A. (1950). Analysis of choreoid hyperkinesia in the rhesus monkey. *Journal of Comparative Neurology, 92*, 293–322.

Clarkson, E. D., Zawada, W. M., Adams, F. S., Bell, K. P., & Freed, C. R. (1998). Strands of embryonic mesencephalic tissue show greater dopamine neuron survival and better behavioral improvement than cell suspensions after transplantation in parkinsonian rats. *Brain Research, 806*, 60–68.

Collins, S. J., Ahlskog, J. E., Parisi, J. E., & Maraganore, D. M. (1995). Progressive supranuclear palsy: Neuropathologically based diagnostic clinical criteria. *Journal of Neurology, Neurosurgery, and Psychiatry, 58*, 167–173.

Colton, R. H., & Casper, J. K. (1996). *Understanding voice problems: A physiological perspective for diagnosis and treatment.* Baltimore: Williams & Wilkins.

Connor, N. P., Abbs, J. H., Cole, K. J., & Gracco, V. L. (1989). Parkinsonian deficits in serial multiarticulate movements for speech. *Brain, 112*(Pt. 4), 997–1009.

Contreras-Vidal, J., & Stelmach, G. (1995). A neural model of basal ganglia-thalamocortical relations in normal and parkinsonian movement. *Biological Cybernetics, 73*, 467–476.

Cooper, I. S. (1954). Surgical alleviation of parkinsonism: Effects of occlusion of anterior choroidal artery. *Journal of the American Geriatric Society, 11*, 691–717.

Cooper, I. S., & Bravo, G. (1958). Chemopallidectomy and chemothalamectomy. *Journal of Neurosurgery, 15*, 244–250.

Corboy, D. L., Wagner, M. L., & Sage, J. I. (1995). Apomorphine for motor fluctuations and freezing in Parkinson's disease. *Annals of Pharmacotherapy, 29*, 282–288.

Countryman, S., Hicks, J., Ramig, L., & Smith, M. (1997). Supraglottal hyperadduction in an individual with Parkinson disease: A clinical treatment note. *American Journal of Speech-Language Pathology, 6*(4), 74–84.

Countryman, S., & Ramig, L. O. (1993). Effects of intensive voice therapy on speech deficits associated with bilateral thalatomy in Parkinson's disease: A case study. *Journal of Medical Speech-Language Pathology, 1,* 233–249.

Countryman, S., Ramig, L. O., & Pawlas, A. A. (1994). Speech and voice deficits in Parkinsonian Plus syndromes: Can they be treated? *Journal of Medical Speech-Language Pathology, 2,* 211–225.

Countryman, S., Spielman, J., Hinds, S., Ramig, L., Sapir, S., & Fox, C. (2000, November). *Articulatory changes in ataxic dysarthria following the LSVT®: A case study.* Poster presented at the annual conference of the American Speech-Language-Hearing Association, Washington, DC.

Critchley, E. M. (1976). Letter: Peak-dose dysphonia in parkinsonism. *The Lancet, 1,* 544.

Critchley, E. M. (1981). Speech disorders of Parkinsonism: A review. *Journal of Neurology, Neurosurgery, and Psychiatry, 44,* 751–758.

Cummings, J., Benson, D., Houlihan, J., & Gosenfeld, L. (1983). Mutism: Loss of neocortical and limbic vocalization. *Journal of Nervous and Mental Disease, 171,* 255–259.

Darley, F. L., Aronson, A. E., & Brown, J. B. (1975). *Motor speech disorders.* Philadelphia: Saunders.

Davis, P., Zhang, S., Winkworth, A., & Bandler, R. (1996). Neural control of vocalization: Respiratory and emotional influences. *Journal of Voice, 10*(1), 23–38.

DeLong, M. R. (1990). Primate models of movement disorders of basal ganglia origin. *Trends in Neuroscience, 13,* 281–285.

Demirci, M., Grill, S., McShane, L., & Hallet, M. (1995). Impairment of kinesthesia in Parkinson's disease. *Neurology, 45,* A218.

Devinsky, O., Morrell, M., & Vogt, B. (1995). Contribution of anterior cingulated cortex to behavior. *Brain, 118,* 279–306.

Diederich, N., Goetz, C. G., Stebbins, G. T., Klawans, H., Nittner, K., Koulosakis, A., et al. (1992). Blinded evaluation confirms long-term asymmetric effect of unilateral thalamotomy or subthalamotomy on tremor in Parkinson's disease. *Neurology, 42,* 1311–1314.

Downie, A. W., Low, J. M., & Lindsay, D. D. (1981). Speech disorders in Parkinsonism: Usefulness of delayed auditory feedback in selected cases. *British Journal of Disordered Communication, 16,* 135–139.

Dromey, C., Kumar, R., Lang, A. E., & Lozano, A. M. (2000). An investigation of the effects of subthalamic nucleus stimulation on acoustic measures of voice. *Movement Disorders, 15,* 1132–1138.

Dromey, C., Ramig, L. O., & Johnson, A. (1995). Phonatory and articulatory changes associated with increased vocal intensity in Parkinson disease: A case study. *Journal of Speech and Hearing Research, 38,* 751–763.

Dubois, B., Danze, F., Pillon, B., Cusimano, G., Lhermitte, F., & Agid, Y. (1987). Cholinergic-dependent cognitive deficits in Parkinson's disease. *Annals of Neurology, 22,* 26–30.

Duffy, J. (1995). *Motor speech disorders.* New York: Thieme.

Eccles, J. (1980). The emotional brain. *Bulletin et Memoires de L'Academie Royale de Medicine de Belgique, 135,* 697–711.

El Sharkawi, A., Ramig, L., Logemann, J., Pauloski, B., Rademaker, A., Smith, C., et al. (2002). Swallowing and voice effects of Lee Silverman Voice Treatment: A pilot study. *Journal of Neurology, Neurosurgery, and Psychiatry, 172,* 31–36.

Engberg, G., Elebring, T., & Nissbrandt, H. (1991). Deprenyl (selegiline), a selective MAO-B inhibitor with active metabolites: Effects on locomotor activity, dopaminergic neurotransmission and firing rate of nigral dopamine neurons. *Journal of Pharmacological Experimental Therapy, 259,* 841–847.

Espejo, M., Cutillas, B., Arenas, T. E., & Ambrosio, S. (2000). Increased survival of dopaminergic neurons in striatal grafts of fetal ventral mesencephalic cells exposed to neurotrophin-3 or glial cell line-derived neurotrophic factor. *Cell Transplant, 9*(1), 45–53.

Factor, S. A., McAlarney, T., Sanchez-Ramos, J. R., & Weiner, W. J. (1990). Sleep disorders and sleep effect in Parkinson's disease. *Movement Disorders, 5,* 280–285.

Fahn, S. (1986). Parkinson's disease and other basal ganglion disorders. In A. K. Asbury, G. M. McKhann, & W. I. McDonald (Eds.), *Diseases of the nervous system: Clinical neurobiology* (pp. 1217–1228). Philadelphia: Ardmore Medical Books.

Fahn, S. (1989). The history of parkinsonism. *Movement Disorders, 4*(Suppl. 1), S2–S10.

Favre, J., Burchiel, K. J., Taha, J. M., & Hammerstad, J. (2000). Outcome of unilateral and bilateral pallidotomy for Parkinson's disease: Patient assessment. *Neurosurgery, 46,* 344–353.

Felten, D. L., Felten, S. Y., Steece-Collier, K., Date, I., & Clemens, J. A. (1992). Age-related decline in the dopaminergic nigrostriatal system: The oxidative hypothesis and protective strategies. *Annals of Neurology, 32,* S133–S136.

Fetoni, V., Genitrini, S., Monza, D., Soliveri, P., Testa, D., Caraceni, T., & Girotti, F. (1997). Variations in axial, proximal, and distal motor response to L-dopa in multisystem atrophy and Parkinson's disease. *Clinical Neuropharmacology, 20,* 239–244.

Fine, J., Duff, J., Chen, R., Chir, B., Hutchison, W., Lozano, A., et al. (2000). Long-term follow-up of unilateral pallidotomy in advanced Parkinson's disease. *New England Journal of Medicine, 342,* 1708–1714.

Forrest, K., Weismer, G., & Turner, G. (1989). Kinematic, acoustic and perceptual analysis of connected speech produced by Parkinsonian and normal geriatric adults. *Journal of the Acoustical Society of America, 85,* 2608–2622.

Fox, C., Morrison, C., Ramig, L., & Sapir, S. (in press). Current perspectives on the Lee Silverman Voice Treatment (LSVT) for individuals with idiopathic Parkinson disease. *American Journal of Speech-Language Pathology.*

Fox, C., & Ramig, L. (1997). Vocal sound pressure level and self-perception of speech and voice in men and women with idiopathic Parkinson disease. *American Journal of Speech-Language Pathology, 6,* 85–94.

Fox, C. M., Ramig, L. O., Countryman, S., Spielman, J., & Sapir, S. (2000, November). *Intensive voice therapy for speech disorders following stroke: Two cases.* Poster presented at the annual conference of the American Speech-Language-Hearing Association, Washington, DC.

Freed, C. R., Greene, P. E., Breeze, R. E, Tsai, W., DuMouchel, W., Kao, R., et al. (2001). Transplantation of embryonic dopamine neurons for severe Parkinson's disease. *New England Journal of Medicine, 344,* 710–719.

Froeschels, E., Kastein, S., & Weiss, D. A. (1955). A method of therapy for paralytic conditions of the mechanisms of phonation, respiration and glutination. *Journal of Speech and Hearing Disorders, 20,* 365–370.

Fronterra, W. R., Meredith, C. N., O'Reilly, K. P., Knuttgen, H. G., & Evans, W. J. (1988). Strength conditioning in older men: Skeletal muscle hypertrophy and improved function. *Journal of Applied Physiology, 64,* 1038–1044.

Frucht, S., Rogers, J. D., Greene, P. E., Gordon, M. F., & Fahn, S. (1999). Falling asleep at the wheel: Motor vehicle mishaps in persons taking pramipexole and ropinirole. *Neurology, 52,* 1908–1910.

Galvin, J. E., Lee, V. M., & Trojanowski, J. Q. (2001). Synucleinopathies: Clinical and pathological implications. *Archives of Neurology, 58,* 186–190.

Gelb, D. J., Oliver, E., & Gilman, S. (1999). Diagnostic criteria for Parkinson disease. *Archives of Neurology, 56,* 33–39.

Gentil, M., Garcia-Ruiz, P., Pollak, P., & Benabid, A. L. (2000). Effect of bilateral deep-brain stimulation on oral control of patients with parkinsonism. *European Neurology, 44,* 147–152.

Glover, V., Clow, A., & Sandler, M. (1993). Effects of dopaminergic drugs on superoxide dismutase: Implications for senescence. *Journal of Neural Transmitters, 40*(Suppl. 199), 37–45.

Goetz, C. G., Stebbins, G. T., III, Klawans, H. L., Koller, W., Grossman, R., Bakay, R., et al. (1991). United Parkinson Foundation Neurotransplantation Registry on adrenal medullary transplants: Presurgical, and 1- and 2-year follow-up. *Neurology, 41*, 1719–1722.

Golbe, L. I., Lieberman, A. N., Muenter, M. D., Ahlskog, J., Gopinathan, G., Neophytides, A., et al. (1988). Deprenyl in the treatment of symptom fluctuations in advanced Parkinson's disease. *Clinical Neuropharmacology, 11*, 45–55.

Greene, H. C. L. (1980). *The voice and its disorders.* London: Pitman Medical.

Gross, C., Rougier, A., Gueh, D., Boraud, T., Julien, J., & Bioulac, B. (1997). High-frequency stimulation of the globus pallidus internalis in Parkinson's disease: A study of seven cases. *Journal of Neurosurgery, 87*, 491–498.

Gupta, S. R., Mlcoch, A. G., Scolaro, C., & Moritz, T. (1995). Bromocriptine treatment of nonfluent aphasia. *Neurology, 45*, 2170–2173.

Hamada, I., & DeLong, M. R. (1992). Excitotoxic acid lesions of the primate subthalamic nucleus result in reduced pallidal neuronal activity during active holding. *Journal of Neurophysiology, 68*, 1859–1866.

Hammen, V. L., & Yorkston, K. M. (1996). Speech and pause characteristics following speech rate reduction in hypokinetic dysarthria. *Journal of Communication Disorders, 29*, 429–444.

Hanson, D., Gerratt, B., & Ward, P. (1984). Cinegraphic observations of laryngeal function in Parkinson's disease. *Laryngoscope, 94*, 348–353.

Hanson, D. J., Ludlow, C. L., & Bassich, C. J. (1983). Vocal fold paresis in Shy-Drager syndrome. *Annals of Otology, Rhinology & Laryngology, 92*(1, Pt. 1), 85–90.

Hardie, R. J., Malcolm, S. L., Lees, A. J., Stern, G. M., & Allen, J. G. (1986). The pharmacokinetics of intravenous and oral levodopa in patients with Parkinson's disease who exhibit on-off fluctuations. *British Journal of Clinical Pharmacology, 22,* 429–436.

Hardy, J. (1967). Suggestions for physiological research in dysarthria. *Cortex, 3,* 128–156.

Hariz, M. I., Johansson, F., Shamsgovara, P., Johansson, E., Hariz, G. M., & Fagerlund, M. (2000). Bilateral subthalamic nucleus stimulation in a parkinsonian patient with preoperative deficits in speech and cognition. Persistent improvement in mobility but increased dependency: A case study. *Movement Disorders, 15,* 136–139.

Hartelius, L., & Svensson, P. (1994). Speech and swallowing symptoms associated with Parkinson's disease and multiple sclerosis: A survey. *Folia Phoniatrica et Logopaedica, 46*(1) 9–17.

Hauser, R. A., Freeman, T. B., Snow, B. J., Nauert, M., Gauger, L., Kordower, J., et al. (1999). Long-term evaluation of bilateral fetal nigral transplantation in Parkinson disease. *Archives of Neurology, 56,* 179–187.

Hauser, R. A., Molho, E., Shale, H., Pedder, S., & Dorflinger, E. E. (1998). A pilot evaluation of the tolerability, safety, and efficacy of tolcapone alone and in combination with oral selegiline in untreated Parkinson's disease patients. *Movement Disorders, 13,* 643–647.

Hayase, N., Miyashita, N., Endo, K., & Narabayashi, H. (1998). Neuronal activity in GP and Vim of parkinsonian patients and clinical changes of tremor through surgical interventions. *Stereotactic Functional Neurosurgery, 71,* 20–28.

Helm, N. (1979). Management of palilalia with a pacing board. *Journal of Speech and Hearing Disorders, 44,* 350–353.

Herrera, E. J., Viano, J. C., Caceres, M., Costello, G., Suarez, M., & Suarez, J. C. (2000). Posteroventral pallidotomy in Parkinson's disease. *Acta Neurochirurgica., 142,* 169–175.

Ho, A. K., Bradshaw, J. L., & Iansek, T. (2000). Volume perception in parkinsonian speech. *Movement Disorders, 15,* 1125–1131.

Hughes, A. J., Daniel, S. E., Kilford, L., & Lees, A. J. (1992). Accuracy of clinical diagnosis of idiopathic Parkinson's disease: A clinico-pathological study of 100 cases. *Journal of Neurology, Neuro-surgery, and Psychiatry, 55,* 181–184.

Hughes, R. C., Polgar, J. G., Weightman, D., & Walton, J. N. (1971). L-dopa in Parkinsonism and the influence of previous thala-motomy. *British Medical Journal, 1,* 7–13.

Hunter, P. C., Crameri, J., Austin, S., Woodward, M. C., & Hughes, A. J. (1997). Response of parkinsonian swallowing dysfunction to dopaminergic stimulation. *Journal of Neurology, Neurosurgery, and Psychiatry, 63,* 579–583.

Hutton, J. T., Koller, W. C., Ahlskog, J. E., Pahwa, R., Hurtig, H. I., Stern, M. B., et al. (1996). Multicenter, placebo-controlled trial of cabergoline taken once daily in the treatment of Parkinson's disease. *Neurology, 46,* 1062–1065.

Intemann, P. M., Masterman, D., Subramanian, I., DeSalles, A., Behnke, E., Frysinger, R., et al. (2001). Staged bilateral palli-dotomy for treatment of Parkinson disease. *Journal of Neuro-surgery, 94,* 437–444.

Jankovic, J., Cardoso, F., Grossman, R. G., & Hamilton, W. J. (1995). Outcome after stereotactic thalamotomy for parkinsonian, es-sential, and other types of tremor. *Neurosurgery, 37,* 680–686.

Jellinger, K. (1987). Lisuride in the combination treatment of Par-kinson disease. *Wiener Medizinische Wochenschrift, 137,* 155–159.

Jiang, J., Lin, E., Wang, J., & Hanson, D. G. (1999). Glottographic measures before and after levodopa treatment in Parkinson's disease. *Laryngoscope, 109,* 1287–1294.

Jobst, E. E., Melnick, M. E., Byl, N. N., Dowling, G. A., & Aminoff, M. J. (1997). Sensory perception in Parkinson disease. *Archives of Neurology, 54,* 450–454.

Johnson, A., Strand, E., & Ramig, L. (2003). *The effect of intensive res-piratory and laryngeal treatment on single word intelligibility and select articulatory acoustics in patients with Parkinson's disease.* Manuscript in preparation.

Jurgens, U., & von Cramon, D. (1982). On the role of the anterior cingulated cortex in phonation: A case report. *Brain and Language, 15,* 234–248.

Kempster, P. A., & Wahlqvist, M. L. (1994). Dietary factors in the management of Parkinson's disease. *Nutrition Review, 52*(2, Pt. 1), 51–58.

Klawans, H. L. (1986). Individual manifestations of Parkinson's disease after ten or more years of levodopa. *Movement Disorders, 1,* 187–192.

Kluin, K. J., Gilman, S., Foster, N. L., Sima, A., D'Amato, C., Bruch, L., et al. (2001). Neuropathological correlates of dysarthria in progressive supranuclear palsy. *Archives of Neurology, 58,* 265–269.

Koller, W. C. (1986). Pharmacologic treatment of parkinsonian tremor. *Archives of Neurology, 43,* 126–127.

Koller, W. C. (2000). Levodopa in the treatment of Parkinson's disease. *Neurology, 55,* S2–S7.

Koller, W. C., & Hubble, J. P. (1990). Levodopa therapy in Parkinson's disease. *Neurology, 40*(10, Suppl. 3), S40–S47.

Koller, W., Pahwa, R., Busenbark, K., Hubble, J., Wilkinson, S., Lang, A., et al. (1997). High-frequency unilateral thalamic stimulation in the treatment of essential and parkinsonian tremor. *Annals of Neurology, 42,* 292–299.

Kompoliti, K., Wang, Q. E., Goetz, C. G., Leurgans, S., & Raman, R. (2000). Effects of central dopaminergic stimulation by apomorphine on speech in Parkinson's disease. *Neurology, 54,* 458–462.

Kornhuber, J., & Weller, M. (1993). Amantadine and the glutamate hypothesis of schizophrenia experiences in the treatment of neuroleptic malignant syndrome. *Journal of Neural Transmission, General Section, 92*(1), 57–65.

Krack, P., Pollak, P., Limousin, P., Hoffman, D., Xie, J., Benazzouz, A., et al. (1998). Subthalamic nucleus or internal pallidal stimulation in young onset Parkinson's disease. *Brain, 121*(Pt. 3), 451–457.

Krause, M., Fogel, W., Heck, A., Hacke, W., Bonsanto, M., Trenkwalder, C., et al. (2001). Deep brain stimulation for the treatment of Parkinson's disease: Subthalamic nucleus versus globus pallidus internus. *Journal of Neurology, Neurosurgery, and Psychiatry, 70,* 464–470.

Kumar, R., Lang, A. E., Rodriguez-Oroz, M. C., et al. (2000). Deep brain stimulation of the globus pallidus pars interna in advanced Parkinson's disease. *Neurology, 55,* S34–S39.

Kumar, R., Lozano, A. M., Kim, Y. J., Lozano, A. M., Limousin, P., Pollack, P., et al. (1998). Double-blind evaluation of subthalamic nucleus deep brain stimulation in advanced Parkinson's disease. *Neurology, 51,* 850–855.

Kurth, M. C., Adler, C. H., Hilaire, M. S., Singer, C., Waters, C., LeWitt, P., Hutchison, W. D., et al. (1997). Tolcapone improves motor function and reduces levodopa requirement in patients with Parkinson's disease experiencing motor fluctuations: A multicenter, double-blind, randomized, placebo-controlled trial. *Neurology, 48,* 81–87.

Langtry, H. D., & Clissold, S. P. (1990). Pergolide: A review of its pharmacological properties and therapeutic potential in Parkinson's disease. *Drugs, 39,* 491–506.

Larson, C. (1985). The midbrain periaqueductal gray: A brainstem structure involved in vocalization. *Journal of Speech and Hearing Research, 28,* 241–249.

Larson, K. K., Ramig, L. O., & Scherer, R. C. (1994). Acoustic and glottographic voice analysis during drug-related fluctuations in Parkinson's disease. *Journal of Medical Speech-Language Pathology, 2,* 227–239.

Leanderson, R., Meyerson, B. A., & Persson, A. (1971). Effect of L-dopa on speech in Parkinsonism: An EMG study of labial articulatory function. *Journal of Neurology, Neurosurgery, and Psychiatry, 34,* 679–681.

Lenz, F. A., Normand, S. L., Kwan, H. C., Andrews, D., Rowland, L., Jones, M., et al. (1995). Statistical prediction of the optimal site for thalamotomy in parkinsonian tremor. *Movement Disorders, 10,* 318–328.

Limousin, P., Krack, P., Pollak, P., Benazzouz, A., Ardouin, C., Hoffman, D., et al. (1998). Electrical stimulation of the subthalamic nucleus in advanced Parkinson's disease. *New England Journal of Medicine, 339,* 1105–1111.

Limousin, P., Pollak, P., Benazzouz, A., Hoffman, D., Le Bas, J., Broussolle, E., et al. (1995). Effect of parkinsonian signs and symptoms of bilateral subthalamic nucleus stimulation. *The Lancet, 345,* 91–95.

Liotti, M., Ramig, L., Vogel, D., New, P., Cook, C., & Fox, P. (2003). Hypophonia in Parkinson disease: Neural correlates of voice treatment with LSVT® revealed by PET. *Neurology, 60*(3), 432–440.

Liotti, M., Vogel, D., New, P., Ramig, L., Mayberg, H., Cook, C., et al. (1999). A PET study of functional reorganization of premotor regions in Parkinson's disease following intensive voice treatment (LSVT®) [Abstract]. *Neurology, 52*(6, Suppl. 2), A348–A349.

Logemann, J. A., & Fisher, H. B. (1981). Vocal tract control in Parkinson's disease: Phonetic feature analysis of misarticulations. *Journal of Speech and Hearing Disorders, 46,* 348–352.

Logemann, J., Fisher, H., Boshes, B., & Blonsky, E. (1978). Frequency and concurrence of vocal tract dysfunctions in the speech of a large sample of Parkinson's patients. *Journal of Speech and Hearing Disorders, 43,* 47–57.

Ludlow, C. L., & Bassich, C. J. (1983). Relationships between perceptual ratings and acoustic measures of lypokinetic speech. In M. R. McNeil, J. C. Rosenbek, & A. E. Aronson (Eds.), *Dysarthria of speech: Physiology-acoustics-linguistics-management* (pp. 163–195). San Diego, CA: College-Hill Press.

Luschei, E. S., Ramig, L. O., Baker, K. L., & Smith, M. E. (1999). Discharge characteristics of laryngeal single motor units during phonation in young and older adults and in persons with Parkinson disease. *Journal of Neurophysiology, 81,* 2131–2139.

Mahler, M., & Cummings, J. (1990). Alzheimer disease and the dementia of Parkinson disease: Comparative investigations. *Alzheimer Disease and Associated Disorders, 4,* 133–149.

Mann, D. C., Pearce, L. A., & Waterbury, L. D. (1971). Amantadine for Parkinson's disease. *Neurology, 21,* 958–962.

Mark, M. H., Sage, J. I., Dickson, D. W., Schwarz, K. O., & Duvoisin, R. C. (1992). Levodopa-nonresponsive Lewy body parkinsonism: Clinicopathologic study of two cases. *Neurology, 42,* 1323–1327.

Markham, A., & Benfield, P. (1997). Pergolide: A review of its pharmacology and therapeutic use in Parkinson's disease. *Central Nervous System Drugs, 7,* 328–340.

Matsumoto, K., Shichijo, F., & Fukami, T. (1984). Long-term follow-up review of cases of Parkinson's disease after unilateral or bilateral thalamotomy. *Journal of Neurosurgery, 60,* 1033–1044.

Mawdsley, C., & Gamsu, C. V. (1971). Periodicity of speech in parkinsonism. *Nature, 231,* 315–316.

Merello, M., Nouzeilles, M. I., Kuzis, G., Cammarota, A., Sabe, L., Betti, O., et al. (1999). Unilateral radiofrequency lesion versus electrostimulation of posteroventral pallidum: A prospective randomized comparison. *Movement Disorders, 14,* 50–56.

Meyers, P. (1976). Comparative neurology of vocalization and speech: Proof of a dichotomy. *Annals of the New York Academy of Sciences, 280,* 745–757.

Meyers, R. (1940). Surgical procedures for postencephalitic tremor, with notes on the physiology of premotor fibers. *Archives of Neurology and Psychiatry, 44,* 455–457.

Meyers, R. (1942). Surgical interruption of the pallidofugal fibers: Its effect on the syndrome of paralysis agitans and technical considerations in its application. *New York State Journal of Medicine, 42,* 317–325.

Middleton, F. A., & Strick, P. L. (2000). Basal ganglia and cerebellar loops: Motor and cognitive circuits. *Brain Research Review, 3,* 236–250.

Montastruc, J. L., Rascol, O., & Senard, J. M. (1993). Current status of dopamine agonists in Parkinson's disease management. *Drugs, 46,* 384–393.

Montastruc, J. L., Rascol, O., & Senard, J. M. (1997). Glutamate antagonists and Parkinson's disease: A review of clinical data. *Neuroscience Biobehavioral Review, 21,* 477–480.

Moriyama, E., Beck, H., & Miyamoto, T. (1999). Long-term results of ventrolateral thalamotomy for patients with Parkinson's disease. *Neurologia Medico-Chirugica, 39,* 350–356.

Muller, J., Wenning, G. K., Verny, M., McKee, A., Chaudhuri, K. R., Jellinger, K., et al. (2001). Progression of dysarthria and dysphagia in postmortem-confirmed Parkinsonian disorders. *Archives of Neurology, 58,* 259–264.

Mutch, W. J., Strudwick, A., & Roy, S. K. (1986). Parkinson's disease: Disability, review, and management. *British Medical Journal, 293,* 675–677.

Myllyla, V. V., Sotaniemi, K. A., Vuorinen, J. A., & Heinonen, E. H. (1993). Selegiline in de novo Parkinsonian patients—The Finnish study. *Movement Disorders, 8,* S41–S44.

Mytilineou, C., Leonardi, E. K., Radcliffe, P. M., Heinonen, E. H., Han, S. K., Werner, P., et al. (1998). Deprenyl and desmethylselegiline protect mensencephalic neurons from toxicity induced by glutathione depletion. *Journal of Pharmacology and Experimental Therapeutics, 284,* 700–706.

Mytilineou, C., Radcliffe, P. M., & Olanow, C. W. (1997). L-(-)-desmethylselegiline, a metabolite of selegiline [L-(-)-deprenyl], protects mesencephalic dopamine neurons from excitotoxicity in vitro. *Journal of Neurochemistry, 68,* 434–436.

Nagaseki, Y., Shibazaki, T., Hirai, T., Kawashima, Y., Hirato, M., Wada, H., et al. (1986). Long-term follow-up results of selective VIM-thalamotomy. *Journal of Neurosurgery, 65,* 296–302.

Nakano, K. K., Zubick, H., & Tyler, H. R. (1973). Speech defects of parkinsonian patients: Effects of levodopa therapy on speech intelligibility. *Neurology, 23,* 865–870.

Naudin, B., Bonnet, J. J., & Costentin, J. (1995). Acute L-dopa pre-treatment potentiates 6-hydroxydopamine-induced toxic effects on nigro-striatal dopamine neurons in mice. *Brain Research, 701*, 151–157.

Netsell, R., Daniel, B., & Celesia, G. G. (1975). Acceleration and weakness in Parkinsonian dysarthria. *Journal of Speech and Hearing Disorders, 40*, 170–178.

Nutt, J. G., Woodward, W. R., Hammerstad, J. P., Carter, J. H., & Anderson, J. L. (1984). The "on-off" phenomenon in Parkinson's disease: Relation to levodopa absorption and transport. *New England Journal of Medicine, 310*, 483–488.

Olanow, C. W. (2000). Tolcapone and hepatotoxic effects. *Archives of Neurology, 57*, 263–267.

Olanow, C. W., & Calne, D. (1992). Does selegiline monotherapy in Parkinson's disease act by symptomatic or protective mechanisms? *Neurology, 42*, 13–26.

Olanow, C. W., & Koller, W. C. (1998). An algorithm (decision tree) for the management of Parkinson's disease: Treatment guidelines. *American Academy of Neurology, 50*, S1–S57.

Olanow, C. W., Schapira, A. H., & Rascol, O. (2000). Continuous dopamine-receptor stimulation in early Parkinson's disease. *Trends in Neuroscience, 23*, S117–S126.

Oliver, L. C. (1949). Surgery in Parkinson's disease: Division of lateral pyramidal tract for tremor. *The Lancet, 1*, 910–913.

Ondo, W., Jankovic, J., Schwartz, K., Almaguer, M., & Simpson, R. K. (1998). Unilateral thalamic deep brain stimulation for refractory essential tremor and Parkinson's disease tremor. *Neurology, 51*, 1063–1069.

Pahwa, R., Wilkinson, S., Smith, D., Lyons, K., Miyawaki, E., & Koller, W. C. (1997). High-frequency stimulation of the globus pallidus for the treatment of Parkinson's disease. *Neurology, 49*, 249–253.

Pal, S., Bhattacharya, K. F., Agapito, C., & Chaudhuri, K. R. (2001). A study of excessive daytime sleepiness and its clinical significance in three groups of Parkinson's disease patients taking pramipexole, cabergoline and levodopa mono and combination therapy. *Journal of Neural Transmitters, 108,* 71–77.

Parkes, J. D., Baxter, R. C., Marsden, C. D., & Rees, J. E. (1974). Comparative trial of benzhexol, amantadine, and levodopa in the treatment of Parkinson's disease. *Journal of Neurology, Neurosurgery, and Psychiatry, 37,* 422–426.

Parkinson Study Group. (1989). DATATOP: Multicenter controlled clinical trial in early Parkinson's disease. *Archives of Neurology, 46,* 1052–1060.

Parkinson Study Group. (1997). Entacapone improves motor fluctuations in levodopa-treated Parkinson's disease patients. *Annals of Neurology, 42,* 747–755.

Parkinson Study Group. (2000). Pramipexole vs levodopa as initial treatment for Parkinson disease: A randomized controlled trial. *Journal of the American Medical Association, 284,* 1931–1938.

Penny, J. B., & Young, A. B. (1983). Speculations on the functional anatomy of basal ganglia disorders. *Annual Review of Neuroscience, 6,* 73–94.

Pezzoli, G., Martignoni, E., Pacchetti, C., Angeleri, V., Lamberti, P., Muratorio, A., et al. (1995). A crossover, controlled study comparing pergolide with bromocriptine as an adjunct to levodopa for the treatment of Parkinson's disease. *Neurology, 45*(3, Suppl. 3), S22–S27.

Pitcairn, T., Clemie, S., Gray, J., & Pentland, B. (1990a). Impressions of parkinsonian patients from their recorded voices. *British Journal of Disorders of Communication, 25,* 85–92.

Pitcairn, T., Clemie, S., Gray, J., & Pentland, B. (1990b). Non-verbal cues in the self-presentation of parkinsonian patients. *British Journal of Clinical Psychology, 29,* 177–184.

Poluha, P. C., Teulings, H. L., & Brookshire, R. H. (1998). Handwriting and speech changes across the levodopa cycle in Parkinson's disease. *Acta Psychologica, 100,* 71–84.

Porges, S. (1995). Orienting in a defensive world: Mammalian modifications of our evolutionary heritage. A polyvagal theory. *Psychophysiology, 32,* 301–318.

Putnam, T. J. (1938). Relief from unilateral paralysis agitans by section of the pyramidal tract. *Archives of Neurologic Psychiatry, 40,* 1049–1050.

Putnam, T. (1940). Treatment of unilateral paralysis agitans by section of the lateral pyramidal tract. *Archives of Neurologic Psychiatry, 44,* 950–976.

Quaglieri, C. E., & Celesia, G. G. (1977). Effect of thalamotomy and levodopa therapy on the speech of Parkinson patients. *European Neurology, 15*(1), 34–39.

Quinn, N. P. (1984). Anti-parkinsonian drugs today. *Drugs, 28,* 236–262.

Rajput, A. H., Rozdilsky, B., & Rajput, A. (1991). Accuracy of clinical diagnosis in parkinsonism—A prospective study. *Canadian Journal of Neurological Science, 18,* 275–278.

Ramaker, C., van de Beek, W. J., Finken, M. J., & van Hilten, B. J. (2000). The efficacy and safety of adjunct bromocriptine therapy for levodopa-induced motor complications: A systematic review. *Movement Disorders, 15,* 56–64.

Ramig, L. O. (1992). The role of phonation in speech intelligibility: A review and preliminary data from patients with Parkinson's disease. In R. D. Kent (Ed.), *Intelligibility in speech disorders: Theory, measurement and management* (119–155). Amsterdam: John Benjamin.

Ramig, L. O., Bonitati, C., Lemke, J., & Horii, Y. (1994). Voice treatment for patients with Parkinson disease: Development of an approach and preliminary efficacy data. *Journal of Medical Speech-Language Pathology, 2,* 191–209.

Ramig, L. O., Countryman, S., O'Brien, C., Hoehn, M., & Thompson, L. (1996). Intensive speech treatment for patients with Parkinson's disease: Short and long term comparison of two techniques. *Neurology, 47,* 1496–1504.

Ramig, L., Countryman, S., Thompson, L., & Horii, Y. (1995). Comparison of two forms of intensive speech treatment for Parkinson disease. *Journal of Speech and Hearing Research, 38,* 1232–1251.

Ramig, L. O., & Dromey, C. (1996). Aerodynamic mechanisms underlying treatment-related changes in SPL in patients with Parkinson disease. *Journal of Speech and Hearing Research, 39,* 798–807.

Ramig, L. O., Dromey, C., Johnson, A., Scherer, et al. (1994, March). *The effects of phonatory, respiratory and articulatory treatment on speech and voice in Parkinson's disease.* Presentation at the Speech Motor Control conference, Sedona, AZ.

Ramig, L. O., Fox, C. M., Countryman, S., Sapir, S., & Spielman, J. (2000, November). Why treat phonation in motor speech disorders? Paper presented at the annual conference of the American Speech-Language-Hearing Association, Washington, DC.

Ramig, L. O., Pawlas, A., & Countryman, S. (1995). *The Lee Silverman Voice Treatment (LSVT): A practical guide to treating the voice and speech disorders in Parkinson disease.* Iowa City, IA: National Center for Voice and Speech.

Ramig, L. O., Sapir, S., Baker, K., Hinds, S., Spielman, J., Brisbie, A., et al. (2000, March). *The "big picture" on the role of phonation in the treatment of individuals with motor speech disorders: Or "what's up with loud?"* Paper presented at the Motor Speech Conference, San Antonio, TX.

Ramig, L. O., Sapir, S., Countryman, S., Pawlas, A. A., O'Brien, C., Hoehn, M., et al. (2001). Intensive voice treatment (LSVT®) for individuals with Parkinson's disease: A 2 year follow-up. *Journal of Neurology, Neurosurgery, and Psychiatry, 71,* 493–498.

Ramig, L. O, Sapir, S., Fox, C., & Countryman, S. (2001). Changes in SPL following intensive voice treatment (LSVT®) in individuals with Parkinson disease: Comparison with untreated patients and with age-matched normal controls. *Movement Disorders, 16,* 79–83.

Rascol, O., Brooks, D. J., Korczyn, A. D., De Deyn, P. P., Clarke, C. E., & Lang, A. E. (2000). A five-year study of the incidence of dyskinesia in patients with early Parkinson's disease who were treated with ropinirole or levodopa. *New England Journal of Medicine, 342,* 1484–1491.

Reynolds, G. P., Elsworth, J. D., Blau, K., Sandler, M., Lees, A. J., & Stern, G. M. (1978). Deprenyl is metabolized to methamphetamine and amphetamine in man. *British Journal of Clinical Pharmacology, 6,* 542–544.

Rigrodsky, S., & Morrison, E. B. (1970). Speech changes in parkinsonism during L-dopa therapy: Preliminary findings. *Journal of the American Geriatric Society, 18,* 142–151.

Rinne, U. K. (1989). Lisuride, a dopamine agonist in the treatment of early Parkinson's disease. *Neurology, 39,* 336–339.

Rinne, U. K., Bracco, F., Chouza, C., Dupont, E., Gershanik, O., Martimasso, J. F., et al. (1998). Early treatment of Parkinson's disease with cabergoline delays the onset of motor complications: Results of a double-blind levodopa controlled trial. *Drugs, 55*(Suppl. 1), 23–30.

Rinne, U. K., Larsen, J. P., Siden, A., & Worm-Petersen, J. (1998). Entacapone enhances the response to levodopa in parkinsonian patients with motor fluctuations. *Neurology, 51,* 1309–1314.

Rinne, U. K., Siirtola, T., & Sonninen, V. (1978). L-deprenyl treatment of on-off phenomena in Parkinson's disease. *Journal of Neural Transmitters, 43,* 253–262.

Robey, R. R., & Schultz, M. (1998). A model for conducting clinical-outcomes research: An adaptation of the standard protocol for use in aphasiology. *Aphasiology, 12,* 787–810.

Rodriguez-Oroz, M. C., Gorospe, A., Guridi, J., Ramos, E., Linazasoro, G., Rodriguez-Palmero, M., et al. (2000). Bilateral deep brain stimulation of the subthalamic nucleus in Parkinson's disease. *Neurology, 55,* S45–S51.

Rosenbek, J. C., & LaPointe, L. L. (1985). The dysarthrias: Description, diagnosis, and treatment. In D. F. Johns (Ed.), *Clinical man-*

agement of neurogenic communicative disorders (2nd ed., pp. 97–152). Boston: Little, Brown.

Rubow, R. T., & Swift, E. (1985). A microcomputer-based wearable biofeedback device to improve transfer of treatment in Parkinsonian dysarthria. *Journal of Speech and Hearing Disorders, 50,* 178–185.

Sabe, L., Salvarezza, F., Garcia, C. A., Leiguarda, R., & Starkstein, S. (1995). A randomized, double-blind, placebo-controlled study of bromocriptine in nonfluent aphasia. *Neurology, 45,* 2272–2274.

Sandyk, R. (1997). Speech impairment in Parkinson's disease is improved by transcranial application of electromagnetic fields. *International Journal of Neuroscience, 92*(1–2), 63–72.

Sapir, S., Pawlas, A. A., Ramig, L. O., Countryman, S., O'Brien, C., Hoehn, M., et al. (in press). Speech and voice abnormalities in Parkinson disease: Relation to severity of motor impairment, duration of disease, medication, depression, gender, and age. *Journal of Medical Speech-Language Pathology.*

Sapir, S., Pawlas, A., Seeley, E., Fox, C., & Corboy, J. (in press). Effects of intensive phonatory-respiratory treatment (LSVT) on voice in individuals with multiple sclerosis. *Journal of Medical Speech-Language Pathology.*

Sapir, S., Ramig, L. O., Hoyt, P., Countryman, S., O'Brien, C., & Hoehn, M. (1999, October). *Phonatory-respiratory effort (LSVT®) vs. respiratory effort treatment for hypokinetic dysarthria: Comparing speech loudness and quality before and 12 months after treatment.* Paper presented to the Academy of Neurology, Vancouver.

Sarno, M. T. (1968). Speech impairment in Parkinson's disease. *Archives of Physical Medicine and Rehabilitation, 49,* 269–275.

Schapira, A. H. (2000). Sleep attacks (sleep episodes) with pergolide. *The Lancet, 355,* 1332–1333.

Schapira, A. H., Obeso, J. A., & Olanow, C. W. (2000). The place of COMT inhibitors in the armamentarium of drugs for the treatment of Parkinson's disease. *Neurology, 55,* S65–S68.

Schmidt, R. A. (1975). A schema theory of discrete motor skill learning. *Psychological Review, 82,* 225–260.

Schmidt, R. A. (1988). *Motor control and learning.* Champaign, IL: Human Kinetics.

Schmidt, R. A., & Lee, T. D. (1999). *Motor control and learning: A behavioral emphasis.* Champaign, IL: Human Kinetics.

Schrag, A., Samuel, M., Caputo, E., Scaravilli, T., Troyer, M., Marsden, C., et al. (1999). Unilateral pallidotomy for Parkinson's disease: Results after more than 1 year. *Journal of Neurology, Neurosurgery, and Psychiatry, 67,* 511–517.

Schulman, R. (1989). Articulatory dynamics of loud and normal speech. *Journal of the Acoustical Society of America, 85,* 295–312.

Schulz, G. M., Greer, M., & Friedman, W. (2000). Changes in vocal intensity in Parkinson's disease following pallidotomy surgery. *Journal of Voice, 14,* 589–606.

Schulzer, M., Mak, E., & Calne, D. B. (1992). The antiparkinson efficacy of deprenyl derives from transient improvement that is likely to be symptomatic. *Annals of Neurology, 32,* 795–798.

Schuurman, P. R., Bosch, D. A., Bossuyt, P. M., Bonsel, G., Someren, E., de Bie, R., et al. (2000). A comparison of continuous thalamic stimulation and thalamotomy for suppression of severe tremor. *New England Journal of Medicine, 342,* 461–468.

Schwab, R. S., Amador, L. V., & Lettvin, J. Y. (1951). Apomorphine in Parkinson's disease. *Transactions of the American Neurological Association, 76,* 251–253.

Scott, S., & Caird, F. L. (1983). Speech therapy for Parkinson's disease. *Journal of Neurology, Neurosurgery, and Psychiatry, 46,* 140–144.

Shea, B. R., Drummond, S. S., Metzer, W. S., & Krueger, K. M. (1993). Effect of selegiline on speech performance in Parkinson's disease. *Folia Phoniatrica, 45,* 40–46.

Smith, M. E., Ramig, L. O., Dromey, C., Perez, K. S., & Samandari, R. (1995). Intensive voice treatment in Parkinson disease: Laryngostroboscopic findings. *Journal of Voice, 9,* 453–459.

Solomon, N. P., & Hixon, T. J. (1993). Speech breathing in Parkinson's disease. *Journal of Speech and Hearing Research, 36,* 294–310.

Solomon, N. P., McKee, A. S., Larson, K. J., Nawrocki, M. D., Tuite, P. J., Eriksen, S., et al. (2000). Effects of bilateral pallidal stimulation on speech in three men with severe Parkinson's disease. *American Journal of Speech-Language Pathology, 9,* 241–256.

Spiegel, E. A., Wycis, H. T., Marks, M., & Lee, A. J. (1946). Stereotactic aparatus for operations in human brain. *Science, 106,* 349–350.

Spielman, J., Ramig, L., & Borod, J. (2001). *Effects of intensive voice therapy on facial expression in Parkinson disease.* Unpublished manuscript.

Spielman, J., Ramig, L. O., Story, B., & Fox, C. M. (2000, November). *Expansion of vowel space in Parkinson's disease following LSVT®.* Poster presented at the annual conference of the American Speech-Language-Hearing Association, Washington, DC.

Stellar, S., & Cooper, I. S. (1968). Mortality and morbidity in cryothalamectomy for parkinsonism: A statistical study of 2868 consecutive operations. *Journal of Neurosurgery, 28,* 459–467.

Stelmach, G. E. (1991). Basal ganglia impairment and force control. In J. Requin & G. E. Stelmach (Eds.), *Tutorial in motor neuroscience* (pp. 216–232). Amsterdam, The Netherlands: Kluwer.

Stemple, J. (1993). *Voice therapy: Clinical studies.* St. Louis, MO: Mosby Year Book.

Stewart, C., Winfield, L., Hunt, A., Bressman, S. B., Fahn, S., Blitzer, A., et al. (1995). Speech dysfunction in early Parkinson's disease. *Movement Disorders, 10,* 562–565.

Tamaki, A., Matsuo, Y., Yanagihara, T., & Abe, K. (2000). Influence of thoracoabdominal movement on pulmonary function in patients with Parkinson's disease: Comparison with healthy subjects. *Neurorehabilitation and Neural Repair, 14*(1), 43–47.

Tasker, R. R., Siqueira, J., Hawrylyshyn, P., & Organ, L. W. (1983). What happened to VIM thalamotomy for Parkinson's disease? *Applied Neurophysiology, 46,* 68–83.

Vaamonde, J., Luquin, M. R., & Obeso, J. A. (1991). Subcutaneous lisuride infusion in Parkinson's disease: Response to chronic administration in 34 patients. *Brain, 114*, 601–617.

Verdolini, K. (1997). Principles of skill acquisition: Implication for voice training. In M. Hampton & B. Acker (Eds.), *The vocal vision: View on voice* (pp. 65–80). New York: Applause.

Volkmann, J., Allert, N., Voges, J., Weiss, P. H., Freund, H. J., & Sturm, V. (2001). Safety and efficacy of pallidal or subthalamic nucleus stimulation in advanced PD. *Neurology, 56*, 548–551.

Ward, E. C., Theodoros, D. G., & Murdoch, B. (2000). *Changes in articulatory pressures following the Lee Silverman Voice Treatment Program.* Paper presented at the Conference on Motor Speech, San Antonio, TX.

Weiner, W. J., & Lang, A. E. (1989). *Movement disorders: A comprehensive survey.* Mount Kisco, NY: Futura.

Wenning, G. K., Ben Shlomo, Y., Hughes, A., Daniel, S. E., Lees, A., & Quinn, N. P. (2000). What clinical features are most useful to distinguish definite multiple system atrophy from Parkinson's disease? *Journal of Neurology, Neurosurgery, and Psychiatry, 68*, 434–440.

Wenning, G. K., Ben Shlomo, Y., Magalhaes, M., Daniel, S. E., & Quinn, N. P. (1995). Clinicopathological study of 35 cases of multiple system atrophy. *Journal of Neurology, Neurosurgery, and Psychiatry, 58*, 160–166.

Wertz, R. T. (1978). Neuropathologies of speech and language: An introduction to patient management. In D. F. Johns (Ed.), *Clinical management of neurogenic communicative disorders* (pp. 1–100). Boston: Little, Brown.

Whittier, J. R., & Mettler, F. A. (1949). Studies on subthalamus of rhesus monkey: Hyperkinesia and other physiological effects of subthalamic lesions, with special reference to the subthalamic nucleus of Luys. *Journal of Comparative Neurology, 90*, 319–372.

Wohlert, A., & Hammen, V. (2000). Lip muscle activity related to speech rate and loudness. *Journal of Speech, Language, and Hearing Research, 43*, 1229–1239.

Yamamoto, T., Katayama, Y., Fukaya, C., Kurihara, J., Oshima, H., & Kasai, M. (2000). Thalamotomy caused by cardioversion in a patient treated with deep brain stimulation. *Stereotactic Functional Neurosurgery, 74,* 73–82.

Yang, H., & Neff, N. H. (1974). The monoamine oxidases of brain: Selective inhibition with drugs and the consequences for the metabolism of the biogenic amines. *Journal of Pharmacological and Experimental Therapy, 189,* 733–740.

Yelnik, J., Damier, P., Bejjani, B. P., Francois, C., Gervais, D., Dormont, D., et al. (2000). Functional mapping of the human globus pallidus: Contrasting effect of stimulation in the internal and external pallidum in Parkinson's disease. *Neuroscience, 101,* 77–87.

Yorkston, K. M. (1996). Treatment efficacy: Dysarthria. *Journal of Speech and Hearing Research, 39,* S46–S57.

Yorkston, K. M., Beukelman, D. R., & Bell, K. R. (1988). *Clinical measurement of dysarthric speakers.* Boston: College-Hill Press.

Young, R. F., Jacques, S., Mark, R., Kopyov, O., Copcutt, B., Posewitz, A., et al. (2000). Gamma knife thalamotomy for treatment of tremor: Long-term results. *Journal of Neurosurgery, 93*(Suppl. 3), 128–135.

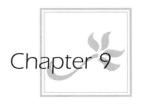

Chapter 9

Systemic Illness

Effects on the Larynx

Glendon M. Gardner and Barbara Jacobson

Gardner and Jacobson state that the most common lesions to affect the voice are benign lesions of the vocal folds, such as nodules, polyps, cysts, and scarring. All of these lesions represent a local laryngeal abnormality of structure and function. According to the authors, a variety of less common illnesses exist that can be systemic or localized to the larynx and may also affect the voice. Gardner and Jacobson stress how important it is for professionals who treat voice disorders to be aware of these diseases so that they may be diagnosed and treated properly and so that the dysphonias are addressed in the right context. In this chapter, the authors define each disease, describe its effect on the larynx and voice, and present treatment options. Specific concerns for speech–language pathologists follow.

1. *How are the symptoms and vocal fold behaviors differentiated among dysphonias associated with systemic disease processes?*

2. *What might the role of the speech–language pathologist be in treating dysphonias associated with systemic disease? Would it be considered short-term or long-term management and why? Choose three disease states to support your thoughts.*

The most common lesions to affect the voice are benign lesions of the vocal folds. Each of these lesions is a local laryngeal abnormality of structure.

Amyloidosis

Amyloid refers to lesions in which there is an extracellular deposit of fibrillar proteins. Von Rokitansky first described the condition in 1842 in a case that involved the liver and spleen (O'Halloran & Lusk, 1994). The first description of amyloidosis of the larynx was in 1873 by Borow. The disease may be localized to one organ or may be systemic, meaning many organs within the body are simultaneously affected. Secondary amyloidosis consists of amyloidosis in association with another systemic illness, such as multiple myeloma, tuberculosis, or an autoimmune disease. Primary amyloidosis does not have that association. The most important aspect of evaluating patients with this condition is ruling out these other associated serious and potentially fatal illnesses. The most common amyloidosis is the systemic form associated with multiple myeloma (Walker, Courey, & Ossoff, 1996). This condition may present in childhood or old age and affects men and women equally (Chen, 1989).

The larynx can be a site for primary localized amyloidosis, but it represents only 1% of all benign laryngeal lesions (Chen, 1989). When laryngeal involvement does occur, it is usually localized. The supraglottis is the most commonly involved structure, followed by the subglottis, ventricle, true vocal folds, and aryepiglottic folds (Lewis, Olsen, Kurtin, & Kyle, 1992).

Many individuals with laryngeal amyloidosis initially complain of change in vocal quality (Mitrani & Biller, 1985). Secondary complaints are frequently associated with airway obstruction, stridor, and shortness of breath. These symptoms may exist as early as 5 years prior to an actual diagnosis (Lewis et al., 1992). Endoscopic examination of the larynx may reveal either a diffuse submucosal swelling with a yellowish or yellowish-gray color or a more discrete submucosal polypoid lesion (Chen, 1989; Graamans & Lubsen, 1985; Lewis et al., 1992; Mitrani & Biller, 1985). Occasionally a thicker, red lesion is seen (Walker et al., 1996; see Figures 9.1A & 9.1B).

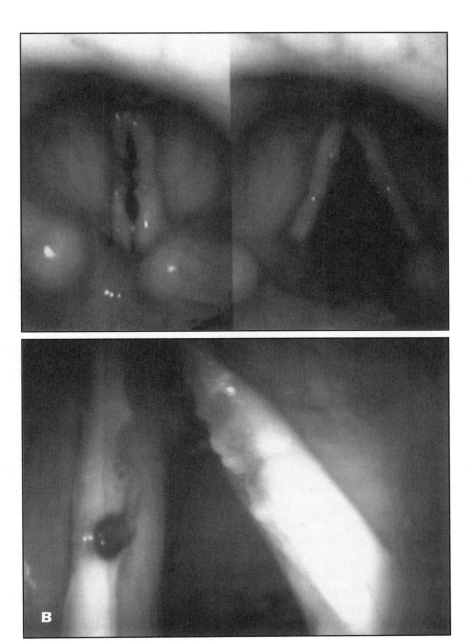

Figure 9.1. Amyloidosis of the true vocal folds. A. View with 70° telescope in clinic (anterior is down in picture). B. Intraoperative view. Note irregularities of the medial edges of both vocal folds. The number of lesions and the asymmetric distribution differentiate them from typical vocal fold nodules (anterior is up in picture).

Following detection, the lesion is excised or, if too widespread to allow for excision via microlaryngoscopy, it is biopsied. Excision occurs if the lesion is discrete and small. Histologic examination will confirm a diagnosis of amyloidosis, and further workup is then conducted to rule out systemic amyloidosis and the other diseases associated with secondary amyloidosis.

Treatment of primary localized laryngeal amyloidosis is surgical and is tailored to the nature of the lesion and the primary complaints of the patient. For a discrete lesion on the vocal folds, a complete but precise excision should be performed, with either a carbon dioxide laser or microdissection instruments. There are no reported cases of malignant degeneration; therefore, wide excision is not indicated. Incomplete excision, however, will often result in recurrence of the lesion and the symptoms. Diffuse lesions may cause airway obstruction and are more difficult to treat. Severe supraglottic involvement has been treated with supraglottic laryngectomy (Mitrani & Biller, 1985). Circumferential glottic or subglottic involvement may be safely treated with an endoscopic staged approach in which a different wedge of tissue is excised at each setting (Walker et al., 1996). Other rarely reported effects of laryngeal amyloidosis include the development of a laryngocele (Aydin, Ustundag, Iseri, Ozkarakas, & Oguz, 1999) and unilateral vocal fold paralysis secondary to mediastinal amyloidosis (Conaghan, Chung, & Vaughan, 2000).

In reviewing case histories of 59 patients with primary systemic amyloidosis, Burroughs, Aronson, Duffy, and Kyle (1991) found that 81% had abnormal voice quality. Twenty-three patients who were endoscopically examined for dysphonia demonstrated no evidence of amyloid deposits in the larynx. In addition to voice changes, dysphagia can be another presenting symptom that is frequently associated with deposits in the supraglottis, larynx, and subglottis (Noguchi et al., 1999). The degree of dysphagia is proportional to the size of the lesion. Patients frequently present with slowly progressing symptoms based on the growth of the deposits.

For patients with amyloidosis, voice therapy is tailored to the extent of the surgical resection. When the lesion is supraglottic, resonance should be evaluated postoperatively to determine if there are significant changes that warrant treatment. When excision of the lesion directly affects the vocal folds, videostroboscopy is critical in determining the degree to which vibratory motion has been affected or preserved. After the foundations for improved voice production (appropriate vocal hygiene, posture, and voice use) have been established, voice therapy may proceed. Realistic goals are to achieve the most vocal fold adduction and vibration while preventing compensatory behaviors that are detrimental to voice quality. As with all postsurgical patients, the prognosis for a return to the premorbid voice level depends on factors such as the extent of the excision, patient motivation, and overall physical health of the patient.

Wegener's Granulomatosis

Wegener's granulomatosis (WG) is a syndrome characterized by necrotizing granulomata and vasculitis (see Figure 9.2). The lesions involve the upper and lower respiratory tracts and the kidneys. The etiology is unknown but may be autoimmune.

In most patients, several systems, including the nasal and sinus cavities, the lungs, and the kidneys, are involved. Laryngeal involvement may be part of this multisystem disease, and the larynx may be the first organ involved or may be the only organ affected (Hellmann et al., 1987; Langford et al., 1996). In systemic WG, the laryngeal component may develop from 3 to 12 years after the initial presentation (Waxman & Bose, 1986). Typically, the subglottis and trachea are involved, but the glottis and supraglottis are spared (McDonald, Neel, & DeRemee, 1982). Subglottic stenosis occurs in 16% of patients with WG and can develop while the remainder of the systemic disease is inactive (Langford et al., 1996). Data from the Langford et al. study indicated that patients with laryngeal WG most commonly complain of shortness of breath (79%), hoarseness (61%), and cough (23%).

Stridor may be present and may be inspiratory or biphasic (inspiratory and expiratory), depending on the severity and location of the stenosis relative to the thoracic cavity. Stenosis in the larynx and cervical trachea will usually cause inspiratory or biphasic stridor, whereas involvement of the thoracic trachea causes expiratory or biphasic stridor. On examination, the airway is noted to be narrowed, usually circumferentially. There is redundant, boggy tissue that may be red and fragile when palpated (Hellmann et al., 1987; McDonald et al., 1982). Diagnosis is made by detecting cytoplasmic patterns of antineutrophilic cytoplasmic autoantibodies (cANCA) in the blood and through a biopsy of the affected tissue, which demonstrates necrotizing granulomata or vasculitis (Yumoto, Saeki, & Kadota, 1997). Pulmonary function tests, specifically the flow-volume loop, are very helpful in measuring the severity of airway stenosis and for documenting progress (McDonald et al., 1982).

Medical treatment with glucocorticosteroids (e.g., prednisone) and cyclophosphamide may be effective for immunosupression of the disease. Surgery to preserve the airway is sometimes necessary despite aggressive medical therapy (McDonald et al., 1982). Dilation of the stenotic region, carbon dioxide laser incisions or excisions, intralesional steroid injections, tracheotomies, and laryngotracheoplasties with or without microvascular reconstructions are all op-

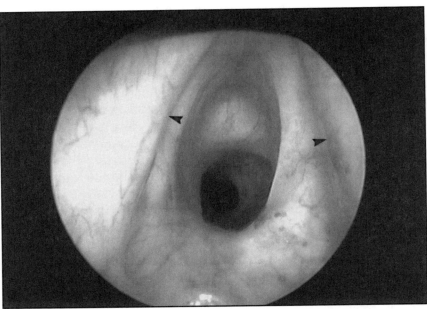

Figure 9.2. Wegener's granulomatosis of the subglottic airway and trachea seen via intraoperative endoscopy. The true vocal folds are in the foreground for reference. Arrows indicate the medial edge of each fold. Beyond the glottis, at least three areas of stenosis are seen (anterior is up in picture).

tions to treat subglottic stenosis due to WG. Many patients will require more than one procedure (Langford et al., 1996; Lebovics et al., 1992; McDonald et al., 1982).

Due to the presentation of most lesions in the subglottis and trachea, the otolaryngologist is the primary care professional for patients with WG. Airway obstruction is of the utmost concern, and the speech–language pathologist works closely with the physician to monitor for symptoms of a narrowing airway. Often, the speech–language pathologist acts supportively to manage voice production in concert with multiple surgical procedures. As with patients with amyloidosis, direct intervention and severity of voice disturbance are dependent on the size of the granuloma or on the extent of the excision if that treatment option is selected.

Sarcoidosis

Sarcoidosis is yet another granulomatous disease of unknown origin. It may be due to an infectious agent, an autoimmune response, or a response to chemicals (Neel & McDonald, 1982). The disease may affect the lungs, skin, lymph nodes, bone, liver, spleen, parotid gland, and lacrimal glands (Adkins & Park, 1989). The larynx is affected in 1% to 5% of all cases (Weisman, Canalis, & Powell, 1980). The disease usually appears in persons in their 30s to 50s and is more common in African Americans and women, but it has been reported in children (Adkins & Park, 1989; Kenny, Werkhaven, & Netterville, 2000). Sarcoidosis is most commonly detected through routine chest X-rays. The chest lymph nodes are broken down into three major areas: the hilar lymph nodes, the mediastinal lymph nodes, and the supraclavicular lymph nodes. In cases of sarcoidosis, the chest X-ray indicates enlarged hilar lymph nodes. Systemic symptoms include weight loss, fatigue, fever, and malaise.

Sarcoidosis is isolated to the larynx only in rare cases, although the patient may initially present with only laryngeal manifestations and later be found to have asymptomatic involvement of other organs. The most common laryngeal symptoms are hoarseness, dysphagia, and shortness of breath (Neel & McDonald, 1982). Globus sensation is also frequently present. Coughing may be due to laryngeal or pulmonary involvement.

In the vocal tract, the most commonly involved site is the supraglottis. An erythematous, edematous, nodular epiglottis with non-ulcerated mucosa is the characteristic appearance (Adkins & Park, 1989; Benjamin, Dalton, & Croxson, 1995; Neel & McDonald, 1982). Enlargement of the epiglottis and other supraglottic structures can lead to airway obstruction (Gerencer, Keohane, & Russell, 1998). Although the glottis itself is rarely involved, isolated masses on the vocal folds have been reported (McLaughlin, Spiegel, Selber, Gotsdiner, & Sataloff, 1999).

Sarcoidosis can also indirectly affect the larynx. Enlarged mediastinal lymph nodes may compress the left recurrent laryngeal nerve, causing a left vocal fold paralysis (el Kassimi, Ashour, & Vijayaraghavan, 1990; Jaffe, Bogomolski-Yahalom, & Kramer, 1994; Tobias, Santiago, & Williams, 1990; see Figure 9.3).

Noncaseating granulomas found on biopsy, accompanied by the appropriate clinical picture and laboratory findings, confirm the diagnosis. The clinical course of sarcoidosis commonly waxes and wanes without any treatment (McLaughlin et al., 1999). When sarcoidosis is symptomatic, systemic steroids are the initial treatment of choice. If the airway obstruction is severe, a tracheotomy may be required until the disease is brought under control (Neel & McDonald, 1982). Laryngeal disease can also be treated with a local, intralesional injection of steroids in an attempt to reduce the size of the lesion (Krespi, Mitrani, Husain, & Meltzer, 1987). Excision of the lesions, when well circumscribed, has also been described, but this procedure is rarely necessary (McLaughlin et al., 1999). Radiation therapy has also been used for localized laryngeal involvement (Fogel, Weissberg, Dobular, & Kirchner, 1984).

The treatment of dysphonia for patients with sarcoidosis can be approached in three ways, depending on the etiology of the dysphonia. Patients with discrete lesions of the vocal folds are managed conservatively, especially as the lesion(s) may resolve with steroid administration. Larger lesions that can compromise the airway require more extensive intervention, but good outcomes, even for professional voice users, may result (Gallivan & Landis, 1993). Patients with vocal fold immobility due to left recurrent laryngeal nerve compression (by mediastinal lymph node) or vagus neuropathy require approaches that concentrate on improving vocal fold adduction through pitch adjustments, modification of the effort for

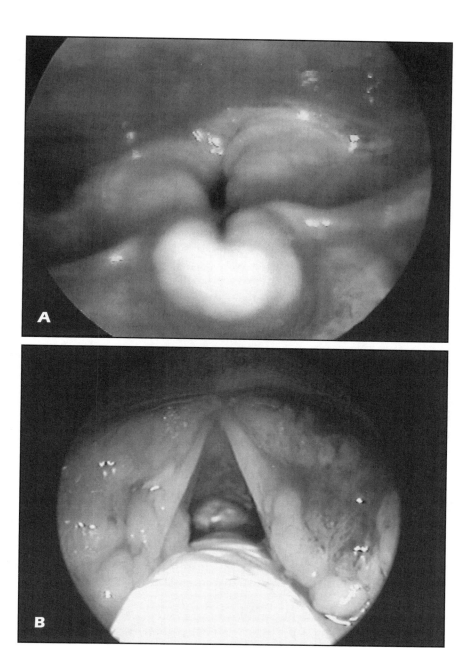

Figure 9.3. Sarcoidosis. A. Typical appearance of the supraglottis with thickening of the epiglottic and arytenoid mucosa and some limitation of the airway (anterior is down in picture). B. Operative view of another patient with sarcoidosis of both the true and false vocal folds (anterior is up in picture).

voice initiation, and environmental modifications during conversation (reducing ambient noise, positioning the listener). Improved vocal fold function depends on the extent of damage the nerve sustains from the mass (Castroagudin, Gonzalez-Quintela, Moldes, Forteza, & Barrio, 1999; Vasan & Allison, 1999). Patients who have late-stage sarcoidosis that affects the lungs exhibit symptoms of restrictive lung disease because the lung parenchyma becomes fibrotic. Functionally, this results in lower total lung capacities and residual volumes. These patients spend more time on inspiration than on expiration and have a higher respiratory rate than do healthy individuals. Consequently, they sound consistently out of breath. Patients with sarcoidosis have shorter inspiratory times than patients with emphysema or asthma and spend the least amount of time without speech during conversation (Lee, Loudon, Jacobson, & Stuebing, 1993). Lee (2000) described a treatment protocol with an asthmatic patient that may be adapted for use with a patient with sarcoidosis. Some modification of speech breathing patterns may be possible in combination with environmental manipulations and monitoring of phrase length.

The three possible causes of dysphonia may occur alone or in combination. The astute clinician carefully considers the underlying pathophysiology before developing a plan of treatment for a dysphonia that may have its origin in more than one site (e.g., lung and larynx) and may be due to structural or neurological causes.

Systemic Lupus Erythematosus

Systemic lupus erythematosus (SLE) is an autoimmune disease of unknown etiology. Antibodies directed against the patient's own nuclear components develop for an unknown reason. These antibodies attack a variety of organs and cause different levels of injury, depending on the stage of the disease. A diagnosis of SLE is made when the antineutrophilic antibody test is positive and a variety of symptoms or signs are present, including arthritis and arthralgias, fever, skin eruptions, lymphadenopathy, renal involvement, anorexia, nausea, vomiting, myalgias, pleuritis, and central nervous system abnormalities. Women are affected nine times as often as men, usually somewhere in their 20s to 50s, but children and the elderly may also be affected. The prevalence is 2 to 3 persons per 100,000, and the disease is often fatal.

The larynx is involved in one third of cases of SLE in many different ways (Teitel, MacKenzie, Stern, & Paget, 1992). Bamboo-joint-like nodules of the true vocal folds and hoarseness may be the only laryngeal manifestation of SLE (Sinclair, Rosen, & Noyek, 1976; Tsunoda & Soda, 1996; Woo, Mendelsohn, & Humphrey, 1995). Excision of these submucosal lesions usually results in improved voice. Edema and ulceration of the mucosa of the glottis and subglottis are the most common findings. These changes cause hoarseness and usually resolve with systemic corticosteroid therapy (Teitel et al., 1992) but can lead to acute airway obstruction from edema or from scarring and to eventual stenosis later in the course of the illness (see Figure 9.4).

The mainstay of treatment is long-term corticosteroid therapy. Although the bamboo-joint-like lesions of the vocal folds have resolved with the use of steroids alone, they more commonly need to

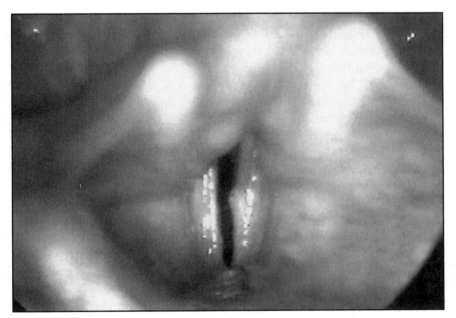

Figure 9.4. Systemic lupus erythematosis.

be excised. More diffuse laryngeal involvement, such as ulceration of multiple mucosal surfaces, requires supportive therapy with improved hydration, mucolytics, and control of gastroesophageal reflux disease and infection. Development of chronic scarring and airway compromise is treated as was described for WG previously.

Vocal fold paralysis, either unilateral or bilateral, can also occur in SLE (Saluja et al., 1989). Pulmonary hypertension with dilation of the pulmonary artery and pressure on the left recurrent laryngeal nerve has been proposed as the mechanism for left unilateral recurrent laryngeal nerve palsy. Another possibility is that vasculitis of the vasa nervosum (the vessels supplying blood to the nerve) causes the nerve injury, although this has never been proven (Teitel et al., 1992). In the majority of cases, the palsy responds to systemic corticosteroids. If the paralysis does not resolve, the larynx is treated as it would be for unilateral or bilateral vocal fold immobility of any etiology. For unilateral immobility with an incompetent glottis, the vocal fold is either augmented or medialized to improve closure. In cases of bilateral immobility with a limited airway, the airway must be expanded. This treatment must consider respiratory patency along with phonatory function when determining the size of airway expansion.

Before initiating voice therapy with patients with SLE and rheumatoid nodules, the diagnosis must be clear. Although the bamboo-joint-like nodules have a very typical appearance, occasionally patients will be referred for voice therapy with the diagnosis of vocal nodules (arising from voice abuse or misuse). For this case of nodules, medical and surgical treatments are more effective than voice therapy in restoring vibratory integrity (Tsunoda & Soda, 1996; Woo et al., 1995). Voice therapy does play a role in supporting optimum voice production pre- and postoperatively. Patients often complain of generalized fatigue, which may affect the effort used to speak, resulting in a laryngeal focus for voice production (i.e., less frontal voice focus, glottal fry). In our clinic, we have seen several women with lupus who use their voices professionally (e.g., telephone operator and singer). Voice conservation techniques teach judicious voice use to ensure that they can rely on their voices when needed. Finally, patients with SLE also present with cricoarytenoid joint arthritis, which will be addressed in the next section.

Rheumatoid Arthritis

Rheumatoid arthritis is also an autoimmune disease that affects 2% to 3% of the adult population and is sometimes part of SLE. Women are affected three times as often as men. Patients often experience systemic symptoms, such as fatigue, malaise, weight loss, sweating, and tachycardia. Stiffness of the joints of the hand, especially in the morning, is characteristic. Subcutaneous rheumatoid nodules may be present in various locations in the body, particularly in areas of repeated microtrauma, such as the elbows (Brooker, 1988).

Head and neck manifestations include inflammation of the temporomandibular, cervical, vertebral, and laryngeal joints. The cricoarytenoid (CA) joints may be involved in 25% to 53% of patients with rheumatoid arthritis (Brooker, 1988; Miller, Wanamaker, Hicks, & Tucker, 1994). Inflammation of these joints causes impairment of the arytenoid cartilage and, therefore, vocal fold movement. At postmortem examination, up to 87% of patients with rheumatoid arthritis have been found to have CA joint changes, but based on laryngoscopy, only 17% to 33% of such patients have clinical signs of laryngeal involvement, namely, posterior laryngeal inflammation and decreased arytenoid mobility (Jurik, Pedersen, & Nrgard, 1985).

Often one CA joint is involved before the other, resulting in unilateral vocal fold immobility. These patients have a weak, breathy voice and possibly aspiration with thin liquids. Later, when the second CA joint becomes fixed, the glottic space is narrow, and patients will complain mostly of shortness of breath. Patients will also have less specific complaints, such as a feeling of fullness or tension in the throat, odynophagia, odynophonia, or dysphagia (Montgomery, 1963; Montgomery & Goodman, 1980).

Physical findings include decreased motion of one or both vocal folds, edematous and erythematous mucosa over the arytenoid cartilages in the acute phase, or thickened mucosa in the chronic phase (Brooker, 1988). Fixation of the joint(s) is confirmed by palpating the arytenoid cartilages during direct laryngoscopy. The lack of movement of the arytenoids and the stiffness of the arytenoid cartilages are key signs that the joint is fixated. Rheumatoid nodules as described for SLE may also be seen (Brooker, 1988; Tsunoda & Soda, 1996; Woo et al., 1995).

Initial treatment includes a variety of medications, such as nonsteroidal anti-inflammatory drugs, systemic corticosteroids, gold salts, penicillamine, and immunosuppressives, such as methotrexate (Vrabec, Driscoll, & Chaljub, 1997). Some patients will respond to this medical regimen. Intrajoint steroid injection has been shown to help in some documented cases (Dockery, Sismanis, & Abedi, 1991; Habib, 1977).

Once one vocal fold has become immobile due to fixation of the CA joint, it is tempting to treat the condition much like unilateral vocal fold immobility due to any other etiology through medialization of the vocal fold to improve closure and voice. It must be assumed, however, that the contralateral vocal fold will eventually cease moving also, and any permanent and irreversible procedure that medializes one vocal fold will be detrimental to the airway. When both vocal folds are immobile, the primary issue becomes restoration of the airway. This usually involves an arytenoidectomy or partial cordectomy. Although these procedures improve the airway, the voice usually becomes weaker and breathy. Arthritic involvement of the cervical vertebrae must also be considered when proceeding with these procedures, which are usually done via direct laryngoscopy with extension of the neck. Reinnervation or electronic pacing of one of the immobile vocal folds is not an option, due to the mechanical fixation of the CA joint.

Dysphonia that results from CA joint arthritis in rheumatoid arthritis (or SLE) can be quite difficult to manage. After ensuring that general vocal health is good, the voice therapist works with the patient to identify patterns of dysphonia that correspond to exacerbations of rheumatoid arthritis, identify appropriate environmental manipulations, and select modifications of voice production that result in the least amount of discomfort. Intervention with the patient with CA joint fixation is restricted to searching for and establishing voice production that results in the best voice possible, considering the limited movement and potential bilateral involvement.

Relapsing Polychondritis

Relapsing polychondritis is a rare systemic disorder that affects cartilaginous structures and connective tissue. The etiology has not been absolutely determined but is thought to be autoimmune, with antibodies to collagen found in one third of patients and 25% of patients having another autoimmune disease (Batsakis & Manning, 1989). Men and women are affected equally, usually between 40 and 60 years of age (Lerner & Deeb, 1993). This disorder can mimic rheumatoid arthritis, and it sometimes occurs in patients with other autoimmune diseases, such as Sjögren's syndrome, systemic lupus erythematosus, and psoriatic and rheumatoid arthritis (Koufman, 1996).

In the head and neck, cartilage of the ears and nose is typically involved, but the eyes and inner ear may also be involved. The airway is involved in up to 50% of cases (Okuyama et al., 1998; Spraggs, Tostevin, & Howard, 1997). The middle and lower respiratory tracts may be involved at the supraglottis, the glottis, the trachea, and the primary or secondary bronchi. Presenting symptoms include cough, hoarseness, aphonia, choking sensation, shortness of breath, and tenderness over the larynx and trachea (Mohsenifar, Tashkin, Carson, & Bellamy, 1982; Spraggs et al., 1997). Respiratory distress has been reported as the initial presenting symptom in 18% of cases (Lerner & Deeb, 1993).

As with other autoimmune and inflammatory conditions, corticosteroids are the primary treatment method. Most patients require maintenance therapy with increased dosage during flare-ups. Other anti-inflammatory and immunosuppressant drugs have also been used.

When the integrity of the cartilage of the larynx and trachea has been destroyed, surgical intervention is required. Tracheotomy is the simplest approach, but intraluminal stents have also been used. The Montgomery T-tube allows for maintenance of the airway and acts as a conduit for air to reach the larynx, thus preserving voice, the quality of which depends on the extent of involvement of the larynx (Rogerson, Higgins, & Godfrey, 1987).

Reconstruction of the airway has not been very successful. Resection of the involved segment with primary anastamosis and reconstruction with a variety of flaps have been reported (Eliachar, Marcovich, & Har Shai, 1984; Rogerson et al., 1987). Patients who have undergone these procedures require aggressive medical therapy and sometimes still require stents to maintain the airway (Spraggs et al., 1997).

The natural history of this disease is quite variable. As with many systemic diseases, voice therapy is supportive and short term. Patients with relapsing polychondritis can present with severe symptoms that may resolve spontaneously (Younis & Casson, 2001); however, once there is airway compromise, there is little the voice therapist can do.

References

Adkins, H., & Park, Y. W. (1989). Pathologic quiz case 1. Sarcoidosis of the larynx. *Archives of Otolaryngology—Head & Neck Surgery, 115,* 1476–1478.

Aydin, O., Ustundag, E., Iseri, M., Ozkarakas, H., & Oguz, A. (1999). Laryngeal amyloidosis with laryngocele. *Journal of Laryngology & Otology, 113,* 361–363.

Batsakis, J., & Manning, J. (1989). Pathology consultation: Relapsing polychondritis. *Annals of Otology, Rhinology & Laryngology, 98,* 83–84.

Benjamin, B., Dalton, C., & Croxson, G. (1995). Laryngoscopic diagnosis of laryngeal sarcoid. *Annals of Otology, Rhinology & Laryngology, 104,* 529–531.

Borow, A. (1873). Amyloide degeneration von larynxtumorer; Canule sieber jahre lang getrager. *Arch Klin Chir* [Archives of Clinical Chiropractry], *15,* 242–246.

Brooker, D. S. (1988). Rheumatoid arthritis: Otorhinolaryngological manifestations. *Clinical Otolaryngology & Allied Sciences, 13,* 239–246.

Burroughs, E. I., Aronson, A. E., Duffy, J. R., & Kyle, R. A. (1991). Speech disorders in systemic amyloidosis. *British Journal of Disorders of Communication, 26,* 201–206.

Castroagudin, J. F., Gonzalez-Quintela, A., Moldes, J., Forteza, J., & Barrio, E. (1999). Acute reversible dysphagia and dysphonia as initial manifestations of sarcoidosis. *Hepato-Gastroenterology, 46,* 2414–2418.

Chen, K. T. (1989). Amyloidosis presenting in the respiratory tract. *Pathology Annual, 24* (Pt. 1), 253–273.

Conaghan, P., Chung, D., & Vaughan, R. (2000). Recurrent laryngeal nerve palsy associated with mediastinal amyloidosis. *Thorax, 55,* 436–437.

Dockery, K. M., Sismanis, A., & Abedi, E. (1991). Rheumatoid arthritis of the larynx: The importance of early diagnosis and corticosteroid therapy. *Southern Medical Journal, 84,* 95–96.

Eliachar, I., Marcovich, A., & Har Shai, Y. (1984). Rotary door flap in laryngotracheal reconstruction. *Archives of Otolaryngology— Head & Neck Surgery, 110,* 580–585.

el Kassimi, F. A., Ashour, M., & Vijayaraghavan, R. (1990). Sarcoidosis presenting as recurrent left laryngeal nerve palsy. *Thorax, 45,* 565–566.

Fogel, T. D., Weissberg, J. B., Dobular, K., & Kirchner, J. A. (1984). Radiotherapy in sarcoidosis of the larynx: Case report and review of the literature. *Laryngoscope, 94,* 1223–1225.

Gallivan, G. J., & Landis, J. N. (1993). Sarcoidosis of the larynx: Preserving and restoring airway and professional voice. *Journal of Voice, 7,* 81–94.

Gerencer, R. Z., Keohane, J. D., Jr., & Russell, L. (1998). Laryngeal sarcoidosis with airway obstruction. *Journal of Otolaryngology, 27,* 90–93.

Graamans, K., & Lubsen, H. (1985). Clinical implications of laryngeal amyloidosis. *Journal of Laryngology & Otology, 99,* 617–623.

Habib, M. A. (1977). Intra-articular steroid injection in acute rheumatoid arthritis of the larynx. *Journal of Laryngology & Otology, 91,* 909–910.

Hellmann, D., Laing, T., Petri, M., Jacobs, D., Crumley, R., & Stulbarg, M. (1987). Wegener's granulomatosis: Isolated involvement of the trachea and larynx. *Annals of the Rheumatic Diseases, 46,* 628–631.

Jaffe, R., Bogomolski-Yahalom, V., & Kramer, M. R. (1994). Vocal cord paralysis as the presenting symptom of sarcoidosis. *Respiratory Medicine, 88,* 633–636.

Jurik, A. G., Pedersen, U., & Nrgård, A. (1985). Rheumatoid arthritis of the cricoarytenoid joints: A case of laryngeal obstruction due to acute and chronic joint changes. *Laryngoscope, 95,* 846–848.

Kenny, T. J., Werkhaven, J., & Netterville, J. L. (2000). Sarcoidosis of the pediatric larynx. *Archives of Otolaryngology—Head & Neck Surgery, 126,* 536–539.

Koufman, J. A. (1996). *Infectious and inflammatory diseases of the larynx.* In J. J. Ballenger & J. B. Snow (Eds.), *Otorhinolaryngology* (15th ed., pp. 535–555). Philadelphia: Williams & Wilkins.

Krespi, Y. P., Mitrani, M., Husain, S., & Meltzer, C. J. (1987). Treatment of laryngeal sarcoidosis with intralesional steroid injection. *Annals of Otology, Rhinology & Laryngology, 96,* 713–715.

Langford, C. A., Sneller, M. C., Hallahan, C. W., Hoffman, G. S., Kammerer, W. A., Talar-Williams, C., et al. (1996). Clinical features and therapeutic management of subglottic stenosis in patients with Wegener's granulomatosis. *Arthritis & Rheumatism, 39,* 1754–1760.

Lebovics, R. S., Hoffman, G. S., Leavitt, R. Y., Kerr, G. S., Travis, W. D., Kammerer, W., et al. (1992). The management of subglottic stenosis in patients with Wegener's granulomatosis. *Laryngoscope, 102,* 1341–1345.

Lee, L. (2000). *Modification of speech breathing in a patient with chronic asthma.* In J. C. Stemple (Ed.), *Voice therapy: Clinical studies* (2nd ed., pp. 335–341). San Diego, CA: Singular.

Lee, L., Loudon, R. G., Jacobson, B. H., & Stuebing, R. (1993). Speech breathing in patients with lung disease. *American Review of Respiratory Disease, 147,* 1199–1206.

Lerner, D. M., & Deeb, Z. (1993). Acute upper airway obstruction resulting from systemic diseases. *Southern Medical Journal, 86,* 623–627.

Lewis, J. E., Olsen, K. D., Kurtin, P. J., & Kyle, R. A. (1992). Laryngeal amyloidosis: A clinicopathologic and immunohistochemical review. *Archives of Otolaryngology—Head & Neck Surgery, 106,* 372–377.

McDonald, T. J., Neel, H. B., III, & DeRemee, R. A. (1982). Wegener's granulomatosis of the subglottis and the upper portion of the trachea. *Annals of Otology, Rhinology & Laryngology, 91,* 588–592.

McLaughlin, R. B., Spiegel, J. R., Selber, J., Gotsdiner, D. B., & Sataloff, R. T. (1999). Laryngeal sarcoidosis presenting as an isolated submucosal vocal fold mass. *Journal of Voice, 13,* 240–245.

Miller, F. R., Wanamaker, J. R., Hicks, D. M., & Tucker, H. M. (1994). Cricoarytenoid arthritis and ankylosing spondylitis. *Archives of Otolaryngology—Head & Neck Surgery, 120,* 214–216.

Mitrani, M., & Biller, H. F. (1985). Laryngeal amyloidosis. *Laryngoscope, 95,* 1346–1347.

Mohsenifar, Z., Tashkin, D., Carson, S., & Bellamy, P. (1982). Pulmonary function in patients with relapsing polychondritis. *Chest, 81,* 711–717.

Montgomery, W. W. (1963). Cricoarytenoid arthritis. *Laryngoscope, 73,* 801–836.

Montgomery, W. W., & Goodman, M. L. (1980). Rheumatoid cricoarytenoid arthritis complicated by upper esophageal ulcerations. *Annals of Otology, Rhinology & Laryngology, 89,* 6–8.

Neel, H. B., III, & McDonald, T. J. (1982). Laryngeal sarcoidosis: Report of 13 patients. *Annals of Otology, Rhinology & Laryngology, 91,* 359–362.

Noguchi, T., Minami, K., Iwagaki, T., Takara, H., Sata, T., & Shigematsu, A. (1999). Anesthetic management of a patient with laryngeal amyloidosis. *Journal of Clinical Anesthesia, 11,* 339–341.

O'Halloran, L. R., & Lusk, R. P. (1994). Amyloidosis of the larynx in a child. *Annals of Otology, Rhinology & Laryngology, 103,* 590–594.

Okuyama, C., Ushijima, Y., Sugihara, H., Okitsu, S., Ito, H., & Maeda, T. (1998). Increased subglottic gallium uptake in relapsing polychondritis. *Journal of Nuclear Medicine, 39,* 1977–1979.

Rogerson, M., Higgins, E., & Godfrey, R. (1987). Tracheal stenosis due to relapsing polychondritis in rheumatoid arthritis. *Thorax, 42,* 905–906.

Saluja, S., Singh, R. R., Misra, A., Gairola, A. K., Prasad, K., Ahuja, G. K., et al. (1989). Bilateral recurrent laryngeal nerve palsy in systemic lupus erythematosus. *Clinical & Experimental Rheumatology, 7,* 81–83.

Sinclair, D. S., Rosen, P. S., & Noyek, A. M. (1976). Systemic lupus erythematosus with a vocal cord granulomatous nodule. *Journal of Otolaryngology, 5,* 337–342.

Spraggs, P. D., Tostevin, P. M., & Howard, D. J. (1997). Management of laryngotracheobronchial sequelae and complications of relapsing polychondritis. *Laryngoscope, 107,* 936–941.

Teitel, A. D., MacKenzie, C. R., Stern, R., & Paget, S. A. (1992). Laryngeal involvement in systemic lupus erythematosus. *Seminars in Arthritis & Rheumatism, 22,* 203–214.

Tobias, J. K., Santiago, S. M., & Williams, A. J. (1990). Sarcoidosis as a cause of left recurrent laryngeal nerve palsy. *Archives of Otolaryngology—Head & Neck Surgery, 116,* 971–972.

Tsunoda, K., & Soda, Y. (1996). Hoarseness as the initial manifestation of systemic lupus erythematosus. *Journal of Laryngology & Otology, 110,* 478–479.

Vasan, N. R., & Allison, R. S. (1999). Sarcoidosis presenting as hoarseness and dysphagia. *Australian and New Zealand Journal of Surgery, 69,* 751–753.

Vrabec, J. T., Driscoll, B. P., & Chaljub, G. (1997). Cricoarytenoid joint effusion secondary to rheumatoid arthritis. *Annals of Otology, Rhinology & Laryngology, 106,* 976–978.

Walker, P. A., Courey, M. S., & Ossoff, R. H. (1996). Staged endoscopic treatment of laryngeal amyloidosis. *Archives of Otolaryngology—Head & Neck Surgery, 114,* 801–805.

Waxman, J., & Bose, W. J. (1986). Laryngeal manifestations of Wegener's granulomatosis: Case reports and review of the literature. *Journal of Rheumatology, 13,* 408–411.

Weisman, R. A., Canalis, R. F., & Powell, W. J. (1980). Laryngeal sarcoidosis with airway obstruction. *Annals of Otology, Rhinology & Laryngology, 89,* 58–61.

Woo, P., Mendelsohn, J., & Humphrey, D. (1995). Rheumatoid nodules of the larynx. *Archives of Otolaryngology—Head & Neck Surgery, 113,* 147–150.

Younis, N., & Casson, I. F. (2001). Joint pains, hoarseness, and deafness. *Postgraduate Medical Journal, 77,* 270, 280–281.

Yumoto, E., Saeki, K., & Kadota, Y. (1997). Subglottic stenosis in Wegener's granulomatosis limited to the head and neck region. *Ear, Nose, & Throat Journal, 76,* 571–574.

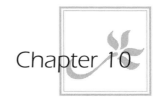

Chapter 10

Gastroesophageal/ Extraesophageal Reflux Disease

Medical, Behavioral, and Pharmacological Perspectives

Savita Collins and Robin Samlan

Collins and Samlan review the pathophysiology, clinical manifestations, diagnosis, and treatment of gastroesophageal reflux disease (GERD) and extraesophageal reflux disease (EERD). Emphasis is placed on the management of patients with these disorders and the importance of a team approach involving otolaryngologists, speech–language pathologists, gastroenterologists, pulmonologists, primary care specialists, and general surgeons.

1. *Identify four main parts that serve as a barrier to reflux. Define each.*

2. *What are the common findings on a laryngeal examination that are associated with GERD?*

3. *What are some of the limitations of the* dual pH probe *for detecting GERD?*

4. *How do the symptoms of EERD and GERD differ?*

5. *The role of the speech–language pathologist in the treatment of GERD is more secondary relative to the physician's role. Describe the recommendations of the speech–language pathologist to the patient in regard to prevention of EERD/GERD.*

Otolaryngologists and speech–language pathologists frequently care for patients with clinical problems of the aerodigestive tract that are associated with reflux of gastric contents beyond the stomach. Regurgitation of gastric material may play a role in the pathogenesis of many disorders.

Gastroesophageal reflux (GER) is defined as the movement of gastric material into the esophagus in the absence of belching or vomiting (Gaynor, 1988, 1991; Giacchi, Sullivan, & Rothstein, 2000). *Gastroesophageal reflux disease* (GERD) occurs when GER is associated with symptoms or complications. The consensus panel at the 1991 meeting of the American Bronchoesophagological Association promoted the use of the term *extraesophageal reflux* (EER) when discussing nonesophageal manifestations of regurgitation of gastric contents (Sasaki & Toohill, 2000).

It has been estimated that 30% of Americans suffer from GERD, with 7% to 10% of adults experiencing daily heartburn and 29% to 33% displaying weekly symptoms (Gaynor, 1991; Kaufman, 1991; Koufman, 1998; Shaker & Lang, 1997; Sontag, 1990). Between 25 million and 75 million people in the United States are affected by GERD, with 13% taking indigestion aids at least twice weekly (Sontag, 1990). GERD is not rare in children, and it has been diagnosed in 18% of children, with a higher incidence in children with esophageal atresia, tracheoesophageal fistula, or neurologic impairment (Zalzal & Tran, 2000). Unfortunately, accurate estimates of the incidence of EER are not available.

Pathophysiology

The esophagus is the conduit for the transfer of material from the pharynx to the stomach. It is a muscular tube with the proximal third made up of striated muscle and the distal two thirds composed of smooth muscle. The gatekeepers for ingress and egress of material are the upper and lower esophageal sphincters (UES and LES). The four main constituents of the barrier to reflux are the UES, LES, esophageal acid clearance, and epithelial resistance.

Upper Esophageal Sphincter

The UES is functionally defined as the area of the distal pharynx and proximal esophagus that maintains a closed pharyngoesophageal segment and opens during specific physiologic demands, such as swallowing and belching. Anatomically, it is composed of the cricopharyngeus, thyropharyngeus, and proximal cervical esophagus (Lang & Shaker, 1997; Pope, 1997). Unlike other muscular sphincters, the UES is not a complete muscular circle; instead, it is a C-shaped sling that attaches to the cricoid cartilage. The pharyngeal plexus innervates the UES and receives contributions from the vagus nerve (superior and recurrent laryngeal nerves), glossopharyngeal nerve, and the sympathetic nerves from the superior cervical ganglion (Lang & Shaker, 1997). Vagal stimulation produces relaxation of the UES. UES pressure is increased with acidification of the distal esophagus (Koufman, 1998; Lang & Shaker, 1997). This pressure is reduced in certain states, such as when a person is under general anesthetics or in a sleep state. Cigarette smoking and peppermint consumption are also associated with decreased UES pressure (Kaufman, 1998; Lang & Shaker, 1997). Kaufman (1998) noted that cigarette smoking and peppermint consumption produced a 50% reduction in UES resting pressure in healthy volunteers within minutes. The UES is the final gatekeeper in the antireflux barrier, and UES dysfunction may be associated with head and neck manifestations of EER. Deveney, Brenner, and Cohen (1993) noted an increased incidence of UES hypotonia in patients with pulmonary problems associated with EER.

Lower Esophageal Sphincter

The LES, which is the most critical antireflux defense mechanism (Dent, 1997; Gaynor, 1991), is located at the gastroesophageal junction and is not as anatomically distinct as the UES. Contraction of the UES results in circular closure that prevents egress of gastric contents, while relaxation of the UES occurs during swallowing, belching, and vomiting. The LES is anatomically surrounded by the diaphragmatic crura, which mechanically augments the sphincter mechanism and is believed to contribute to 25% of LES competence

(Koufman, 1998). Manometric measurements at the LES reflect the combined contributions of the esophageal LES and the diaphragmatic crura. The intrinsic resting pressure of the LES varies with the phase of respiratory cycle secondary to differential diaphragmatic contraction (Dent, 1997). During episodes of straining, LES pressure increases secondary to increased diaphragmatic activity, yielding an increased diaphragmatic squeeze of the LES (Dent, 1997; Pope, 1997). Hormonal control of LES activity is complex. Gastrin, pitressin, angiotensin II, and motilin increase contractile tone, whereas secretin, cholecystokinin, glucagon, and vasoactive intestinal peptide decrease LES pressure (Dent, 1997; Koufman, 1998).

In order to prevent GER, the LES must maintain a resting pressure that is higher than the gastric pressure. GER occurs when there is a reversal of this gastric-to-LES pressure gradient (Dent, 1997; Pope, 1997; Reynolds, 1996). Retrograde flow will occur with relaxation of the LES, chronic hypotonia of the LES, or increases in gastric pressure that overcome the LES resting pressure. Transient relaxation of the LES occurs in normal healthy adults and children, and it is the most critical mechanism in the production of GER (Dent, 1997). Dent showed that 63% to 74% of GER episodes were associated with transient LES relaxation. Chronic hypotonia of the LES is thought to be associated with GER episodes in a smaller percentage of patients, but it may be associated with more severe esophagitis. Lower LES resting pressures are seen in patients with CRST syndrome, scleroderma, and isolated Raynaud's phenomenon. Although chronic hypotonia of the LES results in more severe reflux, it is an uncommon mechanism for GERD (Reynolds, 1996). Large hiatal hernias may result in disruption of the relationship of the LES to the diaphragmatic crura. This may impair the ability of the LES to act as an antireflux barrier by removing the additional pressure generated by the squeeze of the diaphragm (Dent, 1997; Reynolds, 1996). Although hiatal hernias may play a role in GERD in some patients, not all patients with hiatal hernias have the disease (Gaynor, 1991). Table 10.1 lists agents that affect the LES pressure.

As stated previously, when gastric pressure exceeds LES pressure, reflux can occur. "Stress reflux" may occur with increased intraabdominal pressure during bending over, heavy lifting, straining, and coughing. Excessive gastric distension resulting in increased

Table 10.1

Factors Associated with Increased
and Decreased Lower Esophageal Sphincter Pressure

Increased LES pressure	Decreased LES pressure
Protein	Fat
Bethanechol	Carbohydrates
Metoclopramide	Alcohol
Antacids	Smoking
Alpha-adrenergic drugs	Carbaminatives (peppermint, spearmint)
	Theophylline
	Calcium channel blockers
	Nitrate drugs
	Atropine
	Beta-adrenergic drugs
	Dopamine
	Sedatives

Note. LES = lower esophageal sphincter.

gastric pressure can occur postprandially after a large meal and with severe gastroparesis. Impaired gastric emptying is more common in patients with GERD (Reynolds, 1996). Pregnancy is a risk factor for GERD secondary to increased abdominal pressure.

Antireflux Barriers

Because some GER is normal, mechanisms that clear and neutralize gastric contents when they pass into the esophagus exist. Esophageal peristaltic waves, along with the effect of gravity, act to mechanically clear the esophagus. Weakened or ineffective peristalsis allows for refluxed materials to come into contact with esophageal tissues for a longer time. Knight, Wells, and Parrish (2000) studied 100 patients with EER and noted that 52% had ineffective esophageal motility. Increased episodes of GER seen in patients with GERD when supine can be partially explained by loss of gravitational effects (Reynolds, 1996). Acidic refluxate left in the esophagus can be neutralized by gastric glandular secretions and buffering agents in saliva (Koufman, 1991, 1998; Reynolds, 1996). Xerostomia (dryness of the mouth) that can be caused by Sjögren's syndrome, certain medications, and previous radiotherapy abolishes this important antireflux barrier (Koufman, 1998; Reynolds, 1996). The low pH of gastric material is damaging to epithelium, and alkaline pH pancreatic and bile juices, when present, may result in tissue injury (Gaynor, 1991; Koufman, 1991).

When the aforementioned antireflux barriers fail, the severity of tissue damage will be determined by epithelial resistance factors. There are preepithelial, epithelial, and intracellular protective mechanisms. The epithelium is preceded by a mucus layer and an aqueous layer with a high bicarbonate content (Koufman, 1998). Mucus resists penetration by large molecules such as pepsin but does not prevent the ingress of acid. The aqueous layer is alkaline and buffers acid material. At the cellular level, the cell membrane and intracellular junctions resist acid and pepsin (Koufman, 1991). Different tissues have variable epithelial resistance, with lower esophageal epithelium being more resistant than respiratory epithelium (Reynolds, 1996). GER to a small degree in the hypopharynx or larynx may cause significant injury, whereas reflux to the same degree in the distal esophagus would be easily resisted (Reynolds, 1996). Hanson and Jiang (2000) postulated that the posterior glottis is especially susceptible to the effect of EER. They theorized that the cilia beat material to the posterior glottis, resulting in increased contact with refluxate and thus more injury to this epithelium.

Direct stimulation of sensory receptors in the larynx by aspirated or refluxed material can result in reflexive vocal fold adduction or laryngospasm (Bauman, Sandler, Schmidt, Maher, & Smith, 1994). This *laryngeal chemoreflex* is associated with bradycardia, central apnea, and hypotension (Zalzal & Tran, 2000). Partial or complete laryngospasm and cough can also be triggered by GER to the distal esophagus via a vagally mediated reflex (Bauman et al., 1994; Cucchiara et al., 1995; Gaynor, 1991; Shaker & Long, 1997). Laryngospasm associated with distal esophageal GER may also be associated with bronchospasm, increased secretions, tachycardia, and hypertension (Zalzal & Tran, 2000). These reflexes have implications for respiratory manifestations of EER and in the mechanisms involved in sudden infant death syndrome and recurrent laryn-gospasm.

Diagnostic Evaluation

History

Obtaining a detailed case history is very critical to both the diagno-sis and treatment of patients with EER. The clinician must identify not only symptoms but also behavioral and medical risk factors for EER. It is also critical to patient compliance with treatment to ac-tively involve the patient in identifying the risk factors that he or she will be able to modify. The second half of this chapter will dis-cuss the case history in greater detail.

Physical Examination and Laryngeal Endoscopy

A physical examination may yield several clues to EER. Observa-tions of the quality of voice, frequent throat clearing, cough, or stri-dor; muscle tension in extralaryngeal musculature; and general body habits are important to the evaluation. The larynx can be eval-uated through indirect laryngoscopy, along with rigid or flexible laryngoscopy. Videoendoscopy and stroboscopy are very useful for documenting treatment effects and for visualizing subtle signs as-sociated with reflux. Further discussion of stroboscopic findings in patients with EER is found later in this chapter.

The majority of laryngeal findings seen in patients with chronic laryngitis associated with EER are seen in the posterior larynx. Pos-terior laryngitis is manifested by edema, increased vascularity, and erythema of the posterior commissure and arytenoids (Haber-mann, Eherer, Lindbichler, Raith, & Friedrich, 1999; Hanson, Kamel, & Kahrilas, 1995; Toohill & Kuhn, 1997). Chronic irritation can re-sult in thickening of the posterior laryngeal mucosa, with hyper-keratosis or "pachydermia laryngeus" (Hanson et al., 1995; Toohill & Kuhn, 1997). Hanson et al. described this posterior mucosal thicken-ing with increased granularity and rough "cobblestone" appear-ance as "granular mucositis." Increased mucus formation and thickness, along with mucus stranding and pooling, may result from chronic irritation (Toohill & Kuhn, 1997). Laryngeal ulceration, granuloma formation, scarring, and stenosis may indicate more severe EER (Hanson & Jiang, 2000). Cherry and Margulies (1968) first identified EER of gastric acid as being associated with contact ulcers.

Hanson et al. (1995) examined 233 patients with chronic laryngitis. Videoendoscopic examination revealed that erythema of the posterior larynx was the most prevalent sign but also the most reversible with treatment of EER. Hanson et al. noted that more severe inflammation or longer duration of symptoms was associated with increasing vascularity and erythema extending into the remainder of the larynx and the supraglottis. In their patient population, posterior glottic mucosa thickening was the second most common finding. In some patients with severe EER and cough, Hanson et al. noted eschar formation over the posterior glottis, which they likened to a "mucosal burn injury." Seven percent of their patients were noted to have ulceration of the vocal processes or ulcer formation between the arytenoids, and 3% had granulomas. Patients with prominent throat-clearing behavior and chronic cough were more likely to demonstrate pachydermia laryngeus. Hanson et al. used the following grading scale: *mild*—mild posterior glottic erythema; *moderate*—marked erythema, stasis of secretions, and mucosal granularity; and *severe*—ulceration, granulation tissue, or hyperkeratosis of the larynx. In another study, Hanson and Jiang (2000) digitized endoscopic examinations of a large group of patients with chronic laryngitis and performed digital color analyses. They found a significant difference between their patients and control group members in the red index, with a significant decrease in this index when patients with chronic laryngitis were treated for EER.

Habermann et al. (1999) reviewed endoscopic findings for 29 patients with chronic dysphonia and chronic laryngitis and showed that alteration of posterior glottic mucosa and reddening of the posterior larynx were the most common findings. The authors noted significant improvement in these alterations with therapy. Alteration and reddening of the true vocal fold mucosa and false vocal folds were also noted to improve with treatment. Shaw and Searl (1997) assessed 96 patients who had symptoms suggestive of

EER and noted that posterior glottic edema, nodularity, and erythema were the most severe and frequent findings. Only 47% were noted to have ulceration, and three patients were noted to have granulomas.

Voice Analysis

Hanson, Chen, Jiang, and Pauloski (1997) reviewed voice quality and measures of jitter, shimmer, and signal-to-noise ratios in 16 patients undergoing treatment for chronic posterior laryngitis. Perceptual analysis did not show any correlation with acoustic measures and did not indicate significant change with treatment. The authors did demonstrate that jitter, shimmer, and signal-to-noise ratio improved significantly with antisecretory and antireflux treatment of the chronic posterior laryngitis. Shaw and Searl (1997) noted significant improvement in jitter, shimmer, habitual frequency, and frequency range after antireflux treatment in their series of patients who had complained of hoarseness.

Esophagram

A barium esophagram is a convenient, an inexpensive, and a noninvasive diagnostic test. It is useful for diagnosing structural and functional abnormalities of the esophagus, including hiatal hernia, erosive esophagitis, strictures, Barrett's esophagitis, esophageal rings, extrinsic compression, motility disorders, diverticula, possible malignancy, cricopharyngeal spasm, aspiration, and esophageal shortening (Hinder, Perdikis, Klinger, & DeVault, 1997; Koufman, 1998; Thompson, Kohler, & Richter, 1994; Toohill & Kuhn, 1997; Zalzal & Tran, 2000). Barium studies have significant utility for planning antireflux surgery. Fluoroscopic evaluation is often used to look for the presence of reflux and is often combined with provocative maneuvers such as valsalva, cough, rolling from supine to right lateral position, and the water siphon test (the patient drinks 60 ml of water through a straw while supine). The sensitivity of barium esophagram to detect GER is between 20% and 60%; its specificity ranges from 64% to 90%, and its accuracy is 69% (Zalzal & Tran, 2000). Thompson et al. (1994) assessed 117 patients with clinical GERD and compared the results of esophageal pH probes and barium esophagrams. The barium studies showed unprovoked reflux in 26% of study participants with positive pH probe studies. The addition of the water siphon test to the barium esophagram increased the sensitivity to 70%, the specificity to 74%, and the positive predictive value to 80%.

The relevance of barium esophagraphy to patients with EER is less clear. In Toohill and Kuhn's (1997) series of 286 patients with dysphonia and various laryngeal disorders, 79.9% had abnormal esophagrams. Rival et al. (1995) showed that 22 of 73 patients with EER symptoms had normal barium swallow evaluations, with 50% of these patients demonstrating GER on subsequent diagnostic testing. Giacchi et al. (2000) reviewed 28 patients with otolaryngologic manifestations of EER and noted that barium esophagrams revealed GER in 45% of patients, whereas 50% had normal examinations.

Esophageal Endoscopy

Esophagogastroscopy is useful for direct visualization of the esophagus, along with biopsies and cultures, for patients with esophagitis and gastritis. In patients with GERD, it may be valuable in the search for esophageal mucosal irritation and to rule out Barrett's esophagitis. Deveney et al. (1993) evaluated a small series of patients with laryngeal inflammatory lesions and found that three out of seven (43%) had esophagitis, with none having Barrett's. The necessity of esophageal endoscopy in patients with EER without GERD is unclear and may be unnecessary (Koufman, 1998).

Manometry

The utility of manometric evaluation for patients with GERD has been well documented. Knight et al. (2000) documented the significance of esophageal dysmotility in patients with EER. They used manometric studies of 100 patients with EER to show that 29% had normal motility, 48% had ineffective motility, 10% had a hypertensive LES, 9% had a nutcracker esophagus, and 4% had esophageal achalasia. Rival et al. (1995) noted low LES pressure in 60% of the patients that they studied who had cervical symptoms of EER. Esophageal manometric evaluation is critical in planning for antireflux surgery (Hinder et al., 1997), but although it is valuable for use with a certain subset of patients with EER, it may not be useful as a diagnostic test for EER. Because manometry is only one measurement in time, and transient relaxations of the LES are important in the pathogenesis of EER, manometry may not accurately assess patients for the absence of relaxations of the LES (Zalzal & Tran, 2000).

pH Probe

Continuous pH monitoring studies are thought to be the "gold standard" study for GERD and EER (Koufman, 1991; Postma, 2000; Zalzal & Tran, 2000). Probes that sense pH changes can be placed in different locations in the esophagus, pharynx, or hypopharynx. Probe placement can be verified through manometry, endoscopy, or fluoroscopy, but manometric localization is the most commonly used technique. Single pH probe techniques in which probes placed 5 cm above the manometrically determined site of the LES are commonly used to evaluate patients with GERD. With the recognition of the extraesophageal symptoms of EER, the importance of adding a second probe above the UES has been proved. Postma described a review of patients with otolaryngological complaints associated with EER who underwent dual pH probe testing at Wake Forest University. Findings indicated that 59% of patients would have been inappropriately assumed to have a negative pH probe when diagnosed based solely on the esophageal probe. In these patients, the pharyngeal sensor was needed to document EER (Postma, 2000). In a similar study, Koufman (1991) showed that 11% of patients had a positive upper probe with normal esophageal pH probe acid exposure time. Little et al. (1997) demonstrated the importance of the proximal probe in children and noted that 46% (78 of 168) of their study participants displayed positive EER by proximal probe in the face of negative esophageal probe studies.

Although the introduction of dual pH probe studies has added significantly to our diagnostic armamentarium, these studies are not without limitations. The dual pH probe is an invasive test, and its sensitivity is no more than 75% to 80% (Sasaki & Toohill, 2000). Hanson et al. (1995) stated that the false negative rate may be up to 50%. Small variations in technique for probe placement or calibration can significantly affect accuracy (Postma, 2000). Careful documentation of a patient's position (supine or upright) during the test, diet, and symptoms are equally important. The patient should maintain his or her usual dietary and smoking habits and activity level during the period of a study (Postma, 2000; Shaw, 2000).

Although there is consensus concerning norms for the distal esophageal pH probe, considerable controversy exists with regard to findings in the proximal pharyngeal probe. Postma (2000), Sasaki and Toohill (2000), and Shaw (2000) reported that a single pharyngeal reflux event as determined by a drop in the pH level to 4 or below was diagnostic of EER. Unfortunately, several studies have documented that a small percentage of individuals without any problems have proximal probe pH drops below 4 (Shaker et al., 1995; Ulualp, Toohill, Hoffman, & Shaker, 1999; Vincent, Garrett, Radionoff, Reussner, & Stasney, 2000). In the Vincent et al. study, control group participants were positive for reflux to the proximal probe (median of one event), with 80.4% of these occurring while the individual was upright. In addition, these authors examined the reflux area index (RAI), which incorporates the number and duration of events of pH less than 4.0, and indicated that the RAI is a useful parameter of measuring the severity of laryngopharyngeal reflux.

Normative data for pediatric patients are also lacking, and there appears to be considerable age-related variation (Zalzal & Tran, 2000). Contencin and Narcy (1992), Hanson, Conley, Jiang, and Kahrilas (2000), and Koufman (1998) argued that the criteria of a pH level below 4 may be too stringent. Contencin and Narcy showed that pH drops to 6 or below at the proximal probe in children with laryngotracheitis may be significant. Pepsin, which has been shown to be critical in the pathogenesis of tissue damage, is active at pH levels up to 5 (Koufman, 1998). Hanson and Jiang (2000) cautioned against stringent use of the pH to 4 criterion in patients who have had prior radiotherapy, because irradiated tissue may be less resistant to reflux trauma.

Although many researchers have shown the importance of a positive proximal pH probe, one must be careful in interpreting a negative study in patients with EER. Many patients with respiratory tract manifestations of EER may not have reflux into the proximal esophagus but have symptoms secondary to a vagally mediated reflex, as discussed previously in this chapter (Shaw, 2000). In addition, there is a potential for sampling error, as EER may potentially cause pathology but be infrequent and therefore not documented in a 24-hour study period.

The empiric treatment of EER prior to obtaining a pH probe study has been supported by many studies (Habermann et al., 1999; Hanson et al., 2000; Toohill & Kuhn, 1997; Wo, Grist, Gissack, Delgaudio, & Waring, 1997). Treatment efficacy is also well documented (Habermann et al., 1995; Hanson et al., 1995; Koufman, 1998; Rival et al., 1995; Wo et al., 1997). These authors have noted that routine pH probe studies in patients who have laryngitis only may be unnecessary but may be reserved for the following indications: symptoms of GERD, partial responses to therapy (to assess for adequacy of acid suppression), continued moderate-to-severe laryngitis despite an adequate trial of therapy, when considering antireflux surgery, evaluation of patients who after fundoplication have recurrent or persistent symptoms, and intubated patients with an altered state of consciousness (Deveney et al., 1993; Gaynor, 1988; Hanson et al., 2000). A positive study may be clinically helpful, but a negative study does not rule out EER.

Fraser, Morton, and Gillibrand (2000) are proponents of routine pH probe testing prior to initiating empiric antireflux therapy. In their study, the presence of posterior laryngitis did not predict treatment response. They argued that a positive pH probe study may better select patients who will respond to therapy and avoid unnecessary treatment in some patients. Further evaluation of pH probe testing in patients with chronic laryngitis is needed to further elucidate norms and its utility in identifying patients who will benefit from therapy.

Reflux Scan

Radionuclide scanning involves the oral administration of saline with technetium, followed by gamma scanning looking for reflux. The reflux scan can also be used to quantify delayed gastric emptying (Zalzal & Tran, 2000). The sensitivity of this test has been stated as between 14% and 90%, and it is considered to have low sensitivity in patients with EER (Koufman, 1998).

Acidification Tests

Acidification tests, such as the Tuttle and Bernstein tests, are rarely used in clinical practice today. The Bernstein test is used with adult patients and involves delivering saline and variable concentrations of hydrochloric acid to the distal esophagus via a nasogastric tube until symptoms are reproduced or 45 minutes have passed (Koufman, 1998). The Bernstein acidification test is a qualitative test that can be used to establish a causal relationship between GER and specific symptoms. The sensitivity of this test for the detection of GERD has been reported to be 32% to 95% (Gaynor, 1991; Koufman, 1998; Rival et al., 1995; Zalzal & Tran, 2000). It is not as useful in the diagnosis of EER because only a fraction of these patients have concurrent symptoms of GERD (Rival et al., 1995). Rival et al. studied 146 patients who underwent acid stimulation testing and found that 16% had positive results, but when they analyzed patients with only cervical symptoms, none had a positive result. The Tuttle test is performed in children. It involves installing an age-dependent concentration of hydrochloric acid into the stomach and measuring pH in the distal esophagus. Two episodes of a pH below 3 are seen as indicative of reflux (Zalzal & Tran, 2000).

Bronchoalveolar Lavage

Bronchoalveolar lavage samples tracheal aspirates, is utilized to look for lipid-laden macrophages, and is a test for aspiration into the lower respiratory tract. It is 85% sensitive, becomes positive within 6 hours of the reflux event, and stays positive for up to 3 days (Zalzal & Tran, 2000). Lipid-laden macrophages increase in children with pulmonary complications of EER (Koufman, 1998). The advantage of this test is that it allows for tracking of EER days after the event, but the disadvantage is that it requires bronchoscopy to acquire the sample.

Treatment

Behavioral Modification

Behavioral changes that are aimed at reducing episodes of reflux are critical to the successful management of EER. Specific suggestions and the background behind them will be discussed in the second half of this chapter. Hanson and colleagues (2000) have shown that nocturnal reflux precautions alone will result in symptomatic improvement in approximately 50% of patients with posterior laryngitis and chronic dysphonia. Giacchi et al. (2000) evaluated patient compliance with treatment for EER and found that compliance with behavior modification varied widely. The degree of symptomatic improvement positively correlated with both medical therapy and behavior modification. The changes that most significantly correlated with symptom reduction were avoidance of food and liquid before bedtime and elevation of the head of the bed.

Medications

Antacids. Multiple antacids are commonly available, are inexpensive, and are used by many persons prior to seeking medical attention. Antacids are effective due to their acid-neutralizing properties. They neutralize the pH of the refluxate and can thereby prevent the tissue damage caused by bile salts and deactivate pepsin at the higher pH levels (Sontag, 1990). Antacids have been shown to increase LES resting pressure (Gaynor, 1991; Sontag, 1990). Gaviscon contains alginic acid and is effective in reducing GER, but it does not appear to change LES pressure. Gaviscon's mechanism of action is not fully understood (Gaynor, 1991).

H$_2$ Blockers. Several H$_2$ (histamine type 2) blockers are currently available by prescription and over the counter. These drugs act at the H$_2$ receptor by competitive binding and reduce gastric acid secretion along with pepsin production (Gaynor, 1991; Sontag, 1990). Some of the H$_2$ blockers affect hepatic metabolism of other drugs; therefore, patients should consult with their physician and pharmacist to avoid drug-to-drug interactions.

Proton Pump Inhibitors. Proton pump inhibitors act against the enzyme hydrogen-potassium adenosine triphosphatase in the parietal cell, thus blocking the final step in gastric acid production (Gaynor, 1991). These drugs are more effective than H_2 antagonists for the long-term reduction of basal and stimulated levels of gastric acid production. The efficacy and dosing regimens for EER will be discussed later in this chapter.

Promotility Agents. Metoclopramide is a dopamine antagonist and is effective against GER. It increases LES pressure, improves gastric emptying, and may increase esophageal clearance (Gaynor, 1991; Orihata & Sarna, 1994). Metoclopramide is the only prokinetic agent currently available on the market. Unfortunately, up to a third of patients may experience side effects (Gaynor, 1991). Patients with diabetes mellitus, dystrophia myotonica, and anorexia nervosa may have significantly delayed gastric emptying and would benefit from prokinetic agents (Orihata & Sarna, 1994).

Other Medications. Sucralfate has been shown to enhance mucosal resistance to trauma, is effective in promoting healing of duodenal ulcers, and has been shown in animal studies to protect esophageal mucosa against injury from acid (Gaynor, 1991). Sucralfate is a salt of sucrose and is well tolerated by patients. Its value as a treatment in patients with EER has not been well elucidated. Bethanechol is an anticholinergic agent that has been shown to increase LES pressure, decrease GER, and improve salivary flow (Gaynor, 1991).

Surgical Treatment. Antireflux surgery involves moving the LES into the abdomen and then augmenting the LES as an antireflux barrier. The Nissen fundoplication utilizes a 360-degree wrap of the gastric fundus around the intraabdominal esophagus. Ten-year success rates for the treatment of GERD have been quoted to be approximately 90%, with a mortality rate of 1% (Hinder et al., 1997). Fundoplication can be performed with an open or laparoscopic approach. Complications of fundoplication are rare and include bleeding, the need for a splenectomy, dysphagia, slippage of the fundoplication into the chest, early satiety, bloating, diarrhea, pneumothorax, and gastric ulceration. Deveney et al. (1993) assessed

13 patients with persistent laryngeal inflammatory lesions and voice disorders who underwent Nissen fundoplication and found that 85% (11 patients) showed resolution of symptoms and endoscopic changes.

Chronic Laryngitis

Chronic laryngitis has been defined as a 3-month or longer history of one or more of the following: hoarseness that worsens with voice use, persistent or recurrent sore throat without throat infection, or sensation of postnasal drip with throat clearing or cough in the absence of lower respiratory tract or pulmonary disease (Hanson et al., 1995). Hanson et al. reported that the sensation of chronic postnasal drip is the most common and earliest manifestation of chronic irritative laryngitis, with throat discomfort and dysphonia as the second and third most common symptoms, respectively. The sensation of constant secretions in the back of the throat is thought to be secondary to ciliary dysfunction in the posterior larynx and pharynx (Hanson & Jiang, 2000). Hanson et al. (1995) studied 182 patients with chronic laryngitis felt to be associated with EER. Ninety-six percent of patients experienced relief with antireflux treatment within 12 weeks. Fifty-one percent (93 patients) responded to nocturnal antireflux management alone. Forty-eight patients required the addition of an H_2 blocker nightly, and 34 patients needed 20 mg of nightly omeprazole. Higher doses were required for 7 patients, all of whom had severe laryngeal changes at their pretreatment examinations. Symptomatic relapse was common with discontinuation of therapy. Habermann et al. (1999) showed that in patients with chronic laryngitis, the symptoms of hoarseness, globus pharyngeus, sore throat, heartburn, and coughing improved significantly with the empiric 6-week use of a proton pump inhibitor. Rival et al. (1995) found that 84% of patients with cervical symptoms associated with EER had improvement of these symptoms with antireflux therapy. Koufman (1998) and Fraser et al. (2000) pointed to the need for a longer duration of treatment, stating that as much as 6 months may be necessary. Koufman's study showed that with 6 months of antireflux treatment, 85% of the participants who had chronic laryngitis displayed improvement. Koufman noted that for half of these responders, effects occurred between 3 weeks and 3 months, with the remaining patients responding by 6 months.

The Role of Speech Pathology

There is substantial evidence that many otolaryngological and respiratory symptoms can be associated with EER; therefore, the evaluation and management of these patients must be individualized. No single available diagnostic test offers a definitive gold standard. These patients are best served by a team approach in which both physicians and voice therapists play integral roles.

Across the clinical care spectrum, speech–language pathologists work with physicians to evaluate and manage a patient's communication, laryngeal, and swallowing disorders associated with reflux. In a voice and laryngeal disorders clinic, patients commonly present with EER. The symptoms, etiology, evaluation, and behavioral treatment of EER and GERD will be described in this portion of the chapter.

Patient Symptoms

The symptoms reviewed earlier in the chapter may be the primary complaint that brings the patient to a clinic or may be secondary symptoms that are brought up during the case history interview. All patients seen for voice evaluation should be questioned about EER and GER symptoms, either through a preappointment questionnaire or during a case history interview.

The following symptoms are associated with EER and are often discovered during the case history or interview:

- hoarseness
- feeling of a lump in the throat (globus sensation)
- chronic cough
- voice fatigue
- intermittent voice loss
- feeling of throat closing
- throat pain

- burning sensation from the throat to the ear
- chronic throat irritation
- chronic throat clearing
- increased time to warm up the voice (singers)
- worse voice in the morning
- increased hoarseness by midafternoon
- excess saliva
- thick phlegm
- food sticking in the throat when swallowing

The following are the typical "esophageal" symptoms of GERD:

- heartburn
- substernal pain
- regurgitation
- frequent belching
- night chokes

Determining Etiology

Patients should be questioned regarding lifestyle factors that increase the likelihood of reflux, including diet, eating habits, exercise habits, and factors inherent to specific professions. As previously discussed, items such as tobacco, ethanol, fatty foods, acidic foods and beverages, coffee and other caffeinated beverages, carbonated beverages, mints, and cinnamon have been linked to increased reflux. Exercise, bending, reclining, or sleeping after eating has also been linked to increased reflux.

Other lifestyle factors that might contribute to reflux include time pressures. People often eat hurried meals and pre-prepared meals that are high in fat. Some of our patients travel frequently, eating quickly in airports and hotels and late at night in restaurants. Students often ingest food that is acidic or spicy during late-night study sessions or might drink alcohol before bed. Some patients eat on the way to the gym, and others finish work late at night and eat just before going to sleep. Patients in hospitals and nursing homes might have physical therapy sessions scheduled after lunch, remain recumbent for meals, or recline shortly after meals.

Discussing exercise regimens with patients is also recommended. Exercise induces reflux in nonsymptomatic individuals, and more reflux occurs with increased body agitation. Clark, Kraus, Sinclair, and Castell (1989), for example, found more reflux occurred with running than cycling. Yazaki, Shawdon, Beasley, and Evans (1996) measured reflux in asymptomatic athletes after fasting or a light meal. They identified reflux in 70% of rowers who fasted, 45% of runners who fasted, and 90% of runners who exercised after a light meal. In contrast, Avidan, Sonnenberg, Schnell, and Sontag (2001) described decreased esophageal acid contact time in persons with reflux when they walked after a meal rather than sat. The effect lasted only while the individuals were walking. Hydration has been one of the mainstays of vocal hygiene recommendations, but hydration during exercise is also important. Van Nieuwenhoven, Brummer, and Brouns (2000) investigated whether sports drinks or caffeinated water induced more reflux than water during a cycling task. They found no differences in reflux or gastric pH.

Although the effects of smoking and alcohol consumption are fairly clear, the effects of caffeine are less absolute. Dennish and Castell (1972) found an increase in gastric acid secretion with caffeine consumption, but Wendl, Pfeiffer, Pehl, Schmidt, and Kaess (1994) found no difference in LES pressure with ingestion of caffeinated water versus decaffeinated water. Alcohol ingestion was found to lead to decreased primary peristalsis (Hogan, Viegas de Andrade, & Winship, 1972).

Lying flat after a meal has been known to cause increased clearance time of refluxed contents. We often counsel patients to elevate the head of their bed because doing so decreases the esophageal clearance time and decreases the number of reflux episodes. Stanciu and Bennett (1977) identified shorter and fewer reflux episodes with head-of-bed elevation versus lying flat, whereas Johnson and DeMeester (1981) found that elevating the head of the bed decreased acid clearance time but did not decrease the number of reflux episodes. Patients should be advised to remain upright for 3 hours after a meal to capitalize on the improved esophageal clearance. Most GER occurs within 3 hours of a meal (Dent et al., 1980), and the acid exposure has been shown to be higher than at 1 hour after a meal (Becker, Sinclair, Castell, & Wu, 1989).

A full dietary history is important. Gastric juices contain hydrochloric acid and pepsin. The injury they cause to the epithelium is variable and depends, in part, on how well the particular mucosa can resist the refluxed material (Gaynor, 1991). Some beverages, such as citrus juices, tomato products, and coffee—all of which have high acidic contents—tend to cause more injury to epithelial tissues (Richter & Castell, 1981b). Alcohol damages the esophageal mucosa and sensitizes it to further damage (Bujanda, 2000).

For some foods that clearly cause reflux, the mechanism is not fully understood. Coffee is one of these foods. Recommendations to decrease or eliminate coffee consumption are often futile or met with dismay. Is it necessary? Many researchers have tried to explain the effects of coffee on the gastrointestinal system. Drinking coffee often leads to heartburn in patients prone to it (Feldman & Barnett, 1995) and causes reflux (Wendl et al., 1994), but the mechanism is unclear. One possibility is the acidity of coffee, which has a pH level of approximately 5 to 6 (Boekema, Samsom, van Berge Henegouwen, & Smout, 1999). When the pH level is raised to 7, however, coffee sensitivity to a Bernstein test is realized (Price, Smithson, & Castell, 1978) and decreases LES pressure (Thomas, Steinbaugh, Fromkes, Mekhjian, & Caldwell, 1980). Caffeine is another possible etiology for coffee-induced reflux. Decaffeinated coffee also causes reflux, but to a lesser degree than caffeinated coffee (Pehl, Pfeiffer, Wendl, & Kaess, 1997; Wendl et al., 1994). Some researchers have found decreased LES pressure with coffee ingestion (Cohen, 1980; Wendl et al., 1994), but Salmon, Fedail, Wurzner, Harvey, and Read (1981) found similar LES decreases following a meal, regardless of whether or not the participant drank coffee. Cohen and Booth (1975) reported increased LES pressure with coffee intake—with a similar acid response for caffeinated and decaffeinated coffees—and also noted that coffee increased gastric acid secretion. Boekema, Samsom, and Smout (1999) found no effect on reflux time or number of reflux episodes when coffee was consumed as part of a meal or 1 hour after a meal. Coffee intake did increase reflux time when consumed by patients with GERD after fasting. The conflicting results of the various studies presented here indicates that the mechanism of coffee's influence on EER or GERD is not clear. Because coffee is a diuretic, we suggest that reductions in coffee consumption be recommended as a part of the vocal health regime to reduce any potential influence on EER or GERD symptoms.

When taking the history, it is important to look for health and medical history factors that predispose patients to reflux disease or increased risk for laryngeal damage from EER. Patients should be interviewed regarding medications, past or present gastrointestinal complaints, history of intubation, diseases that are associated with gastrointestinal disorders, and history of radiation therapy. Psychological stress is a risk factor for GERD (Stanghellini, 1999) and should also be investigated during the case history.

The symptoms of EER are also symptoms of other medical conditions and must be evaluated by the otolaryngologist. A list of the patient's current medications is essential. Several medications, listed earlier in this chapter, are known to induce reflux. In addition to medications that cause reflux, the knowledge of other medications the patient may be taking that mitigate or prevent reflux is valuable. Frequency and type of over-the-counter antacid and H_2 blocker use, as well as the extent to which these medications control the symptoms, should be documented.

Any past history of reflux symptoms and gastrointestinal disorders is important. Some patients will report that they had an ulcer or GERD but the problem is "all better now." Such a history warrants careful evaluation of the current symptoms, because patients often adapt to the presence of symptoms and no longer notice their frequency or severity. Patients commonly experience EER symptoms even if they no longer identify esophageal symptoms of reflux. Many voice clinic patients have already seen a gastroenterologist and will report a known hiatal hernia or esophageal disorder.

Intubation and reflux are common causes for contact granuloma (Delahunty & Cherry, 1968; Gaynor, 1988; Kaufman, 1991). The symptoms of a granuloma include throat pain or discomfort, pain radiating to the ear, a feeling of something in the throat, and chronic throat clearing or coughing. Hoarseness and vocal fatigue can occur (Colton & Casper, 1990). Gaynor (1988) found that GER occurs in at least 40% of intubated patients in intensive care units and questioned whether concurrent reflux makes a patient more likely to experience a laryngeal or tracheal complication from intubation.

Several diseases can affect the gastrointestinal system and lead to reflux. One mechanism is through decreased saliva. Saliva is an important esophageal acid clearance mechanism for two reasons: It is an antacid, and swallowing it helps clear refluxed material from the esophagus (Helm et al., 1983). Radiation therapy to the head and neck places a patient at risk for decreased saliva flow, or xerostomia. Patients with xerostomia have abnormal pH levels and abnormal esophageal clearance (Korsten et al., 1991). As was noted previously, xerostomia is also found in patients with Sjögren's syndrome and can be a side effect of medications. Diseases cause reflux through other mechanisms as well. Patients with diabetes are at risk for reflux because of gastric paresis and delayed gastric emptying. Scleroderma often leads to reflux and esophagitis because of decreased peristalsis of the smooth muscles of the esophagus and decreased LES pressure. Scleroderma is also associated with Sjögren's syndrome. Polymyositis causes decreased peristalsis of the striated muscles of the esophagus, dilation of the esophagus, and decreased UES pressure.

Symptoms associated with EER are not specific to it, and other etiologies may be responsible. The case history interview should include questions that identify other potential causes for the symptoms. Allergies, chronic sinusitis, and under-hydration can cause thickened mucus and chronic throat clearing or coughing. Muscle tension in the throat and neck can cause pain or discomfort in the throat and pain radiating to the ear. Temporomandibular joint dysfunction can cause ear pain. Asthma, chronic obstructive pulmonary disease, emphysema, bronchitis, and pneumonia can cause chronic cough. Lesions can cause hoarseness, a feeling of a lump in the throat, cough, throat clearing, and voice fatigue. Medications and inhalers can lead to hoarseness or cough. Documentation of this information and communication with the patient's physician will facilitate the diagnostic process.

Pediatric Considerations

Interview questions should be modified when talking to children. Children should be asked whether they burp a lot, often feel sick to the stomach, or often taste "throw up" in the mouth. Their diets might include reflux-promoting foods such as carbonated beverages, caffeine, chocolate, fatty foods, or fast food. The proximity of meals to exercise, nap time, and bedtime should be investigated. Older children should be asked about smoking and alcohol use. Nelson, Chen, Syniar, and Christoffel (2000) identified the prevalence of symptoms associated with GER in 615 children. According to parents' reports, 1.8% of 556 children ages 3 to 9 years experienced heartburn ("burning/painful feeling in middle of chest"), 7.2% experienced epigastric pain ("stomachache above belly button"), and 2.3% experienced regurgitation ("sour taste or taste of throw up"). For children ages 10 to 17, of 584 parents, 3.5% reported heartburn, 3.0% reported epigastric pain, and 1.4% reported regurgitation symptoms. The 615 children identified the same symptoms more frequently: 5.2%, 5.0%, and 8.2%, respectively. It clearly is important to question children directly about reflux rather than accept the parent's historical information by itself.

Voice Disorders Associated with GERD and EERD

Team Management

Voice disorders are typically assessed and managed by a team composed of an otolaryngologist and a speech–language pathologist, and reflux-related laryngeal complaints are no exception. When reflux is suspected, the team is often expanded to include the patient's primary care physician and a gastroenterologist. Because different kinds of physicians have varied levels of expertise and interest in GERD and EER, any of these physicians might take responsibility for directing the workup and prescribing and monitoring medications. The otolaryngologist's involvement is vital because the differential diagnosis for symptoms such as chronic cough, hoarseness, and throat irritation includes many disorders that require medical and surgical interventions. Several authors have discussed a relationship between reflux and laryngeal disorders, such as contact ulcer, contact granuloma, vocal nodules, dysplasia, laryngeal cancer, and subglottic stenosis (Cherry & Margulies, 1968; Delahunty & Cherry, 1968; Kaufman, 1991; Toohill & Kuhn, 1997; Wiener et al., 1989).

Endoscopy and Stroboscopy

As previously discussed, the classic description of laryngeal findings in EER that affect the voice includes erythema and edema of the posterior glottis, with "cherry-red" arytenoids and thickened tissue of the posterior commissure that has a cobblestone appearance. More subtle findings include prominent vascularity, general vocal fold edema, and mucus pooling in the pyriform sinuses (Hanson et al., 1995).

With videostroboscopy, the closure pattern might be notable for an anterior gap, possibly in response to posterior edema and possibly as a co-occurring factor. Edema and epithelial thickening might also cause reduction in the amplitude of vibration, a mucosal wave, or periodicity. Small lesions and subtle vibratory changes are best identified through stroboscopic exams. Such changes might be associated with the reflux disease but could also be separate findings. Toohill and Kuhn (1997) suggested that nodules and polypoid degeneration are sequelae of reflux.

Videofluoroscopy

Evaluation of swallowing includes a clinical examination and a videofluoroscopic swallowing study. In the latter, the oral, pharyngeal, and esophageal stages of swallowing are assessed. The speech–language pathologist is primarily responsible for assessing the oral and pharyngeal stages. The radiologist diagnoses structural and physiologic abnormalities, including those of the esophagus. Speech–language pathologists should be aware that a commonly referred esophageal symptom is the perception of food sticking high in the throat with swallowing. Ossakow, Elta, Colturi, Bogdasarian, and Nostrant (1987) studied esophageal abnormalities in patients with cervical symptoms (cough, sore throat, globus, intermittent dysphagia, chronic throat clearing, and hoarseness). They found acid reflux in 68% of their patients and esophageal dysmotility in 63%. Acid clearance times were prolonged in 79%. Ossakow et al. concluded that patients with cervical symptoms might have sensitivity of the esophageal body to acid. Diagnosing reflux is important because of its association with Barrett's esophagitis and esophageal cancer, and patients' complaints should never be taken lightly. However, as previously discussed, videofluoroscopy may be limited in its diagnosis of EER. Additional procedures helpful in diagnosing EER were discussed in the first half of this chapter; they do not directly involve a speech–language pathologist.

Treatment

Patients with extraesophageal manifestations of reflux are often reluctant to believe their symptoms are caused by stomach acid irritating the laryngeal tissue. Although the esophageal symptoms that may occur with GERD are commonly known and heavily advertised, the extraesophageal manifestations are not. The patient's belief in the diagnosis is important for ensuring compliance with medication and behavioral recommendations, and it is worth the time to help the patient understand why he or she is being treated for reflux when heartburn is not present.

The patient will often accept the working diagnosis of laryngopharyngeal reflux following a short tutorial about EER, a video demonstration of the laryngeal findings, and a review of the swallowing study. The tutorial should include information about reflux in general and the explanation that the refluxed material probably clears from the esophagus quickly enough to prevent damage to the esophagus and the subsequent appearance of traditional symptoms, such as heartburn, substernal pain, regurgitation, and frequent belching. The material does not clear quickly enough, however, to prevent damage to the larynx, because it has less protection against acid. The patient must understand that a short acid exposure can cause significant effects.

Many patients with a diagnosis of EER begin voice therapy before their first scheduled follow-up appointment with the otolaryngologist or gastroenterologist. The treatment plan should be reviewed with the patient, and the extent of compliance should be determined. The clinician should investigate any reasons given for noncompliance. Some patients experience medication side effects, such as cramping or dyspepsia. Costs of certain medications (especially proton pump inhibitors) are often prohibitive. If any factors are limiting the patient's use of a medication, the speech–language pathologist should encourage the patient to call the prescribing physician's office. Sometimes the patient does not comply with the dietary recommendations because he or she becomes overwhelmed by the list of recommendations and decides to ignore this component of treatment. It might be necessary to suggest foods or even help a patient plan a sample meal schedule. Consultation with a nutritionist would be helpful in such cases.

Behavioral Antireflux Precautions. Many foods, beverages, and medications have been shown to increase reflux or to increase the potential for reflux or esophageal irritation. Elimination of these foods, modifications to decrease reflux, and strategies to improve esophageal clearance form the heart of a behavioral antireflux program. The recommendations should encompass diet, posture, exercise, weight, eating habits, abdominal pressure, stress, and antacid therapy.

Published studies that describe behavioral antireflux precautions for laryngeal manifestations of EER usually combine the behavioral program with medications, but few researchers have reported the incidence of compliance to recommendations. In many of the studies, the investigators requested that the patients follow only one or two precautions. Hanson et al. (1995), for example, reported improvement in 51% of patients treated only with two recommendations—to raise the head of the bed 8 to 10 inches and not to eat or drink 3 hours before bed. Most (94%) of these patients had mild laryngeal findings.

The following recommendations are made in an effort to prevent or mediate reflux. There is no consensus in the literature, however, about which recommendations are necessary or even adequate for laryngeal or vocal fold healing. The effect of the recommendations varies among individuals. Tailoring a behavioral antireflux program takes patience and detective work. Patients are often counseled to adhere strictly to the guidelines until either the symptoms or the laryngeal changes resolve. The next step is to slowly begin to vary the diet or return to old habits, carefully monitoring the effects each addition has. Reflux has been described as a "chronic intermittent" disease (Ulualp & Toohill, 2000). Patients are therefore reminded to tighten their adherence to the precautions at the first sign of symptom relapse or during events that precipitate increased reflux (e.g., stressful times). Some of the precautions may require long-term compliance. The following are lists of recommendations by category.

Things To Be Avoided

- smoking
- fatty or fried foods
- citrus fruits and juices
- coffee (caffeinated or decaffeinated)
- caffeine
- tomato-based products
- spicy foods
- carbonated beverages
- alcohol
- chocolate
- mint (spearmint, peppermint, and cinnamon)
- sedatives

Posture

- Remain upright at least 3 hours after eating a meal.
- Sleep with the head of the bed elevated 4 to 6 inches. This can be done with blocks under the bedposts, blankets between the mattress and boxspring, or a wedge. The goal is a gradual incline. Two pillows are not adequate because they only elevate the neck.

Exercise

- Do not exercise directly after eating.
- When possible, choose activities that agitate the body less.
- Talk to your doctor about taking an antacid before exercise.

Weight and Eating Habits

- Lose weight if you are overweight.
- Eat smaller meals and eat them more frequently.
- Do not eat too much at one sitting.

Abdominal Pressure

- Do not wear clothing or belts that compress the abdomen.
- Avoid bending forward after a meal.
- Singers should not sing after a meal.

Stress

- Learn stress management techniques.
- Consult a mental health professional to help with stress management.

Antacids

- Talk to your doctor about using an antacid when you have heartburn and before bed.

The traditional view (and the one included above) is to avoid exercise after eating. As discussed earlier, moderate exercise (e.g., walking) might be beneficial for decreasing postprandial acid exposure (Avidan et al., 2001). The authors of this study reported another interesting finding that is not yet reflected in the standard behavioral program above: Chewing sugar-free gum for an hour after the meal significantly reduced postprandial acid contact time for 3 hours in participants with reflux, and it significantly reduced acid contact time for 2 hours in control group members.

Pediatric Considerations. Children should be counseled to eat small meals; wait 2 to 3 hours after eating before going to bed, lying down, or exercising; and stay away from tobacco smoke. Parents should be counseled to stop smoking around their children. Children should also be encouraged to avoid chocolate, caffeinated products, carbonated beverages, highly seasoned food, and fried foods. Helping children to coordinate well-balanced meals and good snacks with sports activities can be challenging and requires some creative planning.

Antacid Therapy. The more common antacids have already been mentioned. One effect of antacids is to increase LES pressure, an effect that lasts approximately 1 hour (Higgs, Smyth, & Castell, 1974; Richter & Castell, 1981a). When used in high doses, however, antacids can have serious side effects. Sodium overload can occur with sodium bicarbonate; hypercalcemia, renal impairment, and stimulation of gastric secretion may accompany heavy use of calcium carbonate; and phosphate depletion and muscle weakness, bone resorption, and hypercalciuria are side effects of aluminum hydroxide use (Morrissey & Barreras, 1974). Even at lower doses, these antacids may cause diarrhea or constipation. The physician must coordinate all medications.

Voice Therapy. Voice use patterns must be considered, and voice therapy should be initiated when appropriate. EER may be the predominant factor in the etiology of dysphonia, or it may be a co-occurring factor. Koufman, Sataloff, and Toohill (1996) noted that muscle tension dysphonia is a common product of EER and must be addressed in order to obtain a full vocal recovery. In cases of mild and moderate laryngeal findings, voice use instruction can result in better voice, reduction of fatigue, and decreased effort. When EER occurs with behaviorally reversible laryngeal pathology, voice therapy should be initiated.

Conclusion

Extraesophageal complications of reflux are often assessed and managed by a team that includes, but is not limited to, the otolaryngologist and the speech–language pathologist. The laryngeal manifestations of reflux are vast, and the diagnosis is sometimes not immediately obvious. No one combination of therapies or standard treatment works for every patient. Careful follow-up and individualized treatment plans that include medical, surgical, and behavioral therapies are essential. Voice therapy and reflux management are complementary.

References

Avidan, B., Sonnenberg, A., Schnell, T. G., & Sontag, S. J. (2001). Walking and chewing reduce postprandial acid reflux. *Current Pharmacological Therapy, 15,* 151–155.

Bauman, N. M., Sandler, A. D., Schmidt, D., Maher, J. W., & Smith, R. J. H. (1994). Reflex laryngospasm induced by stimulation of distal esophageal afferents. *Laryngoscope, 104,* 209–214.

Becker, D. J., Sinclair, J., Castell, D. O., & Wu, W. C. (1989). A comparison of high and low fat meals on postprandial esophageal acid exposure. *The American Journal of Gastroenterology, 84,* 782–786.

Boekema, P. J., Samsom, M., & Smout, A. J. (1999). Effect of coffee on gastroesophageal reflux on patients with reflux disease and healthy controls. *European Journal of Gastroenterology and Hepatology, 11,* 1271–1276.

Boekema, P. J., Samsom, M., van Berge Henegouwen, G. P., & Smout, A. J. (1999). Coffee and gastrointestinal function: Facts and fiction. A review. *Scandinavian Journal of Gastroenterology* (Suppl.), 23035–23039.

Bujanda, L. (2000). The effects of alcohol consumption upon the gastrointestinal tract. *The American Journal of Gastroenterology, 95,* 3374–3382.

Cherry, J., & Margulies, S. L. (1968). Contact ulcer of the larynx. *Laryngoscope, 78,* 1937–1940.

Clark, C. S., Kraus, B. B., Sinclair, J., & Castell, D. O. (1989). Gastroesophageal reflux induced by exercise in healthy volunteers. *Journal of the American Medical Association, 261,* 3599–3601.

Cohen, S. (1980). Pathogenesis of coffee-induced gastrointestinal symptoms. *The New England Journal of Medicine, 303,* 122–124.

Cohen, S., & Booth, G. H. (1975). Gastric acid secretion and lower esophageal sphincter pressure in response to coffee and caffeine. *The New England Journal of Medicine, 293,* 897–899.

Colton, R., & Casper, J. (1990). *Understanding voice problems: A physiological perspective for diagnosis and treatment.* Baltimore: Williams & Wilkins.

Contencin, P., & Narcy, P. (1992). Gastropharyngeal reflux in infants and children: A pharyngeal pH monitoring study. *Archives of Otolaryngology—Head & Neck Surgery, 118,* 1028–1030.

Cucchiara, S., Santamaria, F., Minella, R., Alfierei, E., Scoppa, A., Calabrese, F., et al. (1995). Simultaneous prolonged recordings of proximal and distal intraesophageal pH in children with gastroesophageal reflux diseases and respiratory symptoms. *The American Journal of Gastroenterology, 90,* 1791–1796.

Delahunty, J., & Cherry, J. (1968). Experimentally produced vocal cord granulomas. *The Laryngoscope, 78,* 1941–1947.

Dennish, G. W., & Castell, D. O. (1972). Caffeine and the lower esophageal sphincter. *The American Journal of Digestive Diseases, 17,* 993–996.

Dent, J. (1997). Patterns of lower esophageal sphincter function associated with gastroesophageal reflux. *The American Journal of Medicine, 103,* 30S–32S.

Dent, J., Dodds, W. J., Friedman, R. H., Sekiguchi, T., Hogan, W. J., Arndorfer, R. C., et al. (1980). Mechanism of gastroesophageal reflux in recumbent asymptomatic human subjects. *The Journal of Clinical Investigation, 65,* 256–267.

Deveney, C. W., Brenner, K., & Cohen, J. (1993). Gastroesophageal reflux and laryngeal disease. *Archives of Surgery, 128,* 1021–1027.

Feldman, M., & Barnett, C. (1995). Relationships between the acidity and osmolality of popular beverages and reported postprandial heartburn. *Gastroenterology, 108,* 125–131.

Fraser, A. G., Morton, R. P., & Gillibrand, J. (2000). Presumed laryngo-pharyngeal reflux: Investigate or treat? *Journal of Laryngology and Otology, 114,* 441–447.

Gaynor, E. B. (1988). Gastroesophageal reflux as an etiologic factor in laryngeal complications of intubation. *Laryngoscope, 98,* 972–979.

Gaynor, E. B. (1991). Otolaryngologic manifestations of gastroesophageal reflux. *The American Journal of Gastroenterology, 86,* 801–808.

Giacchi, R. J., Sullivan, D., & Rothstein, S. G. (2000). Compliance with anti-reflux therapy in patients with otolaryngologic manifestations of gastroesophageal reflux disease. *Laryngoscope, 110,* 19–22.

Habermann, W., Eherer, A., Lindbichler, F., Raith, J., & Friedrich, G. (1999). Ex juvantibus approach for chronic posterior laryngitis:

Results of short-term pantoprazole therapy. *The Journal of Laryngology and Otology, 113*, 734–739.

Hanson, D. G., Chen, J., Jiang, J. J., & Pauloski, B. R. (1997). Acoustic measurements of change in voice quality with treatment for chronic posterior laryngitis. *Annals of Otology, Rhinology & Laryngology, 106*, 279–285.

Hanson, D. G., Conley, D., Jiang, J., & Kahrilas, P. (2000). Role of esophageal pH recording in management of chronic laryngitis: An overview. *Annals of Otology, Rhinology & Laryngology, 109*(Suppl. 10), 4–9.

Hanson, D. G., & Jiang, J. J. (2000). Diagnosis and management of chronic laryngitis associated with reflux. *The American Journal of Medicine, 108*, 112S–119S.

Hanson, D. G., Kamel, P. L., & Kahrilas, P. J. (1995). Outcomes of antireflux therapy for the treatment of chronic laryngitis. *Annals of Otology, Rhinology & Laryngology, 104*, 550–555.

Helm, J. S., Dodds, W. J., Riedel, D. R., Teeter, B. C., Hogan, W. J., & Arndorfer, R. C. (1983). Determinants of esophageal acid clearance in normal subjects. *Gastroenterology, 85*, 607–612.

Higgs, R. H., Smyth, R. D., & Castell, D. O. (1974). Gastric alkalinization: Effect on lower esophageal sphincter pressure and serum gastrin. *The New England Journal of Medicine, 291*, 486–490.

Hinder, R. A., Perdikis, G., Klinger, P. J., & DeVault K. R. (1997). The surgical option for gastroesophageal reflux disease. *The American Journal of Medicine, 103*, 144S–148S.

Hogan, W. J., Viegas de Andrade, S. R., & Winship, D. H. (1972). Ethanol-induced acute esophageal motor dysfunction. *Journal of Applied Physiology, 32*, 755–760.

Johnson, L. F., & DeMeester, T. R. (1981). Evaluation of elevation of the head of the bed, bethanechol, and antacid form tablets on gastroesophageal reflux. *Digestive Diseases and Sciences, 26*, 673–680.

Kaufman, O. (1991). The controversial aspects of granulomatous inflammation. *Arkhiv-Patologii, 53*(6), 65–66.

Knight, R. E., Wells, J. R., & Parrish, R. S. (2000). Esophageal dysmotility as an important co-factor in extraesophageal manifestations of gastroesophageal reflux. *Laryngoscope, 110,* 1462–1469.

Korsten, M. A., Roseman, A. S., Fishbein, S., Shlein, R. D., Goldberg, H. E., & Beiner, A. (1991). Chronic xerostomia increases esophageal acid exposure and is associated with esophageal injury. *The American Journal of Medicine, 90,* 701–706.

Koufman, J. A. (1991). The otolaryngologic manifestations of gastroesophageal reflux disease (GERD): A clinical investigation of 225 patients using ambulatory 24-hour pH monitoring and an experimental investigation of the role of acid and pepsin in the development of laryngeal injury. *Laryngoscope, 101*(Suppl. 4), 1–78.

Koufman, J. A. (1998). Gastroesophageal reflux disease. In C. Cummings (Ed.), *Otolaryngology, head and neck surgery* (pp. 2411–2429). St. Louis, MO: Mosby.

Koufman, J. A., Sataloff, R. J., & Toohill, R. (1996). Laryngopharyngeal reflux: Concensus conference report. *Journal of Voice, 10,* 215–216.

Lang, I. M., & Shaker, R. (1997). Anatomy and physiology of the upper esophageal sphincter. *The American Journal of Medicine, 103,* 50S–55S.

Little, J. P., Matthews, B. L., Glock, M. S., Koufman, J. A., Reboussin, D. M., Loughlin, C. J., et al. (1997, July). Extraesophageal reflux: 24-hour double probe pH monitoring of 222 children. *Annals of Otology, Rhinology & Laryngology* (Suppl. 169), 1–16.

Morrissey, J. F., & Barreras, R. F. (1974). Drug therapy. Antacid therapy. *The New England Journal of Medicine, 290,* 550–554.

Nelson, S. P., Chen, E. H., Syniar, G. M., & Christoffel, K. K. (2000). Prevalence of symptoms of gastroesophageal reflux during childhood: A pediatric practice-based survey. *Archives of Pediatrics and Adolescent Medicine, 154,* 150–154.

Orihata, M., & Sarna, S. K. (1994). Contractile mechanism action of gastroprokinetic agents: Cisapride, metoclopramide, and domperidone. *American Journal of Physiology, 266,* G665–G676.

Ossakow, S. J., Elta, G., Colturi, T., Bogdasarian, R., & Nostrant, T. T. (1987). Esophageal reflux and dysmotility as the basis for persistent cervical symptoms. *Annals of Otology, Rhinology & Laryngology, 96*, 387–392.

Pehl, C., Pfeiffer, A., Wendl, B., & Kaess, H. (1997). The effect of decaffeination of coffee on gastroesophageal reflux in patients with reflux disease. *Alimentary, Pharmacology and Theraputics, 11*, 483–486.

Pope, C. E. (1997). The esophagus for the nonesophagologist. *The American Journal of Medicine, 24*, 19S–22S.

Postma, G. N. (2000). Ambulatory pH monitoring methodology. *Annals of Otology, Rhinology & Laryngology, 109*(Suppl. 10), 10–14.

Price, S. F., Smithson, K. W., & Castell, D. O. (1978). Food sensitivity in reflux esophagitis. *Gastroenterology, 75*, 240–243.

Reynolds, J. C. (1996). Influence of pathophysiology, severity, and cost on the medical management of gastroesophageal reflux disease. *American Journal of Health-Systems Pharmacists, 53*, S5–S12.

Richter, J. E., & Castell, D. O. (1981a). Current approaches in the medical treatment of oesophageal reflux. *Drugs, 21*, 283–291.

Richter, J. E., & Castell, D. O. (1981b). Drugs, foods, and other substances in the cause and treatment of reflux esophagitis. *The Medical Clinics of North America, 65*, 1223–1234.

Rival, R., Wong, R., Mendelsohn, M., Rosgen, S., Goldberg, M., & Freeman, J. (1995). Role of gastroesophageal reflux disease in patients with cervical symptoms. *Archives of Otolaryngology—Head & Neck Surgery, 113*, 364–369.

Salmon, P. R., Fedail, S. S., Wurzner, H. P., Harvey, R. F., & Read, A. E. (1981). Effect of coffee on human lower oesophageal function. *Digestion, 21*(2), 69–73.

Sasaki, C. T., & Toohill, R. J. (2000). 24-hour ambulatory pH monitoring for patients with suspected extraesophageal reflux: Indications and interpretations. *Annals of Otology, Rhinology & Laryngology, 109*(Suppl. 10), 1–27.

Shaker, R., & Lang, I. M. (1997). Reflux mediated airway protective mechanisms against retrograde aspiration. *The American Journal of Medicine, 103,* 64S–73S.

Shaker, R., Milbrath, M., Ren, J., Toohill, R., Hogan W. J., Li, Q., et al. (1995). Esophagopharyngeal distribution of refluxed gastric acid in patients with reflux laryngitis. *Gastroenterology, 109,* 1575–1582.

Shaw, G. Y. (2000). Application of ambulatory 24-hour multiprobe pH monitoring in the presence of extraesophageal manifestations of gastroesophageal reflux. *Annals of Otology, Rhinology & Laryngology, 109*(Suppl. 10), 15–17.

Shaw, G. Y., & Searl, J. P. (1997). Laryngeal manifestations of gastroesophageal reflux before and after treatment with omeprazole. *Southern Medical Journal, 90,* 1115–1122.

Sontag, S. J. (1990). The medical management of reflux esophagitis: Role of antacids and acid inhibition. *Gastroenterology Clinics of North America, 19,* 683–712.

Stanciu, C., & Bennett, J. R. (1977). Effects of posture on gastroesophageal reflux. *Digestion, 15,* 104–109.

Stanghellini, V. (1999). Relationship between upper gastrointestinal symptoms and lifestyle, psychosocial factors and comorbidity in the general population: Results from the Domestic/International Gastroenterology Surveillance Study (DIGEST). *Scandinavian Journal of Gastroenterology, 231*(Suppl.), 29–37.

Thomas, F. B., Steinbaugh, J. T., Fromkes, J. J., Mekhijian, H. S., & Caldwell, J. H. (1980). Inhibitory effect of coffee on lower esophageal sphincter pressure. *Gastroenterology, 79,* 1262–1266.

Thompson, J. K., Koehler, R. E., & Richter, J. E. (1994). Detection of gastroesophageal reflux: Value of barium studies compared with 24-hr pH monitoring. *American Journal of Radiology, 162,* 621–629.

Toohill, R. J., & Kuhn, J. C. (1997). Role of refluxed acid in pathogenesis of laryngeal disorders. *The American Journal of Medicine, 103*(Suppl. 5A), 100S–106S.

Ulualp, S. O., Toohill, R. J., Hoffman, R., & Shaker, R. (1999). Pharyngeal pH monitoring in patients with posterior laryngitis. *Archives of Otolaryngology—Head & Neck Surgery, 120,* 672–677.

VanNieuwenhoven, M. A., Brummer, R. M., & Brouns, F. (2000). Gastrointestinal function during exercise: Comparison of water, sports drink, and sports drink with caffeine. *Journal of Applied Physiology, 89,* 1079–1085.

Vincent, D. A., Garrett, J. D., Radionoff, S. L., Reussner, L. A., & Stasney, C. R. (2000). The proximal probe in esophageal pH monitoring: Development of a normative database. *Journal of Voice, 14,* 247–254.

Wendl, B., Pfeiffer, A., Pehl, C., Schmidt, T., & Kaess, H. (1994). Effect of decaffeination of coffee or tea on gastroesophageal reflux. *Alimentary, Pharmacology and Therapeutics, 8,* 283–287.

Wiener, G. J., Koufman, J. A., Wu, W. C., Cooper, J. B., Richter, J. E., & Castell, D. O. (1989). Chronic hoarseness secondary to gastroesophageal reflux disease: Documentation with 24-h ambulatory pH monitoring. *The American Journal of Gastroenterology, 84,* 1503–1508.

Wo, J. M., Grist, W. J., Gissack, G., Delgaudio, J. M., & Waring, J. P. (1997). Empiric trial of high-dose omeprazole in patients with posterior laryngitis: A prospective study. *The American Journal of Gastroenterology, 92,* 2160–2165.

Yazaki, E., Shawdon, A., Beasley, I., & Evans, D. F. (1996). The effect of different types of exercise on gastro-esophageal reflux. *Australian Journal of Science and Medicine in Sport, 28*(4), 93–96.

Zalzal, G. H., & Tran, L. P. (2000). Pediatric gastroesphageal reflux and laryngopharyngeal reflux. *Otolaryngology Clinics of North America, 33,* 151–161.

Chapter 11

Pulmonary Function and Breathing for Speech

Paul Davenport and Christine M. Sapienza

Davenport and Sapienza stress that proper respiratory function is very important for the production of normal voice. Depicting the respiratory system as the power source for voicing, Davenport and Sapienza review the components of this system, its processes relative to typical and disordered voice production, and its critical role in the generation and maintenance of subglottal air pressure.

1. *The respiratory system is driven by two mechanisms: passive and active. Define how they are different and what role each plays in producing speech.*

2. *How can knowledge of the relaxation pressure curve be used as a therapeutic aid in educating the patient about the role of the respiratory system in voice production?*

3. *Is every patient with a voice disorder a candidate for respiratory function exercises in therapy? Why or why not?*

The process of moving air requires a driving force. In the respiratory system, this driving force is the pressure gradient between the alveoli and the atmosphere. For inflation of the lung to occur, the inward driving force must be an alveolar pressure that is less than the atmospheric pressure so that a pressure gradient into the lung is created. For expiration to occur, the driving force must be an alveolar pressure that is greater than the atmospheric pressure to generate a pressure gradient out of the lung. In order to produce voice, air is required to move from the alveolar spaces through the conducting airways and the glottis to the pharynx and the oral cavity. The driving force for this air movement is a pressure in the alveolar space that is greater than atmospheric pressure (see Figure 11.1).

Alveolar pressure is changed by two forces: the passive, elastic properties of the respiratory system and the active contraction of the respiratory muscles. The example that can be used to understand and explain these concepts is a balloon. Inflation of the balloon requires an active stretching of it. This increases the volume of the balloon, creating a pressure gradient into the balloon. It takes active muscle force to overcome the balloon's stiffness and force air into the balloon. With the balloon inflated and the opening closed, the balloon retracting toward its resting position produces an inside pressure that causes the air to be compressed. This is an elastic force, which is an inherent, passive property of the balloon that is directly proportional to the stretch of the balloon. The greater the balloon volume (i.e., the greater the stretch of the balloon wall), the greater the elastic recoil of the balloon and the greater the pressure inside it. This pressure can be increased even more if the outside of the balloon is squeezed. The result is an active contraction of muscles and is active pressure. The total pressure within the balloon is the sum of the passive elastic pressure and the active squeeze pressure (see Figures 11.2 and 11.3).

In the lungs and thorax, the elastic forces are the pressure–volume relationship of the two systems. The elastic behavior of the system as a whole is the result of the combination of the elastic forces of the lung and thorax. When the respiratory system is at rest, the lungs are partially inflated to approximately 40% of their total capacity (total lung capacity, or TLC). This resting position is referred to as the functional residual capacity (FRC; see Figure 11.4A).

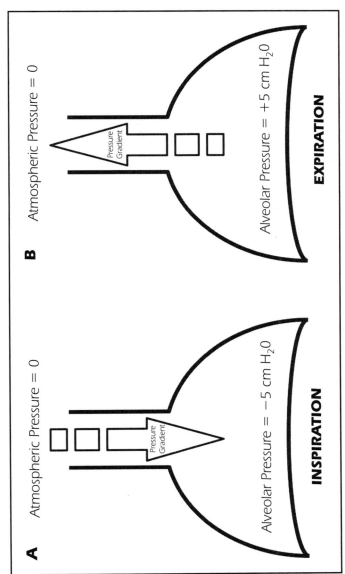

Figure 11.1. Schematic depicting pressure relationships for (A) inspiration and (B) expiration. The arrow indicates the direction of the driving force.

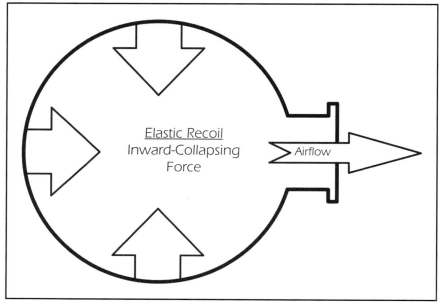

Figure 11.2. Schematic of a balloon showing the direction of elastic recoil forces during passive expiration.

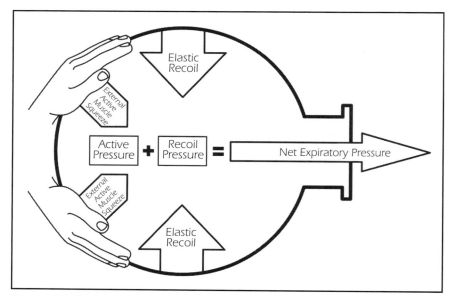

Figure 11.3. Schematic of a balloon depicting active and passive mechanisms during expiration. The passive elastic recoil is the same as in Figure 11.2. The hands squeezing the balloon illustrate the addition of an active expiratory force.

At FRC, neither the lungs nor the thorax is at the respective rest position. Making a hole in the thoracic wall and producing a pneumothorax results in the lung collapsing and the thorax expanding (see Figure 11.4B). The elastic neutral position for the lung thus is a volume much smaller than FRC; therefore at FRC, the lung has a natural tendency to collapse. The thoracic elastic neutral position is a volume much greater than FRC, approximately 70% of TLC, which means the thorax has a natural tendency to expand at FRC.

Measuring the lungs' elastic behavior involves applying various pressures and recording the resultant volume change. This produces a pressure–volume curve for the lung. The slope of the curve is a measure of the elasticity of the lungs, the lung compliance (C_L). The pressure–volume relationship shows that increasing pressures are required to increase lung volume. If the lungs are inflated to a volume above their elastic neutral position and the trachea is closed, the alveolar pressure will be greater than the atmospheric pressure, as in the example of the balloon mentioned earlier. The amount of pressure in the alveolar space will be directly related to the inflation volume (see Figure 11.4C).

The thoracic elastic behavior is similarly measured by a pressure–volume curve. The thorax has a compliance (C_{CW}) that is measured by the slope of the pressure–volume relationship for the thorax. This pressure–volume curve is produced in two parts: by applying collapsing pressure to the thorax, which decreases the thoracic volume, and expanding pressure to increase the thoracic volume. The pressure–volume curve for the thorax therefore extends to volumes above and below the elastic neutral position (see Figure 11.4D).

The outer surface of the lungs is apposed to the inner surface of the thorax by hydrostatic forces. A membrane called the *visceral pleura* covers the lungs. A similar membrane, the *parietal pleura*, covers the thorax. A thin layer of pleural fluid separates these membranes. Placing two smooth surfaces against each other with fluid between them is much like two microscope slides with water between them. The microscope slides can easily move back and forth but are very hard to pull apart. This hydrostatic force "holds" the two smooth surfaces together but allows free sliding between the surfaces. In the respiratory system, the pleural fluid holds the lungs against the thoracic wall while allowing the lungs to slide freely

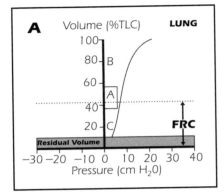

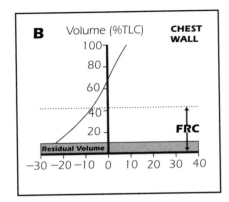

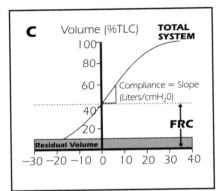

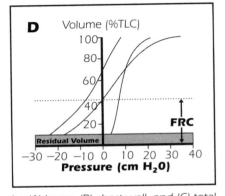

Figure 11.4. Pressure–volume curves for the (A) lungs, (B) chest wall, and (C) total system. The relationship of all three pressure–volume curves is shown in D. Note in D that the passive relaxation point for the total system, FRC (functional residual capacity), is the volume point where the lung and chest wall pressures are equal.

during volume changes. The mechanical linking of the lungs and the chest wall means that the combined systems' elastic behavior is a result of the interaction of their separate elastic forces. The lungs are at a volume above the elastic neutral position and have a collapsing force, whereas the thorax is at a volume smaller than its elastic neutral position and has an expanding force. At FRC, the expanding elastic force of the thorax balances the collapsing elastic force of the lungs.

Application of pressures to the combined system results in a system pressure–volume curve (see Figure 11.4D). The respiratory system compliance (C_{RS}) is the slope of this pressure–volume relationship. If the system's volume is increased above FRC, there is a net collapsing force for the respiratory system. The greater the volume, the greater the collapsing force. Similarly, volumes below FRC will result in an expanding force. The lower the volume below FRC, the greater the expanding force.

Passive and Active Forces of the Respiratory System

The system volume is increased by the action of the inspiratory muscles. At the end of the inflation, the inspiratory muscles relax and the system's elastic forces produce an alveolar pressure greater than atmospheric pressure, which is predicted from the pressure–volume curve. The alveolar pressure will become closer to atmospheric pressure as the volume returns to FRC. The passive pressure–volume nature of the respiratory system thus provides one component of the driving force for expiratory airflow. This passive elastic pressure component is regulated by the magnitude of the active inspiration.

The passive elastic pressure is the foundation driving force that is modified by the action of the expiratory muscles. The respiratory chamber can be viewed as a tube with the top chamber separated from the bottom chamber by a piston (see Figure 11.5). The upper chamber of the tube contains the lung (represented by the balloon) and is the thorax. The volume of the top chamber can be changed by increasing or decreasing its diameter and by moving the piston up or down. Active inspiration is a muscle action that increases the diameter of the tube and pulls the piston down. A portion of the inspiratory muscle energy used to expand the thorax is recaptured by the passive collapsing force of the elastic recoil pressure, which is volume dependent. To this passive elastic expiratory driving force is added an active expiratory pressure generated by contraction of muscles that will decrease the diameter of the tube, or push the piston into the upper chamber. The decrease in upper chamber diameter is achieved by pulling the ribs downward. The ribs are attached at the costochondral joint of the thoracic vertebra and the sternum

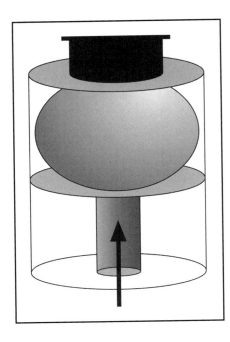

Figure 11.5. Schematic depicting the respiratory chamber. The upper chamber contains the lung/thorax unit, and the bottom chamber represents the pistonlike mechanism of active expiratory force derived from active abdominal movement.

or costal arch. The arch of the ribs is oriented downward. Pulling the ribs up produces a "bucket handle" effect and increases the diameter of the upper chamber (see Figure 11.6).

Pulling the ribs down similarly decreases the diameter of the upper chamber. Any muscle that acts to pull the ribs down will assist in producing an active expiratory driving force. The active expiratory driving force is like squeezing the balloon from the outside: The force of the squeeze generates a pressure that adds to the elastic recoil pressure. The muscles that produce this squeeze pressure are usually identified as the internal intercostal muscles and abdominal muscles. The internal intercostal muscles attach to the inner, lower margin of the cranial rib and the inner, upper margin of the adjacent caudal rib. The fibers are oriented ventrodorsally. When activated during active breathing efforts, the internal intercostal muscles are known to contract in synchrony with expiratory airflow. Contraction of these muscles will decrease the intercostal space width and will pull the ribs down.

The abdominal muscles are the rectus abdominis, external abdominal oblique, internal abdominal oblique, and transversus ab-

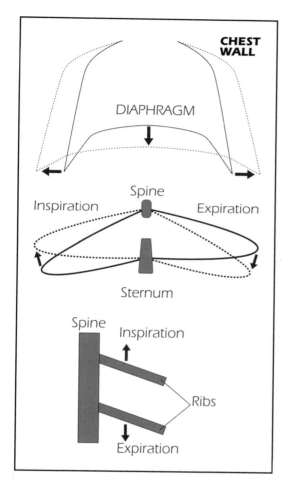

Figure 11.6. Schematic representation of the motion of the diaphragm and ribs during respiratory muscle contraction. The "bucket handle" nature of the parasternal ribs is illustrated with the ends attached to a vertebra and the sternum.

dominis. The rectus abdominis is attached to the lower margin of the sternum and to the lower edge of the lower parasternal ribs a few centimeters lateral to the sternum. The caudal attachment is the ventral pelvic girdle. The internal and external abdominal oblique muscles attach cranially to the caudal edge of the costal ribs. The caudal attachment is the rectus abdominis and the pelvic girdle. The external abdominal oblique fibers are oriented at a cranial to caudal direction, dorsoventral angle. The internal abdominal oblique fibers are oriented cranial to caudal in a ventrodorsal angle. The transversus abdominis fibers are oriented circumferentially between the rectus abdominis and the spine. The action of the rectus abdominis is to stabilize the ventral midline and stiffen the ventral abdominal midline. The external abdominal oblique, internal abdominal oblique, and transversus abdominis act to decrease the diameter of the abdomen and pull the costal ribs down. This increases the abdominal pressure and forces the abdominal contents upward, providing the force that drives the piston action of the diaphragm up into the thorax.

To these muscles must be added any muscle group that attaches to the rib cage with a fiber orientation to pull the ribs downward or to compress the abdomen. The longissimus dorsi, iliocostalis dorsi, iliocostalis lumborum, and serratus posterior inferior muscles in the dorsal side of the back attach to the lower margin of the ribs with the pelvic girdle spine. Portions of the quadratus lumborum on the ventral side of the spine attach the caudal border of the last rib with the pelvic girdle. These muscles are found on the dorsal and ventral sides of the spine. Their orientation provides a downward pull of the ribs, decreasing the diameter of the thorax. The dorsal muscles are also in a position to stabilize the spine during strong ventral contraction of the ventral abdominal muscles, preventing a forward bending action from rectus abdominis contraction. An erect posture thus is important in the action of these muscles, by assisting in the generation of an active compression of the thorax to produce the active expiratory pressure.

The act of breathing on the generation of alveolar pressure thus is an inspiratory action involving contraction of the diaphragm and external intercostal muscles to increase lung volume. The magnitude of the volume determines the static elastic pressure when the inspiration ends and the diaphragm relaxes. The driving force of active expiratory pressure is the coordinated action of a variety of muscles that decrease the diameter of the thorax and compress the abdomen. Abdominal compression increases abdominal pressure and is the driving force for the piston action of stretching the relaxed diaphragm, which is pushed up into the thorax, compressing the lung. This force is added to the static elastic pressure to generate the net alveolar pressure, which is the driving force for expiratory airflow. Active expiratory pressure is the one component of the net expiratory driving force that can be regulated by volitional control of the expiratory muscles (see Figure 11.7).

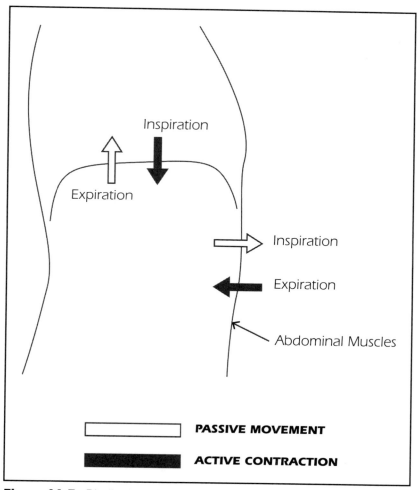

Figure 11.7. Distribution of active and passive forces during inspiratory and expiratory movements.

The alveolar pressure is the pressure source for vocalization and is greater than the subglottal pressure during expiratory airflow because the resistance of the conducting airways dissipates a portion of the pressure. The resistance of the airways actually limits the airflow in an effort-independent manner. The tubes that connect the alveoli to the larynx form a highly branching network, the bronchial tree. The diameter of the individual tubes progressively decreases from the trachea to the alveoli. While the individual tube resistance increases as the tube diameter decreases, the total resistance decreases because of the large increase in the surface area of the tubes. The conducting airways are supported by cartilage from the trachea to the bronchioles, which are the smallest airways. They are surrounded by smooth muscle but do not have cartilage. Thus, the bronchioles are collapsible because there is no cartilage to restrict the collapse of the airway through an external compressing force. The cartilaginous airways are not fully collapsible, but their diameter will decrease in response to an external compressing force. To further understand the relationship between the generation of expiratory airflow and resistance, a few fundamental points must be made:

1. The pressure during expiration is the sum of the elastic recoil and active compression pressures.
2. The expiratory pressure is the greatest in the alveolus (i.e., alveolar pressure).
3. The pressure at the mouth is atmospheric, which is referred to as *zero pressure*.
4. Somewhere between the alveolus and the mouth, all the alveolar pressure is dissipated.
5. It is the resistance of the airways that causes the loss of pressure.
6. When an active pressure is applied, that pressure is pressing on all the alveoli and conducting airways in the thorax.

When an active expiration begins, the alveolar pressure is greater than atmospheric pressure, creating a positive pressure. The elastic recoil portion of the alveolar pressure is determined by the volume of the lungs (see Figure 11.4A). To this elastic pressure is added the external squeeze pressure applied by the action of the expiratory muscles compressing the thorax (see Figure 11.3). This combination of elastic and active pressures in the alveoli is greater than the surrounding active pressure, driving air out of the lungs. The resistance of the conducting airways opposes the expiratory airflow, and pressure is lost along the path to the mouth. As the pressure decreases along the conducting airways, a point is reached at which the pressure inside the airway has decreased sufficiently to equal the active pressure. This is called the *equal pressure point* (see Figure 11.8).

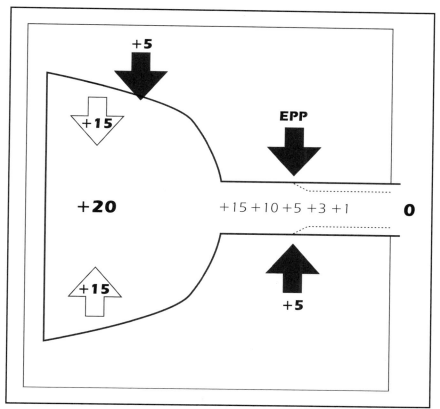

Figure 11.8. Schematic representation of the lung and chest wall. The arrow within the lung and associated number represents the passive recoil pressure. The arrow and number on the outside of the lung is the active expiratory pressure provided by the expiratory muscles. The number in the center of the lung is the sum of the passive and active expiratory pressures and is the P_A expiratory driving pressure. The intraluminal pressure decreases from the maximum pressure, P_A, to zero at the mouth. The arrow labeled EPP (equal pressure point) indicates the point along the airway where the active expiratory pressure equals the intraluminal pressure. The portion of the airway closer to the mouth from this EPP point is associated with further decreases in intraluminal pressure, which will result in a net collapsing force and airway narrowing.

Moving along the conducting airways beyond the equal pressure point and closer to the mouth, pressure continues to be dissipated by the resistance, and the pressure inside the airway becomes less than the outside active pressure. This results in a compression of the conducting airways because there is a net collapsing force from the pressure gradient across the airway wall. The compression of the airway decreases the diameter of the airway, increasing the resistance. The magnitude of the compression of the airway is directly related to the strength of the active expiratory effort, that is, the stronger the active expiratory effort, the greater the active pressure and the greater the compression of the airway after the equal pressure point has been reached. The consequence of this process is a limitation of expiratory airflow due to dynamic airway compression, and the maximum airflow rate at any specific lung volume becomes effort-independent. This means the expiratory airflow rate can increase with effort to a point where there is a balance between the compression of the airway and the expiratory pressure driving force. Increasing the effort will not increase the expiratory airflow rate. Typically the equal pressure point occurs in the cartilaginous airways, which prevent complete collapse of the airway with strong active expiratory efforts. Disease conditions can shift the equal pressure point closer to the bronchioles, which have no cartilage to prevent full collapse. For example, if a patient has a bronchoconstriction, such as that which occurs with an asthma attack, the smooth muscle of the bronchioles contracts, narrowing the bronchiole diameter and increasing the resistance. This means that a greater amount of the alveolar pressure will be dissipated, pushing air across this increased resistance. The pressure in the airway will decrease faster and will reach the external active pressure closer to the alveoli. The equal pressure point is moved away from the mouth, closer to the alveoli and possibly more into the collapsible airways. This will restrict the peak expiratory airflow rate and make the subglottal pressure less than normal. In some cases, the distal airways may fully collapse, trapping gas in the alveoli and producing a lung hyperinflation.

In another type of disease process, such as emphysema, the elastic recoil of the lung is decreased. The alveolar pressure is decreased at each lung volume because there is less elastic recoil pressure. The active pressure is added to this reduced elastic recoil pressure and again provides the driving force for expiratory airflow. The conducting airways still have a resistance, however, that causes the dissipation of the intra-airway pressure. Because there is less alveolar pressure due to the reduced elastic recoil pressure, the pressure in the airway equals the active pressure closer to the alveoli, moving the equal pressure point distally into the more collapsible airways (see Figure 11.9). Again, increased expiratory effort does not increase expiratory airflow, and dynamic airway collapse can occur,

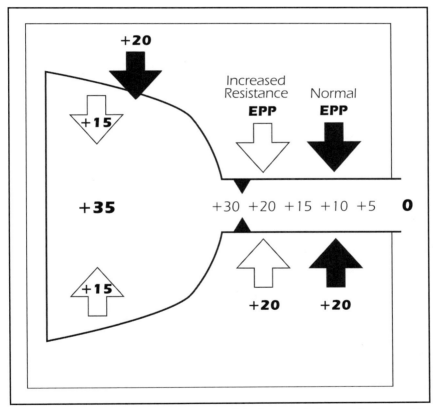

Figure 11.9. Schematic representation of the lung and chest wall when an increased resistance is present in the distal airways. The P_A expiratory driving pressure is the same as in Figure 11.8. The increased resistance causes a greater decrease in intraluminal pressure in the distal airways, moving the equal pressure point (EPP) closer to the alveoli.

with the associated trapping of gas in the alveoli. The subglottal pressure will also be reduced, even with strong expiratory efforts. The significance of the equal pressure point and effort-independent airflow is the limitation of subglottal pressure and airflow for speech.

Speech Production

Adequate control of lung volume and respiratory muscle activity during speech expiration is crucial for the regulation of subglottal pressure (Hixon, Goldman, & Mead, 1973). Subglottal pressure controls a variety of glottal parameters, such as airflow, glottal area, fundamental frequency, and sound pressure level. It is the driving force for the initiation of vocal fold vibration and the key variable that clinicians attempt to manipulate when working to alleviate the breathing symptoms of patients with dysphonia. As stated previously, both active and passive forces regulate the main alveolar pressure. In turn, a certain percentage of the generated alveolar pressure is used for voice production. Passive properties refer to the inherent recoil properties (elasticity) of the chest wall, as well as gravitational forces. The respiratory muscles, both inspiratory and expiratory, supply the active forces.

Understanding the Relaxation Pressure Curve

To educate the patient regarding the mechanisms employed to produce voice/speech, the clinician can use the relaxation pressure curve and explain which parts of speech are active and which are passive during production. Finally, by integrating the concepts of the relaxation pressure curve with the symptoms being presented by the patient, the clinician can determine if a particular breathing technique may or may not work. Simply put, one must understand the mechanics of the respiratory pump and the relationship between volume and pressure in order to establish why (a) a particular technique can or cannot be used to improve voice and (b) a particular patient may be experiencing difficulty producing voice or breathing. Figure 11.4A depicted a relaxation pressure curve produced along the lung volume continuum of 0% lung volume to 100% (TLC). At each lung volume, a pressure is generated by the inherent recoil forces of the lungs, thorax, and abdominal–diaphragm unit. In Figure 11.4A, it can be seen that pressures produced at lung volumes between 35% and 55% TLC produce pressures on the order of 5 cm to 10 cm of water. At these lung volumes, inspiratory or expiratory work needed to produce speech is minimal. For the purposes of this description, *work* is defined as the recruitment of muscular forces used to depart from the relaxation pressure. By recruiting muscular effort, higher pressures can be generated in order to meet the demands of any given speech task. When a higher lung volume is approached, at, for example, 80% TLC, an active inspiratory muscle force must be generated to resist the high recoil forces generated by the lung–thorax unit. Note that this unit's rest position is 0% TLC for the lungs and approximately 55% TLC for the thorax. Therefore, at volumes as high as 80%, the tendency to recoil to those resting volumes is very high. In order to resist the high recoil force, inspiratory muscles must be recruited in a "checking" fashion (Hixon, 1987). At very low lung volumes, on the order of 20% TLC, it is apparent from Figure 11.4A (Point C) that there is not enough pressure to meet the demands required for comfortable-effort speech. This demand is on the order of 4 cm to 5 cm of water and increases if the speech task requires the person's voice to be louder. At 20% TLC, the relaxation pressure is negative. One way to create a positive pressure for speech is recruiting abdominal musculature to decrease the volume within the chest wall by using a piston-like force. This force increases the pressure needed to meet the demands of the speech task. The fact that the abdominal muscles must be "turned on" for speech to occur at low lung volumes requires an active mechanism (i.e., muscle contraction), which is work.

The ability to interpret the relaxation pressure diagram will assist the clinician in providing appropriate recommendations to the voice patient. For example, having a patient take big breaths before he or she starts to voice does not make good physiological sense, because the patient would have to recruit inspiratory muscles to resist high recoil forces. Instead, the clinician should counsel the patient to take a small breath before starting to voice and should try to determine if there are any lower or upper airway limitations that might be preventing him or her from using the lung volumes he or she has generated effectively.

Therapeutic Issues

The goal of therapy is intelligible speech that can be easily perceived by the listener. In the production side of breathing, generation of adequate subglottal pressure is critical to producing volume, varying the frequency of the voice, and sustaining the sound's duration. Although speech demands will vary, constant pressure will be required, regardless of the lungs' volume and the duration of the task.

There are many clinical instances where alveolar pressure cannot be generated effectively. Emphysema and asthma have already been mentioned. Other cases involve low muscular tone such as in a spinal cord injury and neuromuscular degenerative diseases (e.g., multiple sclerosis). In both cases, a lack of muscular integrity results in the inability to generate strong enough muscular forces to deviate from the relaxation pressure.

In individuals with voice disorders, there may be multiple reasons why breathing symptoms might be associated with the laryngeal condition. First, it may be that the patient has low muscular effort due to a primary disease process, such as motor neuron disease. Second, it may be that the patient has a laryngeal disorder that creates strong laryngeal airway resistance. Cases such as abductor spasmodic dysphonia, muscle tension dysphonia, or other dynamic conditions resulting in increased glottal closure can produce strong laryngeal airway resistance, thus restricting airflow. Static laryngeal conditions that result in high laryngeal airway resistance include webbing, stenosis, abductor vocal fold paralysis, and arytenoid joint dislocation. Finally, the patient who presents with low laryngeal airway resistance and cannot control expiratory airflow may also complain of breathing symptoms. These cases of hypofunctional voice disorders include adductor vocal fold paralysis or any other condition that limits the mobility of one or both vocal folds. In each of the conditions mentioned, the voice is often abnormal and the patient presents with a secondary complaint of breathing difficulties, such as a sensation of breathlessness or dyspnea, which is one of the most commonly perceived symptoms. Dyspnea is the conscious awareness of labored breathing, or "air hunger," and occurs in conditions other than during heavy exercise. Conditions about which patients may complain are walking and having to talk simultaneously, or even just walking. Dyspnea is a critical symptom to try to understand because it is common to many pulmonary diseases. It is complex, however, and requires a psychological assessment and a physiological assessment of the upper and lower airways. Physiologically, the origin of dyspnea can be multifaceted. When patients complain of dyspnea, the speech–language pathologist must do two things. First, he or she must understand and explain to the patient the relationships among laryngeal configuration, upper airway resistance, and respiratory mechanics by relying on an understanding of the volume–pressure relationships discussed previously. Second, prior to treating any breathing symptoms, he or she must rule out heart disease, lung disease, or a state of anxiety as possible causes.

Pulmonary Function Testing

Referral to a pulmonologist is recommended to help discern the cause of the dyspnea. The standard pulmonary function tests used to help determine the origin of the dyspnea are the forced vital capacity (FVC), the forced expiratory volume in 1 s (FEV_1) or the maximum voluntary ventilation (MVV), and the maximum inspiratory and expiratory flow-volume loop. These tests are done with spirometry. The flow-volume relationships in particular diagnose the presence of a large (central) airway obstruction and assess its effect. Characteristic patterns of the flow-volume loop also distinguish a fixed obstruction from a variable one and an extrathoracic location from an intrathoracic location. The overall shape of the flow-volume loop is used in interpreting the results of this spirometric test. The speed of air movement in and out of the lungs is assessed by the flow rate, whereas the volume measures the amount of air moved. The major landmark of a flow-volume loop is the peak expiratory flow rate. This is the first peak of air exhaled from the patient. The peak expiratory flow rate measures whether the patient is giving maximal effort and tests the overall strength of the expiratory muscles and the general condition of the large airways, such as the trachea and main bronchi. Forced expiratory flow at 25% of FVC is the flow rate at the 25% point of the total volume exhaled. Assuming maximal effort, this flow rate is still indicative of the condition of fairly large to medium-size bronchi. Forced expiratory flow at 50% of FVC is the flow rate at the 50% point of the total volume exhaled. This landmark is at the midpoint of the FVC and indicates the status of medium to small airways. Forced expiratory flow at 75% of FVC is the flow rate at the 75% point of the total volume exhaled and indicates the status of small airways. Forced inspiratory flow at 25% of FVC is the flow rate at the 25% point of the total volume inhaled. Abnormalities noted here indicate upper airway obstructions. Areas of the mouth, upper and lower pharynx (back of the throat), and the vocal folds affect the inspiratory flow rates. Peak inspiratory flow rate is the fastest flow rate achieved during inspiration. Forced inspiratory flow at 50% of FVC is the flow rate at the 50% point of the total volume inhaled, and forced inspiratory flow at 75% of FVC is the flow rate at the 75% point of the total volume inhaled (see Figure 11.10). Clinical reports that indicate spirometry values are typically presented in absolute numbers and percentage predicted, based on normative values. The normative values are race, gender, and age dependent, and the standards may vary across clinical laboratories. If the spirometric data rule out lower airway disease or the flow-volume loop data indicate upper airway obstruction, appropriate care can be focused on the remediation of the laryngeal condition. With intervention, the sensation of dyspnea should diminish.

Terminology

In the speech–language pathologist's assessment and treatment of voice, many terms related to breathing are used, including *support, diaphragmatic breathing, clavicular breathing, circular breathing*, and *breathing exercises*. The term *support* can be vague, and when used in clinical report writing, frequently does not tell much about the physiological status of the respiratory pump. When used, this term probably relates to the physiological driving force (i.e., pressure) for voicing.

The term *diaphragmatic breathing* is a play on words. Given that the diaphragm is a muscle of inspiration, it doesn't make much physiological sense to use this term when directing instruction of expiration to the patient. If the term is used to indicate the piston-like mechanism of the abdomen, it should be replaced with the term *abdominal force*, which makes more physiological sense with regard to the mechanics of breathing.

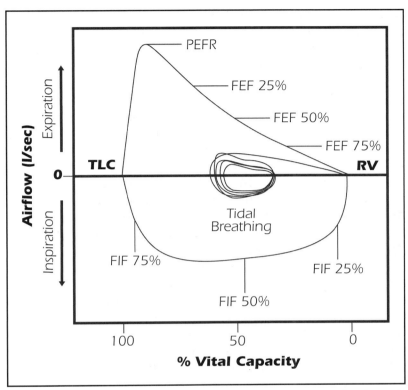

Figure 11.10. Flow-volume loop indicating major flow and volumetric landmarks during expiratory and inspiratory cycle. PEFR = peak expiratory flow; FEF = forced expiratory flow; FIF = forced inspiratory flow; TLC = total lung capacity; RV = residual volume.

Clavicular breathing is usually used when referring to individuals who breathe by raising the pectoral area of the chest wall and the shoulders, but it has become used too often to identify patients with presumed poor breath support. In fact, *clavicular breathing* is often used to classify the way women breathe. This term is also used inaccurately, because individuals who have normal respiratory structure and function of the chest wall wouldn't use a less efficient system voluntarily or reflexively. When the problem is solely laryngeal, and the individual has intact respiratory muscle tone, clavicular breathing is unlikely. The human body likes to work less, not more, for any given task. Therefore, unless they are completely exhausted, patients with voice disorders but no neurological impairment or lower airway disease are unlikely to be clavicular breathers. This term should be used cautiously.

Circular breathing, which is most often associated with musicians (in particular, saxophonists), is difficult to do. Basically, the process begins with half-full lungs. The person then supposedly fills the mouth with an air pocket while still breathing out from the lungs. He or she switches from lungs to mouth air with no interruption and forces air out from the mouth with the cheeks. The person then switches back to the now-full lungs and repeats the process.

Finally, in our clinical treatment of voice patients we have often come across the term *breathing exercises.* This is another broad, categorical phrase that ranges from a spectrum of relaxation exercises to yoga methods. Many of these exercises have merit, particularly those that are focused on teaching coordination of inspiration and expiration, postural alignment, and use of the abdomen to help produce pressure for speech. Exercises that do not offer specific physiological guidelines or that place the patient in the supine position are not based on an understanding of the nature of and relationship between relaxation pressures and gravitational forces, and these exercises are probably being taught in a mystic manner. Some promoted exercise programs have included music therapy for working on breathing patterns in patients with multiple sclerosis (Wiens, Reimer, & Guyn, 1999). Other programs have placed people on their backs to facilitate better breathing or relaxation. With these techniques there has been little study dedicated to understanding the mechanism of breathing. Hoit (1995) examined how breathing differs in the upright and supine positions and discussed in detail the clinical implications of the different postures when treating patients with speech and voice disorders. On the one hand, it would be unfair to say that all breathing exercises do not have merit in some form; in fact, many of these techniques may work by facilitating production of the voice at higher lung volumes or by taking advantage of the appropriate gravitational effects that direct breathing in an expiratory direction. Often, however, we do not know which factors are being manipulated, and quantitative outcome measures to verify the validity of these exercises with singers and patient groups are lacking.

Interventions for Specific Groups

The next section focuses on some specific patient groups and describes the specific respiratory mechanisms used by these patients. The types of interventions that may be helpful when working with a particular group are also listed.

Ventilator Dependency. Mechanical ventilation effectively helps or replaces typical spontaneous breathing by taking over the role that the respiratory muscles usually play in ventilation. A ventilator induces rhythmic inflation and emptying of the lungs to regulate the exchange rate of gases in the blood. The most common type of ventilator delivers inspiratory gases directly into the patient's airway. The patient is connected to the ventilator by an endotracheal tube passed through the nose or mouth into the trachea (windpipe). If prolonged ventilation is likely to be required, a tube is inserted into a stoma.

Individuals with a spinal cord injury at a high cervical level (C2–C5) will typically have some degree of, if not complete, paralysis of the diaphragm and intercostal muscles. These muscle groups are critical to maintaining ventilation and secondarily to providing the activity to engage in forced maneuvers for speech, such as increasing volume, sustaining durations, and varying prosody. Individuals with this type of spinal cord injury are mechanically ventilated, with the equipment setting a certain amount of volume and pressure. This mechanical ventilation sustains their breathing and allows them to speak. Because the speech variations are a function of the ventilator settings, however, there are limitations to the degree of volume and sound duration that can be generated and maintained. In addition, if there is partial paralysis of the diaphragm or other respiratory musculature, the person with the spinal cord injury may be unable to be off the ventilator for long periods of time because the muscles that were once consistently active in ventilation and speech breathing are no longer responsible for generating force. These muscles atrophy over time, creating a vicious circle and a state of chronic mechanical ventilation. The patient who is mechanically ventilated therefore has a reduced pressure-generating capacity due initially to a reduced phrenic motor drive and then to atrophy of inspiratory muscles caused by mechanical ventilation. The process of weaning a patient off the ventilator is complicated, and the reasons for failure may be numerous. However, in the case of spinal cord injury, inspiratory muscle weakness plays a key role.

The decrease in inspiratory muscle strength in a spinal cord injury is caused by a reduction in inspiratory muscle fiber activity. This occurs when the ventilator rests the muscles (causing a decrease in muscle mass and strength) and also because a reduced number of motor units are activated during spontaneous breathing efforts. The primary cause of reduced inspiratory muscle strength usually is reduced brain stem drive caused by a severing of the descending spinal tracts (such as occurs in C1 and C2 injuries) that originate in the brain stem respiratory oscillator and terminate on the inspiratory muscle motor neuron nuclei. A second cause of reduced brain stem drive is direct damage of the phrenic motor nucleus (a C3–C5 spinal cord injury), which is the locus of the muscle drive to the diaphragm. These lesions result in a reduced pressure-generating capacity and cause varying mechanical ventilator dependency. The higher the lesion is in the cervical spinal cord, the greater the respiratory muscle weakness. The greater the inspiratory muscle weakness (larger loss of phrenic motor units), the greater the percentage of the respiratory pump's pressure-generating capability the patient must use to maintain ventilation. This places the patient at risk for inspiratory muscle fatigue and increases the patient's dependency on a mechanical ventilator. This high-level activation of the respiratory pump leads to awareness of respiratory effort, which is perceived as the very distressing sensation of dyspnea or shortness of breath, as discussed previously. Many patients with spinal cord injuries who are dependent on ventilators are able to breathe without ventilator support for short periods of time, but they are unable to sustain the pressure generation needed for comfortable, long-term breathing and cannot communicate because of reduced inspiratory muscle strength. The reduced muscle strength limits the amount of inspiratory volume that can be drawn in for speech, thereby limiting the amount of available subglottal pressure for generating and maintaining adequate speech durations and speech volume.

For these types of patients, reducing the effort of breathing and freeing them from ventilator dependency has been attempted by trying to increase the strength of their inspiratory muscles using inspiratory muscle strength training techniques (IMST) as opposed to conventional weaning methods, which have been shown to produce a maximum increase of only 20% (Leith & Bradley, 1976). IMST methods involve use of a threshold pressure device, which consists of an adjustable, spring-loaded pressure relief valve attached to the tracheotomy tube. For inspiratory air to flow, the patient must generate an inspiratory pressure greater than the pressure set on the threshold device. This provides an isotonic load to the muscle for the entire inspiratory portion of the breath. The magnitude of this inspiratory threshold load is set at a certain percentage of the patient's maximum inspiratory pressure. As the patient's inspiratory strength becomes greater, the pressure setting is progressively increased to further challenge the muscles. IMST is similar to a weight-training program for weak limb muscles that would be conducted for a patient recovering from prolonged bed rest. It is based on two physiological principles: The first principle is *specificity*, which refers to isolating the training of a specific muscle group and the neuromuscular patterns of interest, and the second is *overload*, which states that physiological adaptations will occur in working muscles with the appropriate stimuli. An appropriate stimulus includes workloads that are greater than the workloads encountered in daily life. In study participants without an injury, such a training regimen increases inspiratory muscle strength by an average of 50% within 4 weeks (Kellerman, Martin, & Davenport, 2000; Sapienza, Brown, Martin, & Davenport, 1999). In our experience, an IMST method used with a patient who had a spinal cord injury and was on a mechanical ventilator helped the individual achieve spontaneous breathing periods for up to 80 minutes while maintaining normal oxygen saturation following training at 4.5 years postinjury. Previous to IMST, spontaneous breathing periods lasted no more than 5 minutes. IMST methods are just beginning to be used for weaning patients from ventilators and have been used with a limited number of patients with spinal cord injuries. The results appear to be quite promising.

Chronic Obstructive Pulmonary Disease. As part of the upper airway, the larynx performs a prominent role in the control of expiratory airflow and lung volume. It is not merely a passive conduit to the lung but constitutes an active mechanism relevant to ventilatory control. Although there is little laryngeal compensation in healthy adults, in patients with airway obstruction the larynx is involved in physiologic adjustments to help compensate for the impaired pulmonary mechanics.

Specifically, in patients with chronic airflow limitations, upper airway resistance is significantly greater than in individuals without this problem. Patients suffering from obstructive airway disease have exhibited a greater than twofold increase in expiratory resistance due to exaggerated glottic narrowing (Campbell, Imberger, & Jones, 1976).

Glottal Configuration. When glottal configuration was examined during a dynamic activity of voluntary panting, patients with chronic obstructive pulmonary disease (COPD) did not widen the glottis like their healthy counterparts (Brancatisano, Dodd, & Engel, 1984). The presumably compensatory narrowing of the glottis demonstrated by patients with COPD during quiet breathing persists during dynamic breathing activities, particularly for those individuals whose FEV_1 is 60% or below the predicted value.

Glottal configuration is likely to compensate to slow expiratory airflow and breathing frequency during speech. Upper airway narrowing used as a compensatory mechanism in an attempt to regulate airflow and maintain lung volume during voice and speech production has not been extensively examined in patients with lung disease, although the symptoms reported by patients with COPD have suggested respiratory and laryngeal involvement. These symptoms include dyspnea, reduced vocal volume, and hoarseness.

Lee, Friesen, Lambert, and Loudon (1998) developed a dyspnea questionnaire because although dyspnea as a factor has been well assessed in patients with pulmonary disease, the interaction of speech and dyspnea has been largely ignored in most of the widely used indexes available to clinicians. In addition, speech questionnaires that are useful for individuals with lung disease are not plentiful. Lee et al.'s (1998) results showed that dyspnea is a relevant factor when assessing the speaking abilities of individuals with lung disease from both personal and vocational standpoints. The authors advocated for the development of scales that are sensitive to the variable of dyspnea. The scale developed by Lee et al., although not used specifically with patients with voice disorders, could be used as a supplement to other indexes, such as the *Voice Handicap Index* (Jacobson et al., 1997), and it should be further investigated for that purpose.

In an assessment of speech breathing behavior in patients with lung disease, Lee, Loudon, Jacobson, and Stuebing (1993) examined three different types of groups—patients with sarcoidosis, with asthma, or with emphysema. Their findings showed alterations in speech breathing that were specific to the disease and the task. Respiratory rates were rapid, and inspiratory durations were longer. When clinically treating persons with lung disease, clinicians should be aware of exacerbations, which usually indicate an active infection or inflammation of the bronchial tubes within the backdrop of the patient's chronic lung disease. These exacerbations will again alter breathing patterns and accentuate feelings of breathlessness, and they may be caused by acute bronchitis or pneumonia. Noninfectious exacerbations usually are related to allergies, or to environmental exposures that caused acute brochospasm.

Patients with lung disease do not commonly realize their detriments in communication until it is too late. In a review of personal stories reported by persons with severe COPD, Hajiro, Nishimura, Tsukino, Ikeda, and Oga (2000) found that the eventual impact of this loss is depression and withdrawal similar to that associated with any progressive and debilitating disease process. In such cases, a multidisciplinary wellness rehabilitation program that can enhance communication strategies should be employed.

Voice Disorders. Vocal pathology changes glottal configuration, alters laryngeal function, and deteriorates sound production. Although many researchers have defined the laryngeal physiological parameters associated with vocal pathology, in only a few studies have researchers determined the mechanical and muscle force modifications to the respiratory system that occur when glottal configuration is altered. Evidence of respiratory-related activity in laryngeal afferent fibers, their modification with variations in subglottal pressures, and the drive of the speech system to maintain aerodynamic integrity in spite of significant changes in upper airway resistance would lead one to hypothesize that there are modifications to speech breathing mechanics when changes in glottal configuration occur with voice disorders.

It is not uncommon to hear complaints about breathing from individuals suffering from hyperfunctional or hypofunctional voice conditions. Whether the person has muscle tension dysphonia, vocal fold nodules, or vocal fold paralysis, the cause of the breathing symptoms tends to be related to an alteration in glottal configuration (resulting in increased or decreased laryngeal airway resistance) rather than to primary lung disease.

Figure 11.11 shows laryngeal configuration changes across a vibratory cycle and an example of laryngeal compensation (ventricular fold approximation, anteroposterior laryngeal squeeze). This occurs when the vocal folds are not functioning appropriately. Laryngeal compensation often occurs with reduced glottal closure, difficulty in maintaining subglottal pressure, or hyperfunctional behaviors associated with voicing. Laryngeal compensation can be

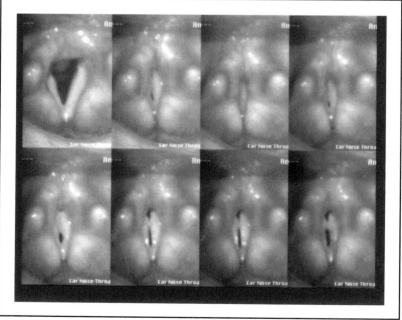

Figure 11.11. Laryngeal endoscopic frames depicting laryngeal compensation during phonation. Note the ventricular fold medialization.

determined through endoscopy. It has also been verified through the use of laryngeal airway resistance measures in persons with vocal nodules (Sapienza & Stathopoulos, 1994) and spasmodic dysphonia (Finnegan, Luschei, Barkmeier, & Hoffman, 1996; Plant & Hillel, 1998; Witsell, Weissler, Donovan, Howard, & Martinkosky, 1994) and has been assumed to be present when there is high laryngeal airway resistance in other hyperfunctional voice conditions, such as muscle tension dysphonia. We also know that decreased laryngeal airway resistance and abnormal flows and breathing patterns exist with hypofunctional voice disorders, such as vocal fold paralysis (Saarinen, Rihkanen, Malmberg, Pekkanen, & Sovijarvi, 2001). Some of the initial work on speech breathing patterns in persons with voice disorders was done by Hixon (1987), Sapienza and Stathopoulos (1994), and Sapienza, Stathopoulos, and Brown (1997). Their studies indicated an interactive role between glottal configuration and speech breathing behavior. Specifically, higher glottal airflows were associated with larger lung volumes used per speech task, lower lung volume terminations (particularly when terminated below functional residual capacity), and deviant phrasing strategies.

Alterations in glottal airflows in cases of vocal fold paralysis and spasmodic dysphonia can change the normal sensory and kinesthetic response of the laryngeal mucosal receptors. It may be that this perturbation to the mechanoreceptors feeds back to the respiratory central controller and alters its impending output. If this is the case, respiratory mechanical changes to the breathing pattern during speech would be altered, and we would expect to see muscle compensations during speech production. We do know that persons with abductor spasmodic dysphonia present with temporal and volumetric deviations during speech. Their speech is characterized by fewer syllables per breath group, smaller lung volume excursions, and inappropriate breaths located at nongrammatical boundaries (Sapienza, Cannito, & Erickson, 1996). Recent work by Bidus, Ludlow, Edgar, and Sapienza (2001) determined whether the respiratory-related symptoms are merely a response to the altered glottal configuration or if the speech breathing pattern has a more central origin related to the overall dystonic condition of the disease process. Some researchers have suggested that airflow stability in speech disorders is lower prior to treatment and that when the spasms are reduced with botox treatment, the stability returns to typical levels (Finnegan, Luschei, Gordon, & Hoffman, 1999). If this is the case, any respiratory-related deviances should also diminish. This theory has not been proved but continues to be investigated.

Other movement disorders of the larynx, such as paradoxical vocal fold dysfunction, cause respiratory distress as well. Symptoms can include coughing, wheezing, and stridor. These patients produce normal expiratory limbs on the flow-volume loop, with a reduced or flattened inspiratory limb. These cases often are initially diagnosed as asthma, but a key difference is that their dyspnea is associated with dysphonia and the severity of the symptoms is discordant with the results of the standardized pulmonary function tests described previously. Treatments for the breathing symptoms associated with paradoxical vocal fold dysfunction have varied and have included speech therapy, psychotherapy, and pharmacotherapy—many with limited success. IMST has been tried in one case of a rower with exercise-induced paradoxical vocal fold dysfunction, and a substantial improvement was made in both inspiratory muscle strength and reduction of paradoxical activity during exercise (Hoffman Ruddy, Sapienza, Lehman, Davenport, & Martin, 2003). This is a single case, and more work needs to be done to clearly understand the mechanisms of the result. Power and Howley (2001) suggested that the elimination of the paradoxing in this case might have been related to the principles of neural adaptations and cross-over effects that accompany physical training.

Biofeedback Techniques

Some clinicians use biofeedback techniques to help the patient monitor and control the inspiratory and expiratory cycles of breathing during voice production. Biofeedback is defined as the feedback of biological information to gain control of bodily processes that normally cannot be controlled voluntarily. An example would be muscle tension. An electromyogram is one way to measure muscle tension through the use of strategically placed electrodes. Theoretically, the clinician who is treating a patient with a voice disorder should have him or her monitor both perceptual and physiological processes associated with the voice disorder while implementing a particular treatment regime that attempts to reduce the hyperfunctional behaviors. Likewise, real-time, visually presented feedback, such as in oscillographic displays or online computer monitoring systems, may help the patient enhance breathing patterns. Murdoch, Pitt, Theodoros, and Ward (1999) used biofeedback with the inductance plethysmography to provide real-time and continuous visual biofeedback of rib cage circumference during breathing in a child with a traumatic brain injury. The results indicated very good success with the biofeedback technique when compared to traditional instructions for proper speech breathing, and Murdoch and colleagues believed that the visual biofeedback techniques brought about a far superior outcome. Noeker, von Ruden, Staab, and Haverkamp (2000) employed biological feedback for monitoring respiratory rhythms in children with bronchial asthma. They used a respiratory corrector unit, which visualized patients' external respiration rhythm, and synchronized it with a reference rhythm whose parameters were set by a physician or by the patient. This method reduced symptoms in mild and moderate bronchial asthma, preventing attacks, prolonging remission, and reducing the amount of bronchodilating agents used. In these studies, the device was used two to three times a day, with 15 to 20 minutes for each session. Biofeedback appears to be effective and is easily incorporated into a treatment program for a variety of patient types.

References

Bidus, K., Ludlow, C. L., Edgar, J., & Sapienza, C. M. (2001). *Respiratory motor control during speech and non-speech tasks in spasmodic dysphonia.* Philadelphia: Voice Foundation.

Brancatisano, A., Dodd, D. S., & Engel, L. A. (1984). Respiratory activity of posterior cricoarytenoid muscle and vocal cords in humans. *Journal of Applied Physiology, 19,* 1143–1149.

Campbell, A. H., Imberger, H., & Jones, B. (1976). Increased upper airway resistance in patients with airway narrowing. *British Journal of Diseases of the Chest, 1,* 58–65.

Finnegan, E. M., Luschei, E. S., Barkmeier, J. M., & Hoffman, H. T. (1996). Sources of error in estimation of laryngeal airway resistance in persons with spasmodic dysphonia. *Journal of Speech and Hearing Research, 39,* 105–113.

Finnegan, E. M., Luschei, E. S., Gordon, J. D., & Hoffman, H. T. (1999). Increased stability of airflow following botulinum toxin injection. *Laryngoscope, 109,* 1300–1306.

Hajiro, T., Nishimura, K., Tsukino, M., Ikeda, A., & Oga, T. (2000). Stages of disease severity and factors that affect the health status of patients with chronic obstructive pulmonary disease. *Respiratory Medicine, 94,* 841–846.

Hixon, T. J. (1987). *Respiratory function in speech and song.* San Diego, CA: Singular.

Hixon, T. J., Goldman, M. D., & Mead, J. (1973). Kinematics of the chest wall during speech production: Volume displacement for the rib cage, abdomen and lung. *Journal of Speech and Hearing Research, 19,* 297–356.

Hoffman Ruddy, B., Sapienza, C. M., Lehman, J., Davenport, P. D., & Martin, A. D. (2003). *Inspiratory muscle strength training in a rower with exercise-induced paradoxical vocal fold dysfunction.* Manuscript submitted for publication.

Hoit, J. D. (1995). Influence of body position on breathing and its implication for the evaluation and treatment of speech and voice disorders. *Journal of Voice, 9,* 341–347.

Jacobson, B., Johnson, A., Grywalski, G., Silbergleit, A., Jacobson, Benninger, M., et al. (1997). The Voice Handicap Index (VHI): Development and validation. *American Journal of Speech-Language Pathology, 6,* 66–70.

Kellerman, B. A., Martin, A. D., & Davenport, P. W. (2000). Inspiratory strengthening effect on resistive load detection and magnitude estimation. *Medicine and Science in Sports and Exercise, 32,* 1859–1867.

Lee, L., Friesen, M., Lambert, I. R., & Loudon, R. G. (1998). Evaluation of dyspnea during physical and speech activities in patients with pulmonary disease. *Chest, 111,* 625–632.

Lee, L., Loudon, R. G., Jacobson, B. H., & Stuebing, R. (1993). Speech breathing in patients with lung disease. *American Review of Respiratory Disease, 147,* 1199–1206.

Leith, D. E., & Bradley, M. (1976). Ventilatory muscle strength and endurance training. *Journal of Applied Physiology, 41,* 508–516.

Murdoch, B. E., Pitt, G., Theodoros, D. G., & Ward, E. C. (1999). Real-time continuous visual biofeedback in the treatment of speech breathing disorders following childhood traumatic brain injury: Report of one case. *Pediatric Rehabilitation, 3*(1), 5–20.

Noeker, M., von Ruden, V., Staab, D., & Haverkamp, F. (2000). Processes of body perception and their therapeutic use in pediatrics: From nonspecific relaxation to training to recognize disease-specific symptoms. *Klinische Pediatric, 212,* 260–265.

Plant, R. L., & Hillel, A. D. (1998). Direct measurement of subglottic pressure and laryngeal resistance in normal subjects and in spasmodic dysphonia. *Journal of Voice, 12,* 300–314.

Power, S., & Howley, E. (2001). *Exercise physiology: Theory and application to fitness and performance* (4th ed.). New York: McGraw-Hill.

Saarinen, A., Rihkanen, H., Malmberg, L. P., Pekkanen, L., & Sovijarvi, A. R. (2001). Disturbances in airflow dynamics and tracheal sounds during forced and quiet breathing in subjects with unilateral vocal fold paralysis. *Clinical Physiology, 21,* 712–717.

Sapienza, C. M., Brown, J. B., Martin, A. D., & Davenport, P. D. (1999). Inspiratory pressure threshold training for glottal airway limitation in laryngeal papilloma. *Journal of Voice, 13,* 382–388.

Sapienza, C. M., Cannito, M., & Erickson, M. (1996, November). *Temporal and volume indices associated with adductor spasmodic dysphonia.* Paper presented at the annual conference of the American Speech-Language-Hearing Association, Seattle.

Sapienza, C. M., & Stathopoulos, E. T. (1994). Respiratory and laryngeal measures of children and women with bilateral vocal fold nodules. *Journal of Speech and Hearing Research, 37,* 1229–1243.

Sapienza, C. M., Stathopoulos, E. T., & Brown, W. S., Jr. (1997). Speech breathing during reading in women with vocal nodules. *Journal of Voice, 11,* 195–201.

Wiens, M. E., Reimer, M. A., & Guyn, H. L. (1999). Music therapy as a treatment method for improving respiratory muscle strength in patients with advanced multiple sclerosis: A pilot study. *Rehabilitation Nursing 24*(2), 74–80.

Witsell, D. L., Weissler, M. C., Donovan, M. K., Howard, J. F., Jr., & Martinkosky, S. J. (1994). Measurement of laryngeal resistance in the evaluation of botulinum toxin injection for treatment of focal laryngeal dystonia. *Laryngoscope, 104*(1, Pt. 1), 8–11.

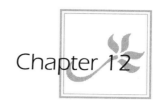

Chapter 12

Pharmatoxicity and Pharmacotherapy

Bari Hoffman Ruddy, Monica Nindra Tipirneni, and Kiran Tipirneni

Hoffman Ruddy, Tipirneni, and Tipirneni note that pharmacological agents are used to treat, prevent, and sometimes cure many illnesses with the purpose of avoiding more invasive treatments. The authors point out that as advancements in research and development continue, many more drugs are becoming available, some with higher potency levels than can be readily administered. Consequently, these drugs may also produce more harmful side effects, which lead to severe impairment of a patient's communicative needs. This chapter addresses many of the drug treatments currently prescribed and discusses their potential side effects. Furthermore, given ongoing advancements in research and development, this chapter provides the most current drug information available at the time of its preparation. Finally, the authors have provided additional sources (see Appendix 12.1) so that the clinician may continue to advance his or her knowledge in this topic area and provide the most current treatment.

1. *Awareness of drug effects, as well as their side effects, is critical knowledge to have when treating patients with medically complex conditions. In general terms, how does the study of pharmokinetics enhance the care of a voice patient?*

2. *What are the potential side effects of antihistamines that should be discussed with a professional singer? Why?*

3. *Many forms of pharmacological therapies for gastroesophageal reflux are available by prescription and over the counter. The major groups are antacids, H_2 receptor antagonists, and proton pump inhibitors. What are the differences among these three drug classifications in how they mediate gastroesophageal reflux disease?*

Virtually all medications have the potential to cause an effect or interaction (Center for Drug Evaluation and Research, 2001). Although some are minor and not significant to the general population of patients seen clinically, other interactions can have a major impact on certain patients by limiting employment opportunities or lifestyle. The challenge to clinicians is to develop the most appropriate treatment plan while taking into account the numerous individual variables. Some of these variables may include mechanisms of drug interactions, disease progression, effects and side effects, activities of daily living, and financial constraints. In addition, within each individual patient, intrinsic variables—such as age, gender, weight, metabolic status, body response times, and use of other drugs—may affect pharmacological treatment. A thorough diagnostic interview that includes obtaining a full list of current medications (prescribed, over-the-counter [OTC], and herbal remedies) thus is vital to a clinician's evaluation process. In addition, the diagnostic interview may also provide significant information regarding the history and progression of the disease and current or past forms of treatment. With this level of understanding, clinicians can work more efficiently in an interdisciplinary manner.

In this chapter, we focus on defining pharmacokinetics and drug administration, followed by an explanation of drug classes, drug mechanisms of action, commonly used medications, effects and side effects, drug interactions, nutritional considerations, drug compliance, and special populations. Coverage of the last item includes geriatrics, pediatrics, spasmodic dysphonia, and persons who use their voice professionally.

Pharmacokinetics

The study of how drugs are absorbed, distributed, metabolized, and excreted is referred to as *pharmacokinetics. Absorption* is the process by which a drug proceeds from the site of administration to systemic circulation. *Distribution* refers to the movement of the drug from one location in the body to another. *Metabolism* is the process by which the drug is chemically altered by the action of enzymes, which typically occurs in the liver. The metabolite may become more active, less active, or as active as the parent compound in the drug. *Excretion* is the process whereby the drug or metabolite is removed from the body. The kidneys are the primary organ of this process (Pronsky, 2001).

Drug Administration

The process of administering a drug can be achieved through invasive or noninvasive means. Examples of invasive administration include *intramuscular,* where the drug is injected into the muscle and absorbed into the blood; *subcutaneous,* in which the drug is injected into the tissue beneath the skin; and *intravenous,* which is the most expedient way to administer a drug to its desired location and has the highest concentration level. The drug is directly injected into the blood stream through a vein and has direct access to most tissues in the body. In *intraventricular* or *intrathecal administration,* the drug is injected into the cerebrospinal fluid. In intraventricular, a catheter is inserted into the cerebral ventricles or the spinal canal by means of a small hole created in the skull. In the latter method, the catheter is then directed into the ventricle and the skin is closed. For intrathecal administration, a pump with a dry reservoir is implanted under the skin. The drug is delivered into the spinal fluid via a small catheter (Craig & Stitzel, 1986; Vogel, Carter, & Carter, 2000).

One noninvasive example is *oral* administration, in which the drug is taken by mouth (either in tablet/capsule form or by liquid) and absorbed in the gastrointestinal tract. The drug is further broken down in the liver and then distributed to the intended tissue. Drugs administered orally include several formulations. *Controlled release tablets* are designed to provide a long period of absorption time through the gastrointestinal tract. These tablets or capsules are taken less frequently, are typically very convenient for patient use, and usually have a good rate of compliance. *Wax tablets* are slowly released to the gastrointestinal tract by gradual melting by body temperature. *Multiple-layer drug tablets* are produced in several different compounds. A common mistake patients make with these tablets is to crush them for oral intake. Doing so destroys the desired drug effects. *Multiple microspheres* are formulated to dissolve at different rates and usually are placed in capsules. Multiple microsphere capsules also should not be crushed. Clinicians working with patients who have dysphagia should caution them against crushing the pills or manipulating the oral intake without investigating the intended mechanism of drug delivery (Craig & Stitzel, 1986; Vogel et al., 2000).

Another noninvasive drug administration technique is *topical,* or *transdermal,* in which the drug is administered on the skin and then absorbed through the body. These types of drugs usually take the forms of creams, ointments, sprays, or patches and have the ability to release the drug over a controlled period of time, ranging from hours to several days. In *rectal administration,* a suppository containing the drug is inserted into the rectum, where it is then absorbed. *Vaginal administration* refers to the drug being administered and absorbed in the vagina. In *sublingual administration,* a drug tablet is placed under the tongue. This method enables a quick absorption rate because of the increased mucosal vascularity. *Buccal administration* is similar but has a slower process and slower absorption rate than sublingual administration. The drug is placed in the buccal cavity, where it dissolves. *Inhalation administration* is the last noninvasive means of administration and refers to drugs that are formulated for nasal and pulmonary absorption. These include steroidal nasal sprays and bronchodilators (Craig & Stitzel, 1986; Vogel et al., 2000).

Drug Classes

Antihistamines

Antihistamines are one of the most common drugs used today. This class of drug is mainly used to treat symptoms resulting from hypersensitivity to environmental allergens. Some antihistamines are available OTC, whereas newer generation antihistamines require a prescription. The newer generation antihistamines are reported to have fewer side effects, such as drowsiness and drying of the mucous membranes. The OTC formulations are known for their sedative effect and should be taken with caution. Antihistamines function by competitively antagonizing histamine at the H_1 receptor sites on mast cells, thereby blocking the cascade of histamine-related symptoms, such as runny nose, nasal congestion, watery eyes, sneezing, and pruritus (itching; Craig & Stitzel, 1986). Because antihistamines offer only symptomatic relief, clinicians should investigate further to determine the underlying environmental allergens and to control exposure.

Clinicians should caution professional voice users of the potential side effects of antihistamine use, which primarily are the drying or thickening of upper respiratory tract secretions, dehydration, and sedation. Antihistamines that are combined with other drugs, such as cough suppressants (codeine, or dextromethorphan), may cause further drying of secretions and sedation. If an antihistamine is combined with a mucolytic agent such as guaifenesin, however, mucosal secretion drying is minimized.

Clinicians who are involved in the care of professional voices should also implement behavioral management, including counseling concerning vocal health and initiation of hygienic voice therapy in order to minimize the side effects from antihistamine use. If laryngeal lubrication is impaired due to alteration of the normal balance of laryngeal mucous secretions, alterations in phonation will occur. For professional voice users, this impairment can significantly affect their livelihood (Sataloff, Hawkshaw, & Rosen, 1998).

Mucolytic Agents

The best mucolytic agent available is water. No medication is considered to be an appropriate substitute for adequate hydration; however, mucolytics and expectorants are helpful in counteracting the drying-out effects of antihistamines. Normal respiratory and laryngeal lubrication is essential for normal function. Respiratory secretions are directly related to the availability of water in the body. Proper hydration decreases the viscosity of mucous secretions. Dehydration may occur as the result of athletics, environment, altitude, or interference from metabolic and pharmacological agents. The most common manufactured mucolytic agents include products that contain guaifenesin, such as Robitussin, Entex, and Humabid. These work to thin and enhance mucosal secretions by increasing respiratory tract fluid and reducing the viscosity of the secretions.

Corticosteroids

Glucocorticoids are the most common class of corticosteroids used to manage acute inflammation. They come in various forms, such as oral tablets, respiratory inhalers, and injectables. Their precise mechanism of action is largely unknown, but they are thought to inhibit the inflammatory response by preventing the synthesis or action of inflammatory mediators (Burham & Short, 1997; Craig & Stitzel, 1986). Oral glucocorticoids are usually administered in the form of a tapered dosing interval to avoid adrenal insufficiency. Signs of adrenal insufficiency include fatigue, anorexia, nausea, vomiting, diarrhea, and weakness (Burham & Short, 1997; Craig & Stitzel, 1986). Because of their anti-inflammatory effect, glucocorticoids are commonly used in asthmatic patients and have also been found to be effective in reducing inflammation associated with laryngitis (Sataloff et al., 1998). Corticosteroids are also effective for short-term use with singers and other professional voice users who experience changes in voice quality due to vocal fold edema. Although this can be an expedited and effective treatment approach, overuse and abuse can be a problem (Sataloff et al., 1998). Corticosteroid therapy should not replace education of the patient regarding vocal abuse and misuse factors. Furthermore, clinicians should advocate vocal health and hygienic voice therapy programs in conjunction with corticosteroid therapy to maximize voice quality improvements. Corticosteroids should be prescribed only after determining that the patient is free of infection because of the ability of this class of drugs to down-regulate the immune response (Burham & Short, 1997; Craig & Stitzel, 1986; Sataloff et al., 1998).

Side effects from long-term use of glucocorticoids may include gastritis, hypertension, hyperglycemia, muscle wasting, and fat redistribution (Burham & Short, 1997; Craig & Stitzel, 1986). Patients requiring long-term inhaled steroid use may also experience excessive laryngeal drying due to direct exposure to a variety of propellants in the steroid formulation. Other side effects include gastric irritation, fluid imbalance, electrolyte disturbances, muscle weakness, ulceration, hemorrhage, insomnia, mild mucosal drying, blurred vision, mood changes, and irritability. These effects usually do not occur in short-term use. Side effects that are not directly related to the use of corticosteroids seen in many asthmatics are hoarseness, throat irritation, and coughing due to the topical release of small drug particles, which lead to localized irritation (Burham & Short, 1997; Craig & Stitzel, 1986; Sataloff et al., 1998; Vogel et al., 2000). See Table 12.1 for a list of commonly prescribed oral corticosteroids.

Many asthma patients may also use bronchodilators, such as Proventil, cromolyn sodium, and epinephrine, which are available as metered-dose inhalers. Patients may also be prescribed oral forms of bronchodilators, such as theophylline and other xanthine derivatives. In general, they all work by promoting the relaxation of the bronchial smooth muscle. Bronchodilators are also used to treat professional voice users. Clinicians should know (a) how impaired pulmonary function can cause serious problems for professional voice users and (b) the proper use of bronchodilators for treatment.

Antihypertensive Agents

Antihypertensive drugs encompass a broad range of medications that are used to control hypertension. They include diuretics, angiotensin-converting enzyme (ACE) inhibitors, beta-blockers, calcium channel blockers, alpha$_2$ agonists, and angiotensin receptor blockers.

Table 12.1
Commonly Prescribed Oral Corticosteroids and Recommended Dosages

Drug name–Generic	Recommended dosage
Prednisone	5 mg to 60 mg per day
Prednisolone	4 mg to 60 mg per day
Methylprednisolone	4 mg to 48 mg per day or can use Medrol dose pak
Solu-Medrol	2 g per vial (dose based on weight)
Dexamethasone	0.75 mg to 9 mg per day

Diuretics work mainly by decreasing the body's plasma volume and thereby decreasing systemic blood pressure (Burham & Short, 1997; Craig & Stitzel, 1986). Dehydration is a common side effect when using medications containing diuretics. Dehydration leads to decreased laryngeal lubrication, increased mucosal drying, and chronic laryngeal edema.

The alpha$_2$ agonists, such as methyldopa and clonidine, work by blocking neurotransmitter release, which results in less sympathetic stimulation (Burham & Short, 1997; Craig & Stitzel, 1986). Consequently, there is a decrease in heart rate and blood pressure. Among the side effects of these drugs are anticholinergic effects. In most cases, patients notice drying of the mucosal membranes of the upper respiratory tract.

Beta-blockers work by blocking the beta-andrenergic receptors, mainly in the heart, which produces a reduction in heart rate and cardiac output and causes a reduction in blood pressure. These cardiac effects have also been useful for professional voice users for reducing performance anxiety; however, some vocalists complain of lackluster performances when they use drugs such as propanolol (Sataloff et al., 1998). Use of any beta-blocker should be discontinued only under medical supervision. Most beta-blockers must be tapered down to avoid potential problems. If a patient is taken off of a beta-blocker abruptly, it may lead to an overstimulation of the beta-receptors that were previously blocked by the drug.

Calcium channel blockers work by blocking the calcium ion movement into the smooth muscle, causing a relaxation of vascular smooth muscle and reducing blood pressure. These also must be tapered down when discontinued, to avoid any problems (Burham & Short, 1997; Craig & Stitzel, 1986).

ACE inhibitors and angiotensin I receptor antagonist (ARB) antihypertensives both work by suppressing the rennin–angiotensin–aldosterone system. ACE inhibitors work by blocking the angiotensin enzyme that converts angiotensin$_1$ to angiotensin$_2$ in smooth muscle (Burham & Short, 1997; Craig & Stitzel, 1986). A very bothersome side effect of ACE inhibitors and some ARBs is a dry, productive cough. In many cases, this leads to a discontinuation of the drug treatment. See Table 12.2 for a list of commonly prescribed antihypertensives.

Table 12.2
Commonly Prescribed Antihypertensives and Recommended Dosages

Drug name–Brand (generic)	Recommended dosage
Norvasc (calcium channel blocker)	5 mg–10 mg per day
Zestril (ACE inhibitor)	20 mg–40 mg per day
Accupril (ACE inhibitor)	20 mg–80 mg every day to twice a day doses
Toprol-XL (beta-blocker)	(Selective) 50 mg–100 mg every day
Prinivil (ACE inhibitor)	20 mg–40 mg per day
Vasotec (ACE inhibitor)	10 mg–40 mg per day every day or in divided doses
Lotensin (combination ACE inhibitor and diuretic)	5/6.25 mg–20/25 mg
Cozaar (angiotensin II receptor antagonist)	50 mg every day
Procardia XL (calcium channel blocker)	30 mg–90 mg every day, depending on the condition
Diovan HCT (angiotensin II receptor antagonist)	80 mg–320 mg every day

Antibiotics

An antibiotic is a chemical substance produced by a microorganism. It has the capacity to inhibit the growth of (*bacteriastatic*), or to kill (*bacteriacidal*), other microorganisms. Antibiotics that are sufficiently nontoxic to the host are used in the treatment of infectious diseases. Antibiotics work in various ways, depending on the class (i.e., penicillins, macrolides, and fluoroquinlones). They cause a bacteriacidal or bacteriastatic action against the bacterial organism via inhibition of basic cellular function in the infecting bacterium (i.e., inhibition of bacterial DNA synthesis, inhibition of cell wall synthesis, or inhibition of protein synthesis; Burham & Short, 1997; Craig & Stitzel, 1986). Antibiotics may be recommended in dosages large enough to produce therapeutic blood levels rapidly. In most cases, choosing an antibiotic should be based on cultures, but if time does not permit a culture, the antibiotic of choice should be a broad-spectrum (effective against a wide range of bacteria) one that is absorbed rapidly and achieves optimal blood levels quickly. The most important rule of antibiotic use is completion of therapy.

Compliance is a significant problem. If the course is not completed, it may have to be repeated due to a reoccurrence of the infection.

Antivirals

Antivirals mainly work by preventing the release of infectious viral nucleic acid into the host cell or by inhibiting viral DNA/RNA replication (Burham & Short, 1997; Craig & Stitzel, 1986). Acyclovir is used most often for cases of oral herpetic recurrent laryngeal nerve paresis or paralysis. The usual dose for an acute attack is 800 mg five times a day for 7 to 10 days. For intermittent therapy, the usual dose is 200 mg five times a day at the first sign or symptom. Amantadine is another antiviral used primarily against influenza. The usual dose is 100 mg twice daily. It can be prescribed if a patient is going to be among a large group of people.

Analgesics

Analgesics are drug agents that are used to relieve pain. Analgesics are available by prescription or OTC. The latter include aspirin, acetaminophen, and ibuprofen. All are presumed safe for short-term use. In cases of pain relief from sore throat and laryngeal irritation, care should be taken to avoid excessive use of aspirin or ibuprofen, because they may cause platelet dysfunction and predispose a performer to vocal fold hemorrhage. The best alternative OTC is acetaminophen. Pain relievers available by prescription include nonsteroidal anti-inflammatory drugs (NSAIDS), narcotics, and a new class of drugs referred to as the Cox-2 inhibitors. NSAIDS work by inhibiting the cycloxygenase$_1$ and cycloxygenase$_2$ isoenzymes and by blocking prostaglandin synthesis. Because NSAIDS affect both isoenzyme 1 and 2, they can have adverse effects, such as ulcers, bleeding, and perforations. It is believed that because the new Cox-2 inhibitor drugs (such as Vioxx and Celebrex; see Table 12.3) are selective, the incidences of these side effects are lowered. Even so, great caution is still advised for all patients who might be at risk of bleeding, especially laryngeal hemorrhage. Cox-2 inhibitors may be useful for voice patients. Their mechanism of action is similar to the NSAIDS in that they block prostaglandin synthesis by blocking the cycloxygenase isoenzymes.

Table 12.3

Commonly Prescribed Anti-Inflammatory Drugs

Drug name–Brand	Recommended dosage
Celebrex	200 mg, prescription only, take every day; use with caution with patients with sulfa hypersensitivity; approved for osteoarthritis and rheumatoid arthritis
Vioxx	12.5 mg–50 mg every day, approved for acute pain and pain associated with dysmenorrhea
Aspirin	325 mg–650 mg, available OTC, 1–2 tablets 4–6 hrs as needed
Tylenol (acetominophen)	325 mg–500 mg, available OTC, 1–2 tablets 4–6 hrs as needed
Motrin (ibuprofen)	200 mg; available OTC, higher strengths available by prescription; 1 tablet every 4–6 hrs as needed
Aleve 200 mg (naproxen)	200 mg; available OTC, higher strengths available by prescription; 1 tablet every 8–12 hrs

Note. ACE = angiotensin-converting enzyme; OTC = over the counter. Most prescription nonsteroidal anti-inflammatory drugs and drugs targeting the Cox-2 (nonsteroidal inhibitor) enzyme are used mainly for arthritis, but some have been used to relieve temporary inflammation and pain caused by trauma.

Although analgesics are helpful for pain relief, care should be taken not to ignore the reason for the pain. Pain is a protective physiological function, and masking it may produce further damage that may not be reversible. Narcotic pain relief should only be prescribed in extreme cases, due to a high incidence of drug dependency and sensory impairment. The side effects of narcotics could lead to an impairment of vocal performance or unconscious vocal abuse.

Hormones

Hormone therapy is used for replacement of hormones no longer biologically produced or to alter hormonal levels in the body. Hormones play a very large role on the body as a whole and can have a dramatic effect on voice quality. Androgenic hormones affect the voice significantly by producing a lowering of the fundamental frequency, especially in women, and a coarsening of the voice (Damste, 1967, 1968; Sataloff et al., 1998). Hormonal therapy is mainly employed to treat breast cancer, endometriosis, and postmenopausal sexual dysfunction. Birth control pills also have an androgen component that is paired with estrogen. In most cases, the balance of estrogen and progesterone is such that the voice changes do not occur. In the few cases where a noticeable change is experienced, discontinuation of the pills will restore normal vocal function (Sataloff et al., 1998). A vocal performer who is a post-menopausal woman should be placed on hormone replacement therapy to avoid the typical voice changes after menopause. The use of hormone replacement theory (HRT) is controversial in regard to its role in heart disease, stroke, and other serious medical side effects. All persons who are on or are prescribed HRT should be made aware of these concerns.

Thyroid replacement is also important for restoring vocal efficiency and the "ring" or resonant voice features lost due to hypothyroidism (Sataloff et al., 1998). Compliance is a very important factor in the efficacy of hormone replacement therapy. A steady state in blood levels should always be maintained to optimize the effectiveness of these drugs. They should be taken at approximately the same time each day as directed by the clinician. See Table 12.4 for a list of commonly prescribed hormone therapy drugs.

Gastroenterologic Medications

Many forms of pharmacological therapies for gastroesophageal reflux are available by prescription and OTC. The major groups in-

Table 12.4
Commonly Prescribed Drugs Used in Hormone Replacement Therapy

Drug name–Brand (generic)	Recommended dosage
Premarin (estrogen)	0.3 mg, 0.625 mg, 0.9 mg, 1.25 mg, 2.5 mg every day, replaces estrogen
Provera (medroxyprogesterone)	2.5 mg, 5 mg, 10 mg
Synthroid (levothyroxine)	Comes in many strengths, used for thyroid replacement
Nolvadex (Tamoxifen, antiestrogen)	10 mg to 20 mg twice a day
Prempro combination product of premarin and provera	Combination product of Premarin and Provera .625–2.5 mg
Various birth control pills	

clude antacids, H$_2$ receptor antagonists, and proton pump inhibitors. Antacids typically consist of a single ingredient or a combination of aluminum hydroxide, magnesium hydroxide, and calcium carbonate. Some antacids may also include simethicone, which helps with bloating discomfort. These products can cause diarrhea, constipation, bloating, and possibly a drying effect (Burham & Short, 1997; Craig & Stitzel, 1986). The problem of diarrhea is most often noted with magnesium hydroxide, and constipation is associated with aluminum hydroxide. Finding an antacid with the right balance of each of the ingredients will eliminate most of the bothersome side effects. If OTC medications do not offer adequate relief, the next step is an H$_2$ blocker.

The H$_2$ blockers (histamine H$_2$-receptor antagonists) work by inhibiting histamine H$_2$-receptors. The primary component of pharmacological activity for these types of drugs is inhibition of gastric secretion. Some H$_2$ blockers are now available OTC. Some drug companies have even begun to combine antacids with the H$_2$ blockers for a more complete relief of gastrointestinal symptoms. Stronger versions of these blockers are still available by prescription. These also may cause an overall drying effect that may be bothersome to a vocal performer.

Gastric proton pump inhibitors (H+/K+ATPase) do not exhibit anticholinergic or histamine H$_2$-receptor antagonist properties. They suppress gastric acid secretion by specific inhibition of the H+/K+ATPase enzyme system at the secretory surface of the gastric parietal cell (Burham & Short, 1997; Craig & Stitzel, 1986). Although they work extremely well, they are not free of side effects, which include diarrhea, abdominal pain, nausea, and depression. Other side effects have included dry mouth, esophageal stenosis, esophageal ulcer, esophagitis, and constipation, but the occurrence rate has been less than 1% (Burham & Short, 1997; Craig & Stitzel, 1986).

Gastrointestinal stimulants, such as metoclopramide, stimulate motility of the upper gastrointestinal tract without stimulating gastric, biliary, or pancreatic secretions (Burham & Short, 1997; Craig & Stitzel, 1986). They have had some serious side effects, such as extrapyramidal symptoms, which is seen very early in therapy, usually within 24 to 48 hours. Drugs such as diphenhydramine IM or beztropine IM may be used to reverse these reactions. The only other drug in this class is cisapride, or Propulsid. It is no longer available, however, due to its cardiac side effects when mixed with other drugs that inhibit cytochrome P-450, such as ketoconazole, erythromycin, fluconazole, and clarithromycin. In some cases where this occurred, the results were fatal.

Other gastrointestinal medications include the antispasmodics/anticholinergics, such as belladonna tincture, dicyclomine, Clindex, Levsin, and Phenerbel-S tablets. All of these agents have had a high rate of dryness on sections of the vocal tract. See Table 12.5 for a list of drugs commonly used to treat gastroesophageal reflux.

Psychoactive Medications

Antipsychotic drugs are a large group, and they include antidepressants, antianxiolytics, anticonvulsants, mood stabilizers, and

Table 12.5
Commonly Prescribed Drugs To Treat Gastroesophageal Reflux

Drug name–Brand	Recommended dosage
H$_2$ Blockers	
Pepcid AC	10 mg, available OTC, every day to twice a day
Pepcid RX	20 mg and 40 mg, every day to twice a day
Zantac 75	75 mg, available OTC, every day to twice a day
Zantac RX	150 mg and 300 mg, every day to twice a day
Tagamet HB	200 mg, available OTC, every day to twice a day
Tagamet RX	300, 400, and 800 mg tablets, every day at bedtime
Axid	150 mg and 300 mg, every day to twice a day
Proton Pump Inhibitors	
Prevacid	15 mg–30 mg, every day
Prilosec	10 mg, 20 mg, and 40 mg, every day
Gastrointestinal Stimulants	
Propulsid	No longer available on the market
Reglan	10 mg–15 mg, every day

Note. OTC = over the counter.

sedatives. They work through various mechanisms and produce many side effects. Antipsychotic medications have proven to be extremely helpful for most patients. With the large number of available drugs in this class, the clinician can modify the drug therapy to provide greater effectiveness and the least amount of side effects.

Antidepressants are a large class of antipsychotic drugs. Older generation drugs still in use include tricyclic antidepressants and monoamine oxidase (MAO) inhibitors. Among the new generation are selective serotonin reuptake inhibitors (SSRIs). Tricyclic and tetracyclic antidepressants include, but are not limited to, imipramine (Tofranil), amitriptyline (Elavil), doxepin (Sinequan), nortriptyline (Pamelor), and desipramine (Norpramin). They work by inhibiting the reuptake of norepinephrine or serotonin at the presynaptic neuron (Burham & Short, 1997; Craig & Stitzel, 1986). The side effects of these drugs include tardive dyskinesia, a syndrome consisting of potentially irreversible and involuntary dyskinetic movements; anticholinergic effects, such as urinary retention, constipation, and dry mouth; and cardiovascular disturbances, such as paroxysmal tachycardia and electrocardiogram abnormalities. All of these side effects may be dose-related and agent-specific.

MAO inhibitors are not commonly used due to their complicated side effects. Their use is confined to cases in which the patient does not respond to the other classes of antidepressants. MAO inhibitors work exactly as their name implies—by inhibiting the monoamine oxidase enzyme system, causing an increase in the concentration of endogenous epinephrine, norepinephrine, and serotonin in storage sites throughout the nervous system (Burham & Short, 1997; Craig & Stitzel, 1986; Sataloff et al., 1998). Some MAO inhibitors include phenelzine (Nardil), tranylcypromine (Parnate), and isocarboxazid (Marplan). These drugs have their own side effects, such as dizziness and orthostatic hypotension, but they also react with many other drugs, such as meperidine (Demerol), epinephrine, local anesthetics containing sympathomimetics, and decongestants (Sataloff et al., 1998). They are also very reactive with certain foods that are rich in tyramine, such as cheese and dairy products; certain meats and fish (meat organs, meat prepared with tenderizer, and caviar); alcoholic beverages (such as red wine—especially chianti, beer, and ale); and certain fruits and vegetables (bananas, bean curd, avocados, and figs; Pronsky, 2001; Sataloff et al., 1998). These side effects can linger after discontinuation of therapy. The use of these drugs should be tapered, and new therapy with any other agents should be started only after a sufficient washing-out period.

The SSRIs are the most commonly prescribed antidepressants. In most cases, they are generally prescribed as the first line of therapy. The antidepressant activity of the SSRIs is linked to their inhibition of central nervous system neuronal uptake of serotonin. These drugs include fluoxetine (Prozac), sertraline (Zoloft), and paroxetine (Paxil). Some of their side effects include dizziness, drowsiness, dry mouth, constipation, and sexual dysfunction (Burham & Short, 1997; Craig & Stitzel, 1986; Sataloff et al., 1998).

Antianxiolytic drugs are also commonly prescribed by clinicians. The most common class is the benzodiazepines. The utility of these drugs varies from antianxiolytics to anticonvulsants to sedatives. They include drugs such as alprazolam (Xanax), diazepam (Valium), lorazepam (Ativan), oxazepam (Serax), clonazepam (Klonopin), chlordiazepoxide (Librium), and clorazepate (Tranxene). These drugs work by potentiating the effects of gaba-aminobutyric acid and other inhibitory transmitters by binding to specific benzodiazepine receptor sites (Burham & Short, 1997; Craig & Stitzel, 1986; Sataloff et al., 1998). Benzodiazepine activity may involve many sites, such as muscle relaxation in the spinal cord, anticonvulsant action in the brain stem, and emotional behavior in the limbic and cortical areas. These activities are agent- and dose-specific. Side effects include sedation, weakness, and decreased motor performance. Benzodiazepines can be highly addictive, and patients will present with withdrawal symptoms if use is stopped abruptly. The clinician should advise patients not to combine these drugs with other depressants, such as alcohol; with stimulants, such as cocaine and amphetamines; or even with OTC decongestants without prior approval from the clinician. These combinations can have deleterious effects.

Buspar (buspirone) is an azaspirodecanedione agent not chemically or pharmacologically related to the benzodiazepines. It does not exert anticonvulsant or muscle relaxant effects. It also lacks the sedative effects associated with typical antianxiolytics. It is slower than the benzodiazepines in establishing antianxiolytic effects, but it has no addictive component. Side effects include headache, nausea, and dizziness. Another agent used on occasion is hydroxyzine, an antihistamine. It is also nonaddictive but can cause a fair amount of drowsiness and mucosal dryness, as is seen with other antihistamines.

Anticonvulsant drugs include a variety of agents, all possessing the ability to depress abnormal neuronal discharges in the central nervous system, thus inhibiting seizure activity. Some of the more common ones are phenytoin (Dilantin), carbamazepine (Tegretol), valproic acid (Depakote), and phenobarbital. All of these drugs have very serious side effects. Phenytoin can cause slurred speech, mental confusion, motor twitching, and gingival hyperplasia. Carbamazepine side effects include adverse hematological reactions, confusion, agitation, stomatitis, lymphadenopathy, and drowsiness. Valproic acid can also be used in the manic phase of bipolar disorder (Burham & Short, 1997; Craig & Stitzel, 1986; Sataloff et al., 1998). Its side effects include thrombocytopenia, suicidal ideation, hepatocellular toxicity, and the more commonly seen sedation, edema of extremities, and hair loss. Phenobarbital is one of the oldest anticonvulsants on the market and has also been used as a hypnotic. It has side effects similar to those of other barbiturates and sedatives, including somnolence, confusion, drowsiness, and vertigo.

Mood stabilizers are used with bipolar patients to prevent manic and depressive recurrences. The main drug used, lithium carbonate, alters sodium transport in nerve and muscle cells and effects a shift toward intraneuronal catecholamine metabolism (Burham & Short, 1997; Craig & Stitzel, 1986; Sataloff et al., 1998; Vogel et al., 2000). Because lithium is available in several forms, dosages may be customized to each patient's symptoms and blood levels. Side effects include hand-resting tremor, polyuria, and mild thirst. These effects usually disappear with continued usage. The more common side effects are drowsiness, fatigue, and dehydration. It is extremely important for patients to drink large amounts of water or liquids every day while on this medication. More rare side effects are pseudotumor cerebri and euthyroid goiter or hypothyroidism, usually accompanied by lower triiodothyronine (T_3) and thyroxine (T_4).

Neurologic Medications

Most drugs used for neurological disorders encompass a large number of side effects, some of which may be quite serious. These drugs are also dosed individually and are customized to each patient, depending on disease progression. Any neurological disorder is in itself debilitating, and many times the drugs prescribed for the disorder can have side effects that will lead to voice and speech difficulties (Sataloff et al., 1998). Examples of these disorders include Parkinson's disease, myasthenia gravis, multiple sclerosis, amyotrophic lateral sclerosis, cerebral palsy, Wilson's disease, essential tremor, epilepsy, Tourette's syndrome, and Huntington's disease. Current therapy for these diseases is palliative because no cure is available. The goals of drug therapy are to provide maximum relief from the symptoms, slow the progression of the disease, and help the patient maintain independence and mobility.

Parkinson's Disease. Parkinson's disease is a motor speech disorder that typically leads to speech and voice difficulties. It is a progressive disease of the brain involving the degeneration of nigral cells and destruction of the nigrostriatal pathway, resulting in loss of striatal dopamine (Marsden, 1994). The role of the neural transmitter dopamine is to facilitate the transfer of electrical messages among the nerve cells that control movement. The characteristic movement abnormalities observed in Parkinson's disease include resting tremor, rigidity in muscle tone, bradykinesia, hypokinesia, akinesia, and postural imbalance/gait abnormalities (Marsden, 1994). Associated speech and voice characteristics include imprecise articulation, rapid speech rate with progressive acceleration and short rushes of speech, reduced stress on syllables, reduced volume, hoarseness, tremorous voice, and monotone (Darely, Aronson, & Brown, 1975; Duffy, 1995). Some patients have described these speech problems as the most debilitating of the symptoms because they are unable to effectively communicate, thus limiting employment opportunities (Ramig, 1998; Ramig, Bonitati, Lemke, & Horii, 1995).

Drugs used to treat Parkinson's disease are anticholinergics such as benztropine (Cogentin), biperiden (Akineton), and trihexyphenidyl (Artane). These anticholinergics alleviate tremor. Dopaminergic replacement agents include levodopa (L-dopa) and

L-dopa in combinations with other drug agents such as carbidopa, including Sinemet and Prolopa, or amantadine (Symmetrel). Dopamine agonists are used to enhance the effects of levodopa. Some of these drugs include apomorphine, bromocriptine (Parlodel), pergolide (Permax), ropinerole (Requip), and pramipexole (Mirapex). Catechol-o-methyltransferase (COMT) inhibitors are used to decrease the levodopa metabolism and, in turn, increase levodopa availability. These drug agents include tolcapone (Tasmar) and entacapone. Monoamine oxidase-B (MAO-B) inhibitors are used for relief of symptoms and to slow disease progression by prolonging the availability of dopamine released into the synapse. MAO-B inhibitor drug agents include selegiline and deprenyl (Eldepryl).

These drugs produce a large number of side effects. Anticholinergic side effects include blurred vision, dryness, drowsiness, confusion, memory loss, gastrointestinal disturbance, muscle cramps, skin rash, nervousness, and hallucinations. Side effects most commonly associated with L-dopa are gastrointestinal disturbance, oral dryness, orthostatic hypotension, syncope, cardiac arrythmias, depression, confusion, dyskinesias, and psychosis (Burham & Short, 1997; Craig & Stitzel, 1986; Vogel et al., 2000). Dopamine agonist side effects include nausea, dizziness, dyskinesias, somnolence, and orthostatic hypotension. COMT inhibitor side effects include increased dyskinesias, nausea, and gastrointestinal disturbance. MAO-B inhibitor side effects include sleep disturbance, increased dyskinesias, increased nausea when added to Sinemet, and increased levels of liver enzymes (Burham & Short, 1997; Craig & Stitzel, 1986; Vogel et al., 2000).

Myasthenia Gravis. Myasthenia gravis is an autoimmune disease that affects the neuromuscular junction where the lower motor neurons meet muscle tissue. The autoimmune system produces antibodies that impair transmission of nerve impulses to the muscles. The neurotransmitter involved is acetycholine (Duffy, 1995; Freed, 2000; Vogel et al., 2000). Primary symptoms are rapid weakening of muscular contractions and fatigue over a short period of time (Duffy, 1995; Freed, 2000). Patients display speech and voice symptoms consistent with flaccid dysarthria. These characteristics include hypernasality, impaired articulation, dysphonia, and reduced volume. The drug endrophonium chloride (Tensilon) is used to confirm a diagnosis of myasthenia gravis. It is administered intra-venously, and the patient is monitored for improvement of symp-toms (Vogel et al., 2000). Drugs used to treat myasthenia gravis include acetylcholinesterase inhibitors, such as pyridostigmine (Mestinon). This drug works to increase levels of acetylcholine, which facilitates stimulation of movement and muscular activity. Some of the side effects of acetycholinesterase include excessive salivation, gastrointestinal disturbances, and confusion. Cortico-steroids are also used to treat myasthenia gravis. The side effects of corticosteroids were described previously.

Multiple Sclerosis. Multiple sclerosis is characterized as a progres-sive disease in which there is a degeneration of myelin covering the axons (Duffy, 1995; Freed, 2000; Vogel et al., 2000). Patients with MS produce voice and speech characteristics consistent with mixed dysarthria (flaccid, spastic, and ataxic dysarthria). The speech and voice symptoms associated with MS include imprecise consonants, slow rate of speech, hypernasality, and a harsh and strained/stran-gled voice quality (Duffy, 1995; Freed, 2000; Vogel et al., 2000). Pharmacological therapy for MS is directed at the underlying cause of the disease or at the symptoms that arise during the disease's progression. Corticosteroids, along with other immunosuppresants, such as azathioprine and cyclophosphamide, are often used. Beta-interferon is also used to slow the progression of physical disability and to prevent exacerbations. Because beta-interferon is adminis-tered by subcutaneous injection every other day, side effects include injection site reactions such as redness, swelling, and irritation. Other side effects include flu-like symptoms, a worsening of symp-toms, and depression (Burham & Short, 1997; Craig & Stitzel, 1986; Vogel et al., 2000).

Drug Compliance

Compliance refers to a patient's ability to follow through with a pre-scribed regimen of treatment. Compliance is a major factor in medi-cation failures. Noncompliance, which is more frequently seen in the geriatric population, is due to factors such as financial limita-tions, multiple drug therapies, and issues associated with normal aging (i.e., confusion, memory loss). Compliance directly relates to an individual patient's motivation. For example, a patient is not feeling well, so he or she begins pharmacological treatment. As the person begins to recover, a sharp decline is typically seen in compliance because he or she believes the prescribed medication is no longer necessary. Not only does this affect health status, it is also more costly, because the drug therapy usually will need to be repeated. For individuals on a fixed income, this can have serious consequences.

In general, patients taking multiple doses of a medication in a 24-hour period (i.e., taking a medication four times a day versus one time per day) have been shown to be less compliant. This is due to the increased frequency of dosing. Patients may either forget to take a medication or try to cut back on the frequency (self-directed) so that the medication will last longer and create less of a financial burden. Older patients frequently do this as a way to contain costs. Pharmaceutical companies have been working to address the lack of drug therapy compliance by altering drug delivery systems. For example, a broad-spectrum antibiotic, which is typically taken four times per day, is replaced with a similar broad-spectrum drug that has to be taken only once or twice per day. This does not translate into cost savings for the consumer, however. Another factor in compliance is that an individual may not see a substantial change in physical health status as a result of taking the intended medication. He or she therefore decides to discontinue drug treatment. For example, in many nonsymptomatic conditions, such as hypertension, individuals do not notice a direct cause-and-effect relationship between their drug therapy and general well-being, which leads to high incidences of noncompliance. In older persons or patients on multiple drug regimens (e.g., patients with neurogenic disorders), confusion may interfere with the disease process. The patient either forgets to take the drug or thinks he or she has already taken it. In some instances, patients may be overcompliant by taking medication too frequently or by overmedicating. Clinicians should counsel patients on various strategies to help minimize noncompliance. For example, pill organizers or beepers can be obtained, and spouse or personal care providers can help monitor the drug regimen. Primary care physicians or pharmacists can help by continuing to monitor all drug therapies, including prescriptions, OTC medications, and dietary supplements, on a regular basis, or more frequently as health status changes.

Effects of Nutrients on Drug Absorption

Many foods and nutrients have the potential to interfere substantially with pharmacotherapeutic goals. Nutrition and diet affect how a drug is absorbed, metabolized, and excreted. For example, protein deficiency may lead to impaired drug metabolism. This is illustrated by an increase in sleeping time produced by barbiturates. Fat-free diets or diets that lack essential fatty acids also impair drug metabolism. Excessive intakes of carbohydrates can impair mono-oxygenase activity. The rates of drug metabolism can also be impaired by deficiencies in vitamin A, riboflavin, ascorbic acid, and vitamin E. Iron deficiency, however, has not been shown to have any effect on drug metabolism, even in severe cases.

The effects of alcohol use while on drug therapy differ, depending on a patient's type of alcohol use and consumption. Chronic alcohol consumption increases the hepatic content of mono-oxygenase enzymes and cytochrome P-450 and increases drug clearance from plasma (Burham & Short, 1997; Craig & Stitzel, 1986; Pronsky, 2001). Acute alcohol ingestion, however, inhibits drug metabolism and prolongs the effects of the drugs, especially central nervous system depressants. Wine can elevate the anticoagulant effect of drugs such as Coumadin. Conversely, some vegetables with high vitamin K will lower the anticoagulant effect.

The presence of certain nutrients in the gastrointestinal tract affects the bioavailability and disposition of many oral medications (Pronsky, 2001). Drug–nutrient interactions may also have positive effects that result in increased drug absorption or reduced gastrointestinal irritation. Knowing the significant drug–nutrient interactions can help the clinician identify which nutrients to avoid with certain medications, as well as the therapeutic agents that should be administered with food. For example, the absorption of the antihistamine astemizole (Hismanal) may be decreased by 60% when taken with food (Pronsky, 2001). Another example is the decreased absorption of tricyclic antidepressants such as amitriptyline (Elavil) when a high-fiber diet is consumed. Taking antibiotics with food may delay or prevent absorption, and dairy products are associated with overall impaired absorption in oral drug administration (Pronsky, 2001; Sataloff et al., 1998; Vogel et al., 2000). High-protein diets are associated with interference of L-dopa absorption. L-dopa is an amino acid, and when taken with a protein it must compete with other amino acids from the protein for transport across the gastrointestinal tract lining and into the blood. This in turn decreases absorption and availability of L-dopa to the brain (Holden, 2001; Pronsky, 2001; Vogel et al., 2000). Patients with Parkinson's disease undergoing L-dopa pharmacotherapy should be advised to have their protein as part of the last meal of the day (Holden, 2001).

Food may also alter the metabolism of some drugs. For example, concurrent ingestion of food and propranolol (Inderal) reduces first-pass metabolism of the drug, resulting in higher drug levels. A high-protein, low-carbohydrate diet induces the cytochrome P-450 mixed oxidase system, promoting hepatic metabolism of drugs that are significantly metabolized by this enzyme system, such as theophylline (Theo-Dur). As a result, drug levels may decrease (Pronsky, 2001). Medications can also affect nutrient metabolism. Some drugs may increase the metabolism of nutrients, resulting in higher requirements and danger of deficiency. For example, the anticonvulsants phenobarbital and phenytoin (Dilantin) increase the metabolism of folic acid and vitamins D and K. Drugs may also cause vitamin antagonism. For example, the antituberculosis drug isoniazid inhibits the conversion of vitamin B6 to the active form, which may cause vitamin B6 deficiency and peripheral neuropathy unless a B6 supplement is also prescribed (Pronsky, 2001).

Modification of medication action may be experienced when a medication is combined with foods or additives that have effects that are similar to the desired effect of a drug or that can enhance the effects or toxicity of the drug. For example, high caffeine intake may increase the adverse effects (nervousness, tremor, insomnia) of theophylline. Tyramine, dopamine, or other vasoconstrictors in food enhance the toxic effects of MAO inhibitors, such as tranylcypromine sulfate (Parnate). The result may be hypertension, which can be fatal (Pronsky, 2001). Nutrients or food ingredients may produce an antagonistic effect on medication action. For example, vitamin K aids the production of clotting factors, in direct opposition to the action of warfarin (Coumadin; Pronsky, 2001).

Caffeine is a stimulant and thus counteracts the antianxiety effects of tranquilizers. Grapefruit juice recently has been shown to have some adverse reactions when mixed with particular drugs. Studies are still being conducted in many drug classes. Drugs that interact with grapefruit juice seem to be metabolized via the cytochrome 450 pathway. Grapefruit juice contains various bioflavonoids that can affect this pathway. More studies are needed, but certain drugs, such as the cholestrol-lowering statins, are already dispensed with warning labels concerning the concomitant use of grapefruit juice (Elbe, 2001).

Drugs may also impair salivary flow, causing dry mouth, increased caries, stomatitis, and glossitis. Some drugs, such as the antibiotic clarithromycin (Biaxin), can be secreted into the saliva, causing a bitter taste (Pronsky, 2001). Specific drugs, for example, tetracycline, may also suppress natural oral bacteria, resulting in oral candidiasis.

Herbal Supplements/Alternative Medicines

Alternative therapies, such as herbal products, are being used in increasing numbers in the United States. Approximately 25% of Americans who consult their physician about a serious health problem are employing some form of unconventional therapy, but only 70% of these patients inform their physician of such use (Eisenberg et al., 1993). Herbal remedies are prepared from a variety of plant materials, including leaves, roots, bark, stems, and flowers. They can be prepared fresh or dried and are used primarily for mild or chronic ailments (Gianni & Dreitlein, 1998). The use of herbal remedies can be problematic for several reasons. Herbal products are not tested with the scientific rigor required of conventional drugs, and they are not subject to the approval process of the U.S. Food and Drug Administration. Herbal products therefore cannot be marketed for the diagnosis, treatment, cure, or prevention of disease. Nonetheless, the Dietary Supplement Health and Education Act of 1994 allows these products to be labeled with statements explain-

ing their effects (e.g., alleviation of fatigue) or their role in promoting general well-being (e.g., enhancement of mood or mentation).
Analysis of some of the effects of herbal products has shown that
they sometimes closely resemble claims of clinical efficacy for various diseases or conditions (Klepser & Klepser, 1999). Unlike conventional drugs, herbal products are not regulated for purity and
potency. Some of the adverse effects and drug interactions reported
for herbal products therefore could be caused by impurities (e.g.,
allergens, pollen, and spores) or batch-to-batch variability. In addition, the potency of an herbal product may increase the possibility
of adverse effects (Cupp, 1999).

Many consumers of herbal remedies also believe that because
an herbal product is a "natural" remedy, it must be better for your
body. This is not true. Patients who are implementing alternative
therapies should consult their physician. Unfortunately, patients
often find that medical professionals do not have enough available
information regarding herbal supplements. As a result, physicians
often are unable to predict any interactions that herbal remedies
may have when mixed with traditional medications and may mis-
diagnose or mistreat a patient's medical condition. This is changing,
however, as more publications regarding herbal products are now
becoming available and are being marketed to medical professionals. Patients who are considering or currently taking an herbal supplement should be properly advised of the impact it can have on an
existing medical condition. A physician or other licensed medical
professional specializing in alternative therapies should be advising the patient and overseeing any alternative/herbal treatments.

Because dietary supplements are becoming increasingly popular, clinicians need to ask questions during the diagnostic interview
about the use of these herbal products as part of the medication history. Although herbal products are available without a prescription,
medical guidance is necessary because of the adverse effects of
many of these products and the potential for drug interactions.
Consequently, clinicians need to stay up to date on trends in dietary
supplement use, realizing that for most supplements, the adverse
effects and potential for drug interactions are not well known
(Cupp, 1999). Some questions to ask patients who may be taking
herbal products include the following: Are you taking an herbal
product, herbal supplement, or other "natural remedy"? If so, are

you taking any prescription or nonprescription medications for the same purpose as the herbal product? Have you used this herbal product before? Are you allergic to any plant products? Are you pregnant or breast-feeding? (Cupp, 1999). Nickjeh (1999) and Surrow (2000) listed common herbal qualities and actions of herbs and vitamins, some of which are included in this discussion. (For further information, the clinician should consult a licensed medical professional specializing in alternative therapies.)

Anti-inflammatories include herbs that soothe inflammation or decrease the inflammatory response of the tissue directly. An anti-inflammatory is echinacea, which is extracted from the purple coneflower. It works by increasing the number of immune cells and decreases inflammation, coughs, colds, sore throats, tonsillitis, and external wounds. Its use is advocated within the first 24 hours of the onset of cold symptoms. Echinacea should not be taken for more than 8 weeks at a time because long-term effects are unknown. A patient should avoid using echinacea if he or she is allergic to pollen or if the immune system is compromised. Goldenseal is another popular anti-inflammatory used to stimulate the immune system. This should not be taken for more than 2 weeks at a time because it may kill good bacteria in the digestive tract. Goldenseal is to be avoided if a patient has high blood pressure or is pregnant. Chamomile is an anti-inflammatory used for its soothing and relaxing effects. It relaxes the lining of the digestive tract and promotes healing of nausea, indigestion, gastritis, and colitis. It also relieves allergies and hay fever, much like an antihistamine. Chamomile has also been used for insomnia and drug withdrawal. It may cause a reaction in persons who are allergic to pollen. Slippery elm is used to soothe irritated mucous membranes of the larynx and ulcers.

Antimicrobials help the body destroy disease-causing microorganisms and strengthen its own resistance to infection. Some antimicrobials include echinacea, goldenseal, vitamin C (no more than 1,000 mg every 2 hours), rose hip, licorice (avoid taking with high blood pressure), and garlic (limit use if taking blood-thinning medications).

Herbals are also sold as antispasmodics, which ease cramps in smooth and skeletal muscles. Some antispasmodics include chamomile and valerian. The latter is a natural tranquilizer and is used to relieve pain and muscle spasms. Valerian contains natural compounds that depress the nervous system and relieve anxiety. It should not be taken with alcohol or any medication that causes drowsiness. Long-term use has been linked to headache, insomnia, and stomach upsets.

Astringents reduce irritation and inflammation and create a barrier against infection. They are helpful in healing wounds and burns. Some common astringents include red sage, yarrow, raspberry leaves, white oak bark, saltwater, and cayenne pepper.

Bitters work by triggering a sensory response in the central nervous system that leads to a range of responses, including stimulating appetite, aiding in liver's detoxification, increasing bile flow, toning, and stimulating the mucosal lining. Wormwood is a common bitter.

Demulcents work to soothe and protect irritated or inflamed tissue. Some common demulcents are zinc, slippery elm, vitamin A, and vitamin E. They work to decrease gastric acids, diarrhea, and muscle spasms. See Table 12.6 for a list of herbals and possible effects.

Special Populations

Pediatric and Geriatric Populations

Age is a factor that must be considered in prescribing medications, especially for pediatric and geriatric populations. These two groups have shown very different rates of drug metabolism from those of the typical middle-age adult. Most drug dosing is tested by considering the average metabolism of an adult man between the ages of 20 and 40 years.

When using medications with children, the clinician should not assume that the very young are just "little adults." It is not always appropriate to dose a child based on a fractional adult-recommended dose. From a physiological perspective, drug-metabolizing enzyme activity in early childhood is very low. These rates of biotransformation do increase dramatically to adult levels at, or about the age of, puberty, but prior to that time, the activity levels are low. In older persons, multiple drug usage is common, and it may cause interactions that may lead to increased side effects, subtherapeutic levels, or drug toxicity. As one ages, drug absorption is less complete

Table 12.6

List of Herbals and Possible Concerns and Cautions Regarding Use of These Products

Possible anticoagulant effects	Possible inhalant, allergy cross-sensitivity	Photosensitivity concerns	Diuretic effects	Possible blood pressure effects	Possible hormonal effects
Dong Quai	Chamomile (with Ragweed)	St. John's Wort	Elder	St. John's Wort	Dong Quai
Willow bark	Goldenseal (with Ragweed)	Celery	Feverfew	Ma Huang	Yam
Primrose	Echinacea (with sunflower)	Dong Quai	Dandelion	Goldenseal	Licorice Root
Cowslip		Iyarrow	Nettles	Ginseng	Hops
Jack-in-the-Pulpit				Licorice root	Primrose
Red root					Melatonin
Garlic					Yohimbe
Gingko biloba					
Feverfew					
Ginger					

Note. This list gives only a sample of possible herbal interactions with traditional medicines. Individual patients should be advised to consult with their health-care providers before considering herbal supplementation.

or slower due to altered gastrointestinal motility, reduced blood flow because of decreased cardiac output, and reduction in absorptive surfaces. Drug distribution is also affected due to hypoalbuminemia, changes in the drug-binding sites, reduced muscle mass, increase in the proportion of body fat, and a decrease in total body water. Drug metabolism and excretion are also affected by age. As blood flow decreases in the kidneys and the liver, a higher incidence of drug toxicity is encountered.

Spasmodic Dysphonia

Spasmodic dysphonia was described in Chapter 6 by Woodson and Murry. One of the treatments these authors discussed was botulinum toxin type A (Botox). Botox is a complex protein produced by clostridium botulinum, which is an anaerobic bacteria. The mechanism of its action is to block neuromuscular conduction by binding to the receptor site on the motor nerve terminal, inhibiting the release of acetylcholine and producing muscle paralysis (Craig & Stitzel, 1986). Botox should be used with caution in patients who have a neuromuscular disease to avoid a compounding effect. Patients with a history of anticoagulation will tend to bruise easily and may have a bleeding problem from the actual insertion of the needle. (This side effect holds true for any injectable drug.) The aminoglycoside class of antibiotics has long been linked with neurotoxicities, the most common of which is ototoxicity. Signs and symptoms include numbness, skin tingling, muscle twitching, and convulsion (Craig & Stitzel, 1986). These are mainly seen with high doses and in patients with renal compromise. Botox-A, as described above, also causes nerve block and may have a cumulative effect, causing more serious consequences.

Dysphagia

There are only a few reports concerning drugs that may cause symptoms of dysphagia. These include antiinfective drugs such as demeclocycline (Declomycin), doxycycline (Vibramycin), minocycline (Dynacin), oxytetracycline (Terramycin), and tetracycline (Achromycin), and an autonomic nervous system drug, pilocarpine hydrochloride, which increases secretions of the salivary glands.

Only a few drugs are advocated in treating symptoms of dysphagia. These include buspirone (an antianxiety drug; Hanna, Feibusch, & Albright, 1997), nifedipine (cardiovascular system drug), and cisapride (Propulsid), which has been found to help ease symptoms of Parkinson's disease and other degenerative diseases. It works by stimulating the serotonin receptors, which enhances the release of acetylcholine and increases gastrointestinal motility (Perez, Smithard, Davies, & Kalra, 1998; Vogel et al., 2000).

Recommended Readings

Due to the development of new medications, the following recommended readings include books, peer-reviewed articles, and Web sites that can be used for updating information reviewed in this chapter.

Brown, C. (2001). Overview of drug interactions. *U.S. pharmacist.* Retrieved September 17, 2001, from http://www.uspharmacist .com

This Web site is maintained by the publisher of *U.S. Pharmacist,* a monthly journal providing pharmacists, students, and other health-care professionals with up-to-date, peer-reviewed clinical articles relevant to contemporary pharmacy practice. Pharmacists licensed in the United States can earn continuing education credits approved by the American Council on Pharmaceutical Education.

Harris, S. *Herbal drug interaction handbook.* Retrieved August 11, 2001, from http://www.foodmedinteractions.com

This reference manual covering more than 300 herbs was written from the perspectives of proponents of herbal remedies and pharmaceutical companies.

Holden, K. (2000). *Eat well, stay well with Parkinson's disease.* Fort Collins, CO: Therapy Five Star Living.

Includes information on meal control with levadopa, food–medication interactions, dehydration control, swallowing difficulties, and nutritional supplements.

Physicians' Desk Reference. (2001). Montvale, NJ: Medical Economics Company.

Includes listings for new drugs currently available, drug interaction data, side effects, and certain drugs that are no longer on the market.

Physicians' Desk Reference for Nutritional Supplements. (2001). Montvale, NJ: Medical Economics Company.

Covers more than 300 nutritional supplements and lists possible effects and side effects. This publication also includes a clinical research summary of published findings for each supplement.

The Medicine Corner. Retrieved September 16, 2001, from www. themedicinecorner.com

Provides nationwide assistance in obtaining prescribed medications based on the needs of the individual.

Appendix 12.A
Overview of Current Drug Classes

Drug class	Brand	Generic	Side effects	OTC or RX
Antihistamines	Benadryl	Diphenhydranime	Sedation, dizziness, insomnia, drying effect	OTC
	Tavist	Clemastine	Sedation, dizziness, insomnia, drying effect; should not be used with children under age 12	OTC
	Chlor-Trimeton	Chlorpheniramine	Sedation, dizziness, insomnia, drying effect	OTC
	Phenergran	Promethazine		Rx
	Dimetapp	Brompheniramine		OTC/Rx
	Allegra	Fexofenadine	Mild to nonsedative, nausea, dyspepsia, drying effect, fatigue	Rx
	Claritin		Mild to nonsedative, nausea, dypepsia, drying effect, fatigue	Rx
	Zyrtec		Mild to nonsedative, nausea, dypepsia, drying effect, fatigue	Rx
Mucolytic agents/ expectorants	marketed under such names as:			
	Humabid	guaifenesin	Nausea, vomiting, dizziness, headache	Rx
	Muco-fen	guaifenesin	Nausea, vomiting, dizziness, headache	Rx
	Robitussin	guaifenesin	Nausea, vomiting, dizziness, headache	Rx
Corticosteroids	Deltasone	Prednisone	Long-term use in children can lead to slowed growth and development	Rx
	Prelone	Prednisone		Rx
Medrol	Methylprednisolone		May mask symptoms of infection	Rx
	Decadron	Dexamethasone	May cause gastrointestinal upset; avoid abrupt withdrawal of therapy after long-term use	Rx

(continues)

Appendix 12.A *Continued.*

Drug class	Brand	Generic	Side effects	OTC or Rx
Bronchodilators	Albuterol	Ventolin/Proventil	Tolerance may be seen with long-term use	Rx
	Alupent	Metaproterenol		Rx
	Serevent	Salmeterol	May see an increase in blood pressure	Rx
	Isuprel	Isoproterenol	Restlessness, throat irritation, dry mouth	Rx
	Primatine Mist	Epinephrine	Increase in temporary rigidity and tremor in Parkinson's disease	OTC
	Slo-bid/ Theo-Dur	Theophyllene	Nausea and vomiting, irritability, insomnia, tachycardia	Rx
Antihypertensive agents	Lasix	Furosemide	Dehydration	Rx
	Diuril	Chlorothiazide	Tinnitus	Rx
	HydroDIURIL	Hydrochlorothiazide	Photosensitivity	Rx
	Procardia or Adalat	Nifedipine	Dizziness/lightheadedness, psychiatric disturbances (depression/amnesia)	Rx
	Cardizem	Diltiazem	Anxiety, weakness, jitters	Rx
	Calan or Isoptin	Verapamil		Rx
	Norvasc	Amlodipine		Rx
	Tenormin	Atenolol	Fatigue, drowsiness	Rx
	Lopressor or Toprol XL	Metoprolol	Bronchospasm; may cause mental depression, do not stop abruptly	Rx
	Accupril	Quinapril	Peristent dry cough may occur; notify	Rx
	Zestril or Prinivil	Lisinopril	doctor if having a sore throat, irregular heartbeat, angioedema, excessive perspiration, or dehydration	Rx
	Vasotec	Enalapril		Rx
	Cozaar	Losartan	Diarrhea, dizziness, possible cough	Rx

(continues)

Appendix 12.A *Continued.*

Drug class	Brand	Generic	Side effects	OTC or Rx
Antianxiety	Tranxene	Clorazepate	Drowsiness, depression	Rx
	Valium	Diazepam	Confusion, behavior problems	Rx
	Xanax	Alprazolam	Visual disturbances	Rx
	Ativan	Lorazepam	Suicidal tendencies	Rx
Antidepressants/ trycyclic antidepressants	Elavil	Amitriptyline	In general, tend to cause sedation, drowsiness, weight changes, sexual dysfunction, & photosensitivity; may impair mental or physical abilities; anticholinergic effects	Rx
	Tofranil	Imipramine		Rx
	Effexor	Venlafaxine	Weight changes, anxiety, insomnia, nervousness, dry mouth, headache	Rx
	Serzone	Nefazodone		Rx
SSRI	Prozac	Fluoxetine	Headache	Rx
	Paxil	Paroxetine	Insomnia, nervousness	Rx
	Zoloft	Setraline	Anxiety, anorexia, nausea, diarrhea	Rx
Monoamine oxidase inhibitors	Nardil	Phenelzine	Hypertension, dizziness, edema, dry mouth; take caution with tyramine-containing foods (i.e., cheese/dairy products, alcohol, avocado, yeast extract)	Rx
	Parnate	Tranylcypromine		Rx
Penicillins	Amoxil	Amoxicillin	Make sure patient doesn't have penicillin allergy; glossitis, stomach upset, dry mouth	Rx
	Pen VR	Penicillin		
Cephalosporins	Ceclor	Cefaclor	May be cross-sensitivity with penicillin; gastrointestinal disturbances	Rx
	Cefzil	Cefprozil		Rx
	Keflex	Cephalexin		Rx
Fluoroquinolones	Cipro	Ciprofloxacin	Photosensitivity; drink fluids heavily, take on an empty stomach, if possible.	Rx
	Floxin	Ofloxacin		

(continues)

Appendix 12.A *Continued.*

Drug class	Brand	Generic	Side effects	OTC or Rx
Tetracyclines	Sumycin Vibramycim	Tetracycline Doxycycline	Photosensitivity; dizziness, lightheadedness; take on an empty stomach; don't give to children under age 8 due to teeth damage/decoloration	Rx
Macrolides	Biaxin Zithromax EryPed, E-Mycin	Clarithromycin Azithromycin Erythromycin	Diarrhea, abnormal taste, vomiting, abdominal cramping	Rx
Aminoglycosides	Mycetracin Kantrex	Neomycin sulfate Kanamycin	Nephrotoxicity, ototoxicity; drink plenty of fluids	Rx
Antivirals	Symmetral Zovirax	Amantadine Acyclovir	Blurred vision, dizziness or lightheadedness, mood or mental disturbances	Rx
Analgesics	Bayer, Ecotrin, & various others	Aspirin	Stomach upset, gastrointestinal bleeding, tinnitus	OTC
	Tylenol	Acetaminophen	With large doses—heptotoxicity over a long period of time	OTC
	Motrin Naprosyn, Aleve	Ibuprofen Naproxen	Stomach upset, gastrointestinal bleeding, drowsiness	OTC/Rx
	Celebrex Vioxx		Avoid if allergic to Sulfa compounds; possible gastrointestinal bleeding, diarrhea, abdominal pain, & dizziness	Rx Rx
Hormones	Premarin	Estrogen	Photosensitivity, breakthrough bleeding, nausea, vomiting, mental depression	Rx

(continues)

Appendix 12.A *Continued.*

Drug class	Brand	Generic	Side effects	OTC or Rx
Hormones (*continued*)	Provera	Medroxyprogesterone	Fluid retention, depression, photosensitivity, some adverse opthalmologic effects	Rx
	Oral contraceptives	Various brands	Depression, fluid retention, vomiting/diarrhea, thrombophlebitis, breakthrough bleeding	Rx
	Nolvadex	Tamoxifen	Visual disturbances, hot flashes, nausea & vomiting, weight gain, fluid retention	Rx
	Synthroid	Levothyroxine	Tachycardia, tremors, headache, diarrhea, weight loss, heat intolerance	Rx
Gastrointestinal drugs	Pepcid	Famotidine	Headaches, fatigue, dizziness, confusion, nausea, and vomiting	OTC/Rx
	Zantac	Ranitidine	Mental confusion, depression, many dry interactions	OTC/Rx
	Tagamet	Cimetidine		OTC/Rx
Antacids	Maalox/ Mylanta	Nizatidine	Magnesium-containing antacids have a laxative effect; aluminum-containing antacids have a constipation effect; also, rebound hyperactivity	OTC
		Axid		
	Prevacid	Lansoprazole	Fatigue, vertigo, confusion, rare cases of rash, diarrhea; take before eating, swallow whole, do not crush or chew	Rx
	Prilosec	Omeprazole		Rx
	Reglan	Metoclopramide	Drowsiness, depression, extrapyramidal symptoms (i.e., involuntary movements, tremor, tardive dyskinesia syndrome)	Rx
	Protonix	Pantoprazole	Headache, diarrhea	Rx
	Aciphex	Rabeprazole sodium	Headache	Rx
	Nexium	Esomeprazole	Fatigue, vertigo, confusion, rash, diarrhea	Rx

Note. OTC = over the counter; Rx = prescription.

References

Burham, T. H., & Short, R. M. (Eds.). (1997). *Drug facts and comparisons*. St. Louis, MO: Facts and Comparisons.

Center for Drug Evaluation and Research. (2001). Retrieved September 16, 2001, from http://www.fda.gov/approval/index.htm

Craig, C. R., & Stitzel, R. E. (Eds.). (1986). *Modern pharmacology* (2nd ed.). Boston: Little, Brown.

Cupp, H. J. (1999). *Herbal remedies: Adverse effects and drug interactions*. Retrieved September 16, 2001, from http://www.aafp.org

Damste, P. H. (1967). Voice changes in adult women caused by virilizing agents. *Journal of Speech and Hearing Disorders, 32,* 126–132.

Damste, P. H. (1968). Virilization of the voice due to anabolic steroids. *Folia Phoniatrica, 16,* 10–18.

Darely, F., Aronson, A., & Brown, J. (1975). *Motor speech disorders*. Philadelphia: Saunders.

Dietary Supplement Health and Education Act of 1994, 21 U.S.C. § 343 (1994).

Duffy, J. R. (1995). *Motor speech disorders: Substrates, differential diagnosis and management*. St. Louis, MO: Mosby-YearBook.

Eisenberg, D. M., Kessler, R. C., Foster, C., Norlock, F. E., Calkins, D. R., & Delbanco, T. L. (1993). Unconventional medicine in the United States: Prevalence, costs, and patterns of use. *New England Journal of Medicine, 328,* 246–252.

Elbe, D. (2001). *Grapefruit juice–drug interactions* Web site. Retrieved September 7, 2001, from http://www.powernetdesign.com/grapefruit

Freed, D. (2000). *Motor speech disorders: Diagnosis and treatment*. San Diego, CA: Singular.

Gianni, L. M., & Dreitlein, W. B. (1998). Some popular OTC herbals can interact with anticoagulant therapy. Available at http://www.uspharmacist.com/oldformat.asp?/newlook/files/atte/acf2ce.htm

Hanna, G. L., Feibusch, E. L., & Albright, K. J. (1997). Buspirone treatment of anxiety associated with pharyngeal dysphagia in a four year old. *Journal of Child and Adolescent Psychopharmacology, 7,* 137–143.

Holden, K. (2001). *Parkinson's disease: Guidelines for medical nutrition.* Fort Collins, CO: Therapy Five Star Living.

Klepser, T. B., & Klepser, M. E. (1999). Unsafe and potentially safe herbal therapies. *American Journal of Health-System Pharmacy, 56,* 125–138.

Marsden, C. D. (1994). Parkinson's disease. *Journal of Neurology, Neurosurgery, and Psychiatry, 57,* 672–681.

Nickjeh, D. A. (1999, October). Laryngitis: *Vitamins and herbal remedies.* Seminar on voice and swallowing, Clearwater, Florida.

Perez, I., Smithard, D. G., Davies, H., & Kalra, L. (1998). Pharmacological treatment of dysphagia in stroke. *Dysphagia, 13*(1), 12–16.

Pronsky, Z. (2001). *Food medication interactions.* Retrieved August 11, 2001, from http://www.foodmedinteractions.com

Ramig, L. O. (1998) Treatment of speech and voice problems associated with Parkinson's disease. *Topics in Geriatric Rehabilitation, 14*(2), 28–42.

Ramig, L. O., Bonitati, C. M., Lemke, J. H., & Horii, Y. (1995). Voice therapy for patients with Parkinson's disease: Development of an approach and preliminary efficacy data. *Journal of Medical Speech-Language Pathology, 2,* 191–212.

Sataloff, R. T., Hawkshaw, M., & Rosen, D. (1998). Medications: Effects and side effects in professional voice users. In R. T. Sataloff (Ed.), *Vocal health and pedagogy* (pp. 223–236). San Diego, CA: Singular.

Surrow, J. (2000, November). *Rational use of herbal medicines for singers.* Paper presented at the 13th annual Pacific Voice Conference, San Diego, CA.

Vogel, D., Carter, J., & Carter, P. (2000). *The effects of drugs on communication disorders* (2nd ed.). San Diego, CA: Singular.

Chapter 13

Optimizing Motor Learning in Speech Interventions

Theory and Practice

Katherine Verdolini and Timothy D. Lee

Verdolini and Lee discuss how motor learning research has arisen from at least two different perspectives. The first perspective is oriented to specific principles of motor learning. *The other perspective considers motor learning within more* global *models of brain functioning, addressing both mental and neural substrates. Unfortunately, as the authors point out, proponents of the two traditions have "talked" to each other surprisingly little, if at all. In addition, although at times the information appears contrasting, the two bodies of research can inform each other, enhancing both understanding and application. In their chapter, Verdolini and Lee provide an overview of general models of human information processing, learning, and memory, using it as a framework for understanding the principles of motor learning. The goal is to provide a set of practical, theoretically informed suggestions that can be applied in the speech clinic or voice studio.*

1. *What are the distinctions between experiential learning processes and rational learning processes?*

2. *What are the critical cognitive characteristics of the initial stages of skill acquisition, in comparison to performance, that point to practical training principles?*

3. *What criteria should the speech–language pathologist use when determining the skill a patient has or has not acquired within a treatment plan?*

4. *Continuous augmented feedback is used readily in training environments. Provide an argument for why it may not be the feedback option of choice.*

5. *What are the benefits of blocked versus random practice paradigms?*

The value of theory has to do with the ability, ultimately, to flexibly adapt the principles to diverse clinical situations. Although "lower-level" neuromuscular considerations are certainly important in training, in this chapter we limit ourselves largely to higher-level cognitive considerations. Cognitive science is the framework for many of our comments, and in it everyday terms are often used in a technical sense that is not always obvious. Examples of such terms include *attention, automaticity, consciousness,* and *memory.* We will attempt to provide clear technical definitions of key terms as we proceed.

General Models of Human Information Processing and Learning

Human information processing is not a unitary phenomenon. For centuries, if not millennia, from the time of Plato and before, diverse thinkers—including philosophers, psychologists, psychiatrists, and neurologists—have independently distinguished at least two fundamentally different ways that people process information. Earlier distinctions were based on philosophical speculations and anecdotal observations. However, over the past century, the collective experimental data have been nontrivial. A summary overview is presented in Table 13.1. In that table, some of the more widely referenced models are characterized according to a general distinction between "experiential" and "rational" processes made by Epstein (1994).

Although differences exist across the models, they are most striking for their similarities. The following is a broad picture of the two processes (see Table 13.2). Experiential processes are driven by exposure and repetition. They ultimately lead to stereotypic response biases, or habits—that is, tendencies of the nervous system to respond in reliable, predictable ways—that are slow to form and slow to change. As such, they seem particularly well suited to survival. There is widespread agreement that much experiential learning occurs and is manifested without awareness, despite subjective impressions to the contrary (see the compelling review by Nisbett & Wilson, 1977; see also Verdolini-Marston, 1991; Verdolini-Marston & Balota, 1994). One reason may be that experiential learning involves the rapid, parallel processing of large amounts of mental

Table 13.1

Complementary Information Processing Phenomena as Conceived in Various Traditions

Tradition/proponent	Experiential	Rational
Psychoanalytic		
Freud (1900/1953)	Primary (nonconscious) processes	Secondary (conscious) processes
Experimental–cognitive psychology		
Pavlov (cited in Luria, 1961; Vygotsky, 1934/1962)	Nonverbal conditioning	Verbally mediated processes
Paivio (1986, 1991)	Nonverbal processes	Verbal processes
Posner & Snyder (1975)	Automatic processing	Controlled processing
Anderson (1976, 1982); Winograd (1975); Squire (1986)	Procedural knowledge	Declarative knowledge
Tulving (1984)	Procedural memory	Semantic and episodic memory
Reber (1993); Nissen, Willingham, & Hartman (1989); Broadbent, FitzGerald, & Broadbent (1986); Graf & Schacter (1985)	Implicit knowledge (process)	Explicit knowledge (process)
Developmental psychology		
Piaget (1973)	Cognitive unconscious (similar to procedural knowledge)	(Other)
Labouvie-Vief (1989, 1990)	*Mythos* (intuitive, holistic information processing)	*Logos* (rational, analytical information processing)
Social–cognitive psychology		
Tversky & Kahneman (1974, 1983)	Natural, intuitive reasoning mode; heuristic processing	Extensional, logical reasoning mode

(continues)

Table 13.1 *Continued.*

Complementary Information Processing Phenomena as Conceived in Various Traditions

Tradition/proponent	Experiential	Rational
Social–cognitive psychology *(continued)*		
Schneider & Shiffrin (1977)	Automatic processing mode not requiring consciousness	Reflective, rational, conscious processing mode
Fiske (1981)	Heuristic processing	Effortful processing
Narrative versus analytical processing		
Bruner (1986)	Narrative representations (storylike, concrete, specific)	Propositional representation (public, logical, theoretical, abstract)
McClelland et al. (1989)	Implicit motivation	Self-attributed motivation
Personality theory		
Epstein (1994)	Experiential system	Rational system

Note. Adapted from "Integration of the Cognitive and the Psychodynamic Unconscious," by S. Epstein, 1994, *American Psychologist.*

data that are unavailable to the slow, serial processes associated with consciousness (Posner & Snyder, 1975). Once experientially based behaviors are established, they are run off automatically, without attentional control. In many current schools of psychotherapy, experiential processes are said to include not only physical behaviors and skills but also emotional "habits," which by nature are strikingly resistant to change (see Epstein, 1994). In contrast, rational processes involve comparatively slow, rational, and conscious thought. They depend on logical, abstract operations. As such, they are flexible and transcend modality and physical environment. They are as quick to change as thought itself. Because consciousness appears uniquely suited to cognitive *inhibition* (e.g., Neely, 1977), rational processes may play an important role in the suppression of established, stereotypic habits until new ones can be established to replace them.

Table 13.2
Characteristics of Experiential Versus Rational Processes

Characteristic	Experiential processes	Rational processes
Role of repetition	Grow with exposure and repetition	Sensitive to type of mental process as much or more than repetition
Processing quality	Sensory processes	Semantic, associational processes
Flexibility	Stereotypic response biases	Flexible responding
Acquisition and change speed	Slow to form, slow to change	Quick to form, quick to change
Role of awareness	Conscious awareness not necessary	Conscious awareness critical
Processing speed, mechanics, and data quantities	Rapid, parallel processing of large amounts of data	Slow, serial processing of limited data bits (7 ± 2)
Attention vs. automatic processes	Initially attentional; automatic control in long run	Attentional control characteristic pervasively
Facilitation vs. inhibition	Response facilitation	Response facilitation or inhibition

Note. Adapted from "Integration of the Cognitive and the Psychodynamic Unconscious," by S. Epstein, 1994, *American Psychologist.*

Such descriptions represent an overarching view of the two classes of mental phenomena that people have identified experimentally over the centuries. In this chapter, we are particularly interested in one aspect of the general distinction, which bears on different types of long-term memory: *declarative* versus *procedural* memory (Squire, 1986) or, using other terminology, *explicit* versus *implicit* memory (Graf & Schacter, 1985). Some differences exist between the declarative/procedural and the explicit/implicit memory distinctions. At the broadest level, the former largely have arisen from neuroanatomical observations and emphasize *structural* differences in memory in both the cognitive and neural domains (Cohen & Squire, 1980; Squire, 1986). In contrast, the latter distinction has emphasized *dynamic* or *processing* differences across different memory manifestations. Furthermore, subtle differences exist in the types of phenomena represented by these two kinds of memory. Whereas declarative memory encompasses both episodic memory and semantic memory, its "parallel," explicit memory, refers to episodic memory alone. Procedural memory refers to any operations governed by rules or procedures, including perceptual–motor learning, "priming," and classical conditioning. Implicit memory refers to memorial phenomena that are seen as performance shifts due to prior exposure, even if individuals are not aware of these prior exposures. In this chapter, the term *memory* refers to long-term memory unless otherwise specified. Critical background information for both pertains to observations of persons with anterograde amnesia.

Individuals with anterograde amnesia are unable to form new conscious memories after traumatic events. They readily acquire new motor skills, however, as well as certain cognitive ones (e.g., puzzle solving), even though they are patently unaware that they have ever practiced them before (Beatty, Scott, Wilson, Prince, & Williamson, 1995; Cohen & Squire, 1980; Damasio, 1989; Eslinger & Damasio, 1986; Kaushall, Zetin, & Squire, 1981; Kime, Lamb, & Wilson, 1996; Knowlton, Mangels, & Squire, 1996; Martone, Butters, Payne, Becker, & Sax, 1984; Milner, 1962; Shadmehr, Brandt, & Corkin, 1998; Tranel, Damasio, Damasio, & Brandt, 1994; Vakil et al., 2000; Yamashita, 1993; Zola-Morgan, Squire, & Mishkin, 1982).

Evidence regarding intact skill acquisition in amnesiacs points to a clear distinction between memorial processes that are impaired versus those that have been spared. The former have to do with conscious memories for specific events, which depend on structures typically damaged in amnesia, that is, the hippocampus and amygdala, and possibly some thalamic structures (Damasio, 1989; Milner, 1962; Scoville & Milner, 1957; Victor, Adams, & Collins, 1971; Zola-Morgan et al., 1982; see also Izquierdo et al., 1997; McGaugh, 2000). The other type of learning and memory, which is relatively spared in amnesia, develops without any necessary awareness of the episodes in which the memory was laid down or its contents. Instead, this type of learning and memory depends on practice or exposure and is unaffected by medial temporal destruction. It regulates a variety of phenomena, including skill acquisition, classical conditioning, and specific performance benefits relative to previously encountered stimuli that persons do not remember, or priming (Squire, 1986). The type of learning and memory impaired in amnesia is variously called *declarative* or *explicit* memory, depending on one's theoretical bias (Graf & Schacter, 1985; Squire, 1986), and it belongs to Epstein's (1994) general category of rational processes. The type of learning and memory spared in amnesia, including motor learning, is called *procedural* or *implicit* memory (Graf & Schacter, 1985; Squire, 1986). We will treat declarative memory and explicit memory as equivalent, and procedural memory and implicit memory as equivalent, unless otherwise noted; however, we previously pointed out that some theoretical differences do exist. Because of motor learning's theoretical link to procedural or implicit memory, cognitive processes that regulate this memory type are of utmost relevance for any physical trainer. Knowledge of such processes should deeply inform any physical training model, including speech models. There are three phases of motor learning: the initial skill acquisition phase, habit formation, and habit change (Verdolini, 1997). All phases of motor learning are distinct from performance, which, paradoxically, frequently responds in exact opposite ways to training manipulations useful for learning. We will focus on the early phase of skill acquisition because more information about it is available.

The information that we present in this chapter appears, at times, to be a study in contradictions. We will suggest that motor learning may not necessarily require *awareness* of events surrounding learning or mechanical principles but does require *attention*, that *cognitive effort* is required but *trying* is counterproductive, that *feedback* is essential for learning but *less is more,* and that motor learning is *stereotypic* but *generalizes.* Some of these apparent contradictions arise out of different research traditions. Ultimately, reliable but contradictory findings must have theoretical resolution. Throughout the chapter, we will suggest possible, or even probable, resolutions to the seeming conflicts noted in the data. We will end the chapter with suggestions about practical applications in the clinic or studio.

Initial Phases of Skill Acquisition

Definition

A clear definition of skill acquisition is critical because it affects how motor learning is studied, especially in the early stages, when much training occurs. An old distinction that dates to early research in experimental psychology concerns differences among performance, skill, and skill acquisition or learning (Tolman, 1932). The importance of the distinction is not just academic; in many cases, a manipulation's impact on performance (a temporary change in performance, to be more accurate) is in *direct opposition* to its impact on learning. For our purpose, *performance* may be considered to be an action that results in a directly measurable outcome. For example, word production performed by a stroke patient may be measured in a variety of ways, including (a) chronometically, such as in total time to initiation or completion; (b) qualitatively, such as in the relative asymmetry of oral posture; (c) kinematically, such as in the biomechanical properties of the intersegmental dynamics; (d) acoustically, such as in selected frequency or temporal characteristics; or (e) communicatively, such as in the proportion of trials on which the word is understood by listeners. Regardless of the level at which one measures the activity, the resultant expression of performance reflects an assessment of a single instance of action. Performance is governed by the nervous system's current neurologic status as well as current performance conditions.

The term *skill* is generally used to refer to a certain *capability* to perform. For example, consider two esophageal speakers, A and B. Speaker A averages eight intelligible syllables per aerodynamic implosion (charge), and Speaker B averages two intelligible syllables per charge under similar performance circumstances. We would probably be correct in saying that Speaker A is generally a more skilled speaker than B. Suppose, however, that on one particular utterance, Speaker B actually achieved more syllables than Speaker A. Would it be correct to conclude that Speaker B is now a more skilled speaker than A? Of course not. There may be many reasons why one particular performance score does not accurately portray a true capability to perform (e.g., just ate, distracted, not feeling well). Researchers therefore view performance scores with caution and require that many performances be assessed before assuming that a measure of skill has been portrayed accurately.

Now consider the concept of learning relative to the concepts of performance and skill. *Motor learning* is generally viewed as the *permanent improvement* in skill. Continuing with the example of the esophageal speakers, suppose that Speaker B, who averages a score of two intelligible syllables per charge, has a great utterance and achieves six syllables from a single charge. Does this mean that his or her skill level has suddenly shown a dramatic and permanent improvement? Perhaps, but maybe not. A performance score can be markedly better or worse than expected for many reasons, which may have nothing at all to do with the more important issue of deciding when there has been a change in *skill level*. In order to conclude that learning has occurred, we must be satisfied that one's level of skill has undergone a permanent improvement. All in all, we define *skill acquisition* as described elsewhere (Schmidt & Lee, 1999): as a *process* that is not directly observed but is inferred, leading to relatively *long-term, stable changes* in performance *potential,* following *practice or exposure.*

Distinctions

In the discussion that follows, we will emphasize the distinction between performance and learning in particular. A critical concept is that given the central role of long-term changes in the definition of motor learning, any claims about learning must be based on transfer or retention tests conducted some period after a training session has been concluded. Such tests will often reveal surprising differences in results at the long-term learning assessment interval as compared with short-term performance changes. The difference between performance and learning variables is crucial to any training model. What, then, are critical cognitive characteristics of initial stages of skill acquisition, in comparison to performance, that point to practical training principles?

Skill acquisition does not appear to require conscious awareness of what is being learned. The role of conscious, verbal (or verbalizable) processes in the early stages of skill acquisition has been a hallmark of motor learning theory (Fitts, 1964; Snoddy, 1926). This concept is so entrenched in modern thinking that few, if any, researchers have challenged it. Surprisingly, though, there is little in the way of solid research evidence to support any causal role of conscious, verbal processes in motor learning (which are equatable), and there is actually considerable evidence to the contrary.

Two issues must be noted here. One is conscious access to events surrounding motor learning in general. The other is awareness of mechanical principles that constitute actual motor learning in particular. Some of the evidence concerning both issues has been provided through observations of amnesic study participants, as previously described. Such individuals do not remember prior training episodes, although they demonstrate motor learning from those episodes. Subsumed in this observation is the corollary that amnesics, who readily demonstrate typical or near-typical motor learning, by logical extension are patently unaware of the mechanical principles that constitute the learning itself. The clear implication, which is amply demonstrated empirically (see preceding sections), is that neither awareness of prior learning nor awareness of its contents is required for motor learning to occur.

Other evidence has been derived from studies of individuals without neurological problems. In these studies, evidence was provided that healthy persons can demonstrate motor learning for specific tasks that they do not remember and thus are unaware of the mechanical substrates that constitute the actual learning. An example of this principle is a series of experiments on a rotary tracking learning, pursuit rotor task (Verdolini-Marston, 1991; Verdolini-Marston & Balota, 1994). In those studies, participants demonstrated either (a) a negative relationship between conscious, explicit remembering of specific stimuli that they had practiced and performance benefits for those same stimuli in comparison to novel ones (Experiment 1; Verdolini-Marston & Balota, 1994) or (b) no clear relationship at all between explicit remembering and performance benefits (Experiments 2 and 3; Verdolini-Marston & Balota, 1994). Stated differently, neither conscious memories of information laid down during training in general nor mechanical principles associated with learning, specifically, were necessary to learning and, in some cases, may have even been harmful to it.

These findings for both amnesiacs and healthy individuals are consistent with a view of motor learning as belonging to an experiential process to which learners have little conscious access. Other data from the pursuit rotor studies speak directly to the issue of conscious access. Data are shown in Figure 13.1 (Experiment 3; Verdolini-Marston, 1991). The left-hand side of the figure shows recognition performance (explicit memory) for specific stimuli study participants had practiced during an earlier training phase (filled squares), as a function of mental strategies that had been imposed during earlier practice ("concentrate," "stir," and "album" mental strategies); the figure also shows participants' ratings of the utility of these strategies for recognition. The data show that for conscious recognition, participants appeared relatively insightful about utility. They tended to rate strategies that yielded low recognition scores (e.g., the "concentrate" strategy) as relatively useless for recognition performance and tended to rate strategies that yielded high recognition scores (e.g., the "album" strategy) as relatively helpful. The same results were not seen for motor (implicit) learning. The right-hand side of Figure 13.1 shows these data. Filled squares indicate actual motor performance during a retention test ("Time on Target," in seconds) as a function of mental strategy condition, and unfilled squares show the participants' ratings of the utility of the various strategies for motor performance and learning. Although no differences were seen in motor performance or learning during the retention test, participants rated some strategies as relatively helpful (e.g., the "concentrate" strategy) and other strategies as not helpful (e.g., the "album" strategy) for motor learning. Stated differently, they were not insightful about the relationship between mental strategies and motor learning. Similar findings occurred in another study on motor learning for a vocal

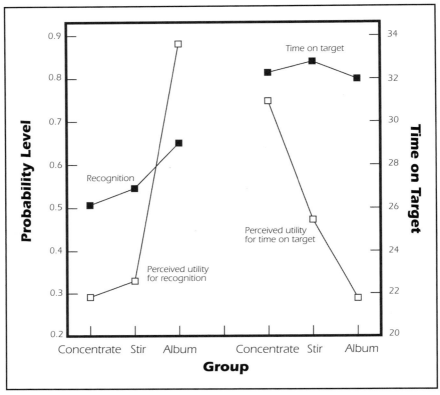

Figure 13.1. Recognition of performance measured by proportion correct, time on target, seconds, and participants' ratings.

task (Verdolini et al., 2003; for data on perceptual learning of a musical sequence without awareness, see also Thompson, Balkwill, & Vernescu, 2000).

Pursuing further the relevance of awareness of the mechanical principles associated with motor learning, several studies have indicated that instructions that specifically directed participants' awareness to mechanical maneuvers, as opposed to the external task goal, interfered with motor learning at the retention interval. Examples include studies on bimanual coordination (Hodges & Lee, 1999), balancing on a stabilometer (C. H. Shea & Wulf, 1999), and slalom-type movements on a ski simulator (Wulf, Höb, & Prinz, 1998; Wulf & Weigelt, 1997).

In sum, observations such as those reviewed here are consistent with the view of motor learning as part of an experientially based process that occurs without any necessary support of conscious awareness of events surrounding learning in general or any awareness of mechanical principles in particular. In fact, there is little evidence that people have reliable access to mechanical principles of learning, even when they think they do.

An important question remains about the role that verbal processes do play in early stages of motor learning: Why do people have the anecdotal impression that verbal processes occur and are relevant for motor learning (Anderson, 1982; Fitts, 1964; Snoddy, 1926)? Possibly, such processes do occur spontaneously for some reason but are counterproductive. Another alternative is that spontaneous or "discovery" verbal awareness is relevant for motor learning, but the types of *imposed* awareness that have been studied are not (e.g., Hodges & Lee, 1999). A third possibility is that verbalizable awareness about the learning process is the *result* rather than the *cause* of learning. In the meantime, a conservative conclusion is that although the question of whether skill acquisition actually requires conscious awareness remains unclear, there is considerable evidence that substantial learning can occur without it.

Skill acquisition requires attention to sensory information. Although awareness is not necessarily involved in early stages of motor learning, paradoxically, apparently attention is. Attention can be defined as a limited capacity mental resource that is applied to certain stimuli and withdrawn from others, increasing the likelihood that the selected stimuli will be further processed—even independent of one's awareness of it (Broadbent, 1958; Cherry, 1953; Deutsch & Deutsch, 1967; Norman, 1969). Attention to a given stimulus can be quantified by measuring the time it takes to respond to a nonattended, secondary stimulus, for example, response time to a flash of light presented to the periphery while attending to a central location on a computer monitor (Posner, 1986). A longer response time to the secondary stimulus implies greater attention to the primary one.

One of the main experiments pointing to the role of attention in early motor learning stages, having to do with a rotary pursuit task (Verdolini-Marston, 1991; Verdolini-Marston & Balota, 1994), was described previously. As noted, in those experiments, when any types of mental strategies were imposed on participants during practice, their later transfer tests revealed poorer learning than when no strategies were imposed. Similar findings were obtained more recently for a voice task involving smooth onset phonation (Verdolini et al., 2003). The most straightforward interpretation is that when mental strategies are imposed, even though individuals may perceive them as helpful to learning, the strategies actually capture their attention, diverting it away from the relevant dimensions of the main task during practice. Motor learning is reduced. It has been assumed that the relevant task dimensions are sensory, not only in motor learning but also in other types of implicit or procedural learning, as demonstrated in word-stem completion, rapid-word identification, and similar tasks (Graf, Mandler, & Haden, 1982; Jacoby & Dallas, 1981).

Skill acquisition requires effort in early stages. Cognitive science has classically linked attention with the concept of cognitive "effort" (e.g., Posner & Snyder, 1975). As such, findings that attention plays a role in early motor learning state that those stages involve cognitive effort. Data from several motor learning studies have indicated that cognitive effort is not only quantitative early in learning—related to attention—but also qualitative, having to do with the actual quality of mental operations. Specifically, beyond attention, three operations appear relevant in cognitive effort: self-generated hypothesis generation and testing, relational processing, and repeated trace activation from baseline. All can be seen in the context of "Hebbian" learning models, which provide a historical basis for many current "connectionist" models of human learning (e.g., Rumelhart, McClelland, & PDP Research Group, 1986). In these models, a core concept is that when Neuron A and Neuron B fire together, synaptic connections are formed that increase the probability that they will fire together again in the future (Hebb, 1949). As discussed in the following text, the use of cognitive effort leading to autologous hypothesis generation and testing, and relational processing, should serve to activate the fullest possible neural traces associated with task performance. Repeated activations of those traces from baseline should continue to increase the likelihood of full-trace activation and thus render stable the interconnected component parts of new behaviors. Evidence for this centers on three specific training variables: augmented feedback, variability of practice, and spacing of practice. A critical note is that these variables are the ones that most clearly distinguish performance from learning variables. Manipulation of the variables in one direction, to reduce cognitive effort, enhances immediate performance during training but depresses learning. Manipulation of the variables in another direction, to increase cognitive effort, compromises immediate performance but enhances learning. The evidence is clear.

Augmented Feedback. Augmented feedback refers to information that learners receive about their performance relative to the target. In motor learning, feedback that a person normally receives as a natural, sensory attribute of an action needs to be distinguished from feedback that is received from sources that have been augmented by an instructor or therapist. Examples of the former are the tension that the speaker perceives in the muscles in and around the larynx prior to speech, or the auditory sounds that the speaker hears during speech. Examples of augmented feedback include verbal reports about a previous performance that are provided by an instructor or various instrumentational methods. If the data from these methods are subsequently made available to the learner, this augmented information has been "fed back" to him or her.

The role of augmented information in motor skills research has a very long history, and its role as a positive influence on learning is not in question (Adams, 1987; Swinnen, 1996). In brief, augmented information can be varied in a number of ways, including frequency (following each performance or following a set of performances) and timing (during performance, immediately after it, or after a lag). Some form of information about one's performance relative to the target is necessary for learning to occur. Without any information about how one is doing, performance does not appear to improve with practice (e.g., Bilodeau, Bilodeau, & Schumsky, 1959). Augmented feedback appears to be a particularly important form of feedback.

Given the value of augmented feedback for motor learning, one would think that the more, the better. Interestingly, this is not the case. In the study by Bilodeau et al. (1959), participants who received the *least frequent* augmented feedback performed the poorest during training; however, the long-term no-feedback retention test showed that those participants actually learned more than the participants who had received frequent feedback during training. More recent studies have indicated similar findings for other motor tasks (e.g., Lee, White, & Carnahan, 1990; Vander-Linden, Cauraugh, & Greene, 1993).

In short, augmented feedback has opposite effects on performance versus learning. The interpretation is that individuals who receive little augmented feedback during training have to exert cognitive effort by way of testing hypotheses, comparing and contrasting results with different strategies, and so forth. (Note that we make no claims about whether these efforts were conscious.) Although their lack of expert guidance during training leads learners to struggle initially, as compared to the more externally supported situations, learners do take the cognitive and neural results of those efforts with them when practice ends. On a return test, they can rely on their own mental wherewithal rather than relying on a trainer or other exogenous sources of support.

Another example of the role of augmented feedback—and its inverse influence on performance versus training—is seen in studies on concurrent augmented feedback. There are many examples in which concurrent feedback can be used to relay information about the progress of an action to the learner. For example, a light can be attached to the head of a putter and used to provide feedback to a golfer about the spatial trajectory. A green light could be used when the putter is on line, and a red light used when the putter's trajectory goes off center. Another example is the illumination of a blue light when the singer's formant is present to a determined criterion level, as opposed to a yellow light when the formant criteria are absent. Such a mechanism for providing augmented feedback would probably be a very effective means for reducing spatial errors in putting and acoustic errors in singing. This commonsense rationale for providing continuous information feedback to the learner serves as the basis for many of the guidance tools that are marketed every day in magazines and on television (physical guidance "tools" are specific types of methods for providing continuous augmented feedback; Schmidt & Lee, 1999). Does this commonsense idea really work? A number of studies in the motor learning literature suggest that not only does it not work, but it is less effective for learning than just about any other method of providing augmented feedback.

Armstrong (1970; described in Schmidt & Lee, 1999, pp. 316–317) reported on an early investigation of the effects of continuous augmented feedback. Armstrong asked his participants to learn a 4-s arm flexion and extension task such that the temporal and spatial characteristics of the action matched a goal template. He compared three practice groups that differed in terms of the augmented feedback provided during practice. For one group, there was a physical restriction in the spatial errors that could be made— participants merely had to learn the temporal characteristics of the task because the spatial trajectories were guided. For another group, there was no mechanical restriction, but group members were provided with a visual feedback trace on a computer monitor that represented the spatial and temporal characteristics of the ongoing movement, together with the template's spatial/temporal characteristics. The participants in this group could easily perceive the difference in the concurrent feedback arising from the movement and the trace showing the intended movement. Last, a group of learners received augmented feedback that was similar to that for the concurrent group, but they received this information as a static feedback display only after the completion of the movement (terminal feedback).

The results of Armstrong's study are illustrated in Figure 13.2. Practice of the task under the various augmented feedback conditions occurred over 3 days and involved 14 blocks of 15 trials per block. A retention test conducted after practice on the 3rd day was performed by all participants. In this test, performance on the learned task was unaccompanied by any augmented feedback. The effects of the various feedback conditions on spatial errors were very dramatic. As can be seen in the left side of Figure 13.2, the guidance condition resulted in very little error during practice. Spatial error for the concurrent feedback group was reduced rapidly during Day 1 of practice, although it never reached the level of performance on Days 2 and 3 that were achieved by the guidance group. The poorest levels of performance were seen for the terminal feedback group. These individuals reduced errors over the

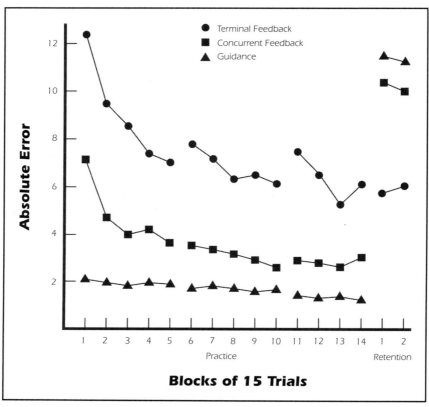

Figure 13.2. Performance during practice and retention testing for three groups of learners given different types of augmented feedback.

entire practice period but still performed with double the number of spatial errors at the end of practice when compared with the concurrent feedback group.

The effects of these feedback conditions on retention, however, were as dramatic as had been their effects on performance, albeit in the *opposite* direction. As can be seen on the right side of Figure 13.2, the terminal feedback group retained the level of performance achieved in practice. Upon removal of the guidance or concurrent feedback, however, the two groups of performers who had previously performed so well in practice now performed at a level of skill that was approximately equivalent to the very early practice trials of the terminal feedback group. Armstrong's results, together with similar findings in a related study by Schmidt and Wulf (1997), suggest that the concurrent methods of providing augmented feedback, although having strong, positive effects on reducing error in performance, actually *degrade* learning compared to other methods that have less of a "guiding-like" influence on immediate changes in performance during practice.

Reviews of the augmented feedback literature (Salmoni, Schmidt, & Walter, 1984; Schmidt, 1991) have suggested that several other methods of providing augmented feedback can also assume "guidance-like" properties that have positive effects in practice but negative consequences on learning. For example, as discussed previously, providing augmented feedback after every performance attempt degrades learning when compared to conditions in which feedback is provided less frequently (Winstein & Schmidt, 1990). Alternatively, there are other methods of utilizing augmented feedback that serve to engage the learner in processing information and that boost the potency of the augmented feedback. For example, requiring learners to estimate how successful their performance had been prior to providing them with that information (as augmented feedback) is very successful in enhancing learning (Swinnen, Schmidt, Nicholson, & Shapiro, 1990).

We believe that the various negative and positive influences of augmented feedback methods occur because of the manner in which they influence the learner's cognitive effort when practicing the task. Remember that in many situations of formalized learning, the instructor or therapist will be available only for a limited period of time. Furthermore, augmented feedback probably will be available to the learner only during this time period. Afterward, it becomes the responsibility of the learner to use internal sources of information to make sense out of performance. For example, the golfer who comes to rely upon an instructor to explain why he or she is slicing the ball in practice will probably be unable to figure out why it suddenly begins to happen again during a round of golf (when the instructor is not available). The speaker who comes to rely upon an instructor to explain why she or he is producing a hyperfunctional sound will probably be unable to figure out why that sound suddenly begins to happen in front of a classroom of students (when the instructor is not available). The learner who uses the augmented feedback as a source of information to further learn to interpret his or her own sources of intrinsically available feedback will be in a much better position to perform when the augmented feedback is not available.

Learning to use augmented feedback to interpret intrinsic sources of information feedback requires cognitive effort, possibly in the form of self-generated hypothesis formulation and testing. Such operations must activate a relatively full set of neural traces that are needed to perform the task. Methods such as physical guidance and concurrent augmented feedback actually minimize this activation, because very good performance can be achieved by relying on powerful external information sources to correct our errors for us or to show us very explicitly how to correct them. In contrast, the augmented feedback methods that provide some information but that also require the learner to effortfully process and relate that information to the intrinsic sources will be more successful in maintaining performance levels following the removal of the feedback.

Variability of Practice. Two key issues in the motor learning literature have emerged regarding the role of practice variability. The first concerns the amount of *task variability* that should be introduced into training. For example, in learning to operate a standard transmission vehicle, is training more effective by using only one vehicle (*nonvariable* practice) or by using more than one vehicle (*variable* practice) in the training sessions? In *Lee Silverman Voice Treatment* (Ramig, Countryman, Thompson, & Horii, 1995), is training more effective by using only a limited word corpus and one physical environment (*nonvariable* practice) or by using an extended word corpus and multiple physical environments (*variable* practice)? Finally, in phonologic training, should training be more effective by using only a single phoneme within a problem distinctive feature class (*nonvariable* practice) or by using multiple phonemes within the class (*variable* practice)?

Many of the research investigations that have addressed this issue have used timing or force production tasks. For example, Mc-Cracken and Stelmach (1977) compared a nonvariable group of learners who were asked to learn to produce an arm movement in exactly 200 ms to a variable group who trained for the same number of trials as the no-variable group but dispersed these trials over varying amplitudes (thus requiring movements of different average velocities). The results indicated a clear performance advantage (mean timing error) that favored the no-variable practice group. A transfer test in which participants were asked to perform the timed movement over an amplitude that neither group had previously practiced clearly favored the variable practice group. In this case, the efficacy of the variable practice conditions did not emerge during the period when formalized training was being assessed. Indeed, during this period, the no-variable practice group performed with less error than did the variable group. It was not until these groups were compared in a transfer test that the true differences in skill levels as a result of the training protocols emerged.

C. H. Shea and Kohl (1990) conducted a similar type of experimental design by using a force production task. In these experiments, however, individuals in the variable practice group were required to perform a retention test on the same task that members of the no-variable group had performed throughout their entire training trials. Similar to the McCracken and Stelmach (1977) results, the no-variable practice group performed with less force production errors than the variable group during training but was much worse in the test for learning (the retention test). This learning effect emerged despite the fact that the retention conditions were clearly more favorable to the no-variable group because the goal used was the same one at which this group had performed *all* of their training trials. Although similar proposals have been made relative to speech therapy, for example, "cyclical training" in developmental language intervention (Cleave & Fey, 2000; Fey, Cleave, Long, & Hughes, 1993), few, if any, data exist.

A variety of explanations are possible to explain the influence of variable practice on motor learning. One of the clearest is described in detail by schema theory (Schmidt, 1975). According to this theory, during practice, learners generate three-dimensional mental "regression plots" that relate initial performance conditions, motor program parameters issued, and movement outcome. Variable practice essentially enriches the regression plot more than no-variable practice, ultimately allowing for the correct prediction of motor program parameters in the face of novel initial conditions that have never been encountered before (generalization). This type of relational processing has similarities to what is called *associational processing* in the conscious verbal learning and memory domains. The difference is that relational processing in motor learning has to do with perception and movement. Associational processing in declarative or explicit memory has to do with processing words' meanings in some way. In any event, both relational and associational processes appear to help make mental representations of events more abstract and thus increase their flexibility and generalizability.

Task Distribution. Another issue related to variable practice—which similarly bears on cognitive issues as well as performance versus learning issues—concerns structuring the order of practice. Working with the assumption that task variability is a more favorable practice condition for retention and transfer than task nonvariability, the question now arises as to the best way to order that practice. In rehabilitation for speech disorders, for example, multiple aspects of speech may need to be addressed. For an adult with dysarthria and aphasia, perhaps articulatory precision and grammar are both relevant. Based on the work presented in the previous section on task variability, one might recommend using multiple speech stimuli for training. If the client thus is required to produce 200 total utterances in a session, that is, 100 relative to articulatory precision and 100 relative to grammar, and 10 repetitions on each of 10 different stimuli are used for each broad goal, how should these practice attempts be ordered? Two extreme orders could be used—one in which all trials corresponding to a single stimulus for a given goal are completed before moving on to the next stimulus × goal condition (e.g., repeating the word *lunchtime* many times, aiming at articulatory precision, followed by repetition of the remaining nine words for precision before proceeding to grammar goals), or another order in which no two consecutive attempts were ever performed using the same condition (*lunchtime* for precision; subject–verb–object [S-V-O] for Sentence 1; *bathroom* for precision; S-V-O for Sentence 2, etc.). In the motor learning literature, the former type of practice order has been termed *blocked practice* (because all of the trials on any particular task are completed at one time, as a "block" of trials). The latter type of practice order has been termed *random practice* (due to the nonrepetitive or unsystematic nature of the practice order).

J. B. Shea and Morgan (1979) performed some of the seminal research in this area, which has been described in detail in many textbooks on motor learning (e.g., Magill, 1993; Schmidt & Lee, 1999). Briefly, J. B. Shea and Morgan compared two groups of individuals who were asked to make distinct patterns of sequential arm movements as fast as possible in response to a visual signal. Three different patterns of arm movements, each paired with specific colored lights, were performed 18 times each. The two groups performed the trials on these three tasks in either a blocked or random practice order, and the time to complete the action was measured. The results were very dramatic. In terms of immediate changes, the blocked group almost immediately performed better (i.e., faster) than did the random group, and this performance advantage was maintained over the entire practice period. However, when J. B. Shea and Morgan examined learning in separate retention and transfer tests (both later in the same day and 10 days after), the random group performed much better than did the blocked group.

The benefit of blocked over random practice during the instructional period, together with the emergence of the random practice superiority when examined later in tests of retention and transfer, captures the essence of what is now known as the *contextual interference effect*. This effect has been replicated and extended many times in experiments involving laboratory tasks and activities of daily living (see reviews by Magill & Hall, 1990; Marley, Ezekiel, Lehto, Wishart, & Lee, 2000; Schmidt & Lee, 1999). Perhaps of more importance, however, is the underlying reason why the effect occurs. In theory, the differences due to random and blocked practice occur because of the cognitive effort that is caused by the interference introduced in each of the practice schedules. For instance, we assume that the preparation to perform a specific task variation involves memory, attentional, and perceptual processes that are specific to that task. An example is placing a phone call to our auto mechanic. We need to recall or look up the number, remember it, examine the telephone display, and plan and execute the sequence of key presses. If the very next phone call that we make is to the same person (e.g., immediately redialing after a busy signal), some of the processes previously performed for the preceding trial can be avoided—we have remembered the number as well as some aspects of the perceptual and motor plan of action. Some or many of the processing demands therefore may be avoided or bypassed because of the fundamental principle that the *repetition of the same action does not necessarily require the repetition of the same processes that resulted in that action* (Lee & Magill, 1983). Compare this situation to the one in which, following the busy signal, you make several other phone calls. Now, returning to call your auto mechanic results in the fact that due to the intervening phone calls, you have forgotten the person's number and the perceptual–motor plan for dialing the number sequence. A repetition of the phone call requires that you perform many more of the same cognitive processes that you did for the original phone call. The former example, of course, is similar to the concept of blocked practice because there is immediate repetition of the same task and, therefore, no need to carry out all of the same cognitive processes on each subsequent occasion. In the latter example, as in random practice, the interference caused by practicing other tasks requires that additional cognitive effort be undertaken by the individual in order to overcome the difficulty that the practice order had created. At minimum, that effort involves repeated activation of the full mental and neural trace for the target behavior, which enhances its later stability (see Aidley, 1998, for discussion of physiology of repeated synaptic activation).

The logic underlying the contextual interference effect is that immediate performance effects (blocked practice benefits) emerge when cognitive processes can be avoided or bypassed. The learning effects in retention and transfer (following random practice) emerge when the cognitive processes must be actively and effortfully undertaken as frequently as possible during practice. In addition, the reversal in performance that is demonstrated by the contextual interference effect is an excellent illustration of the need to carefully distinguish between the effects of various practice methods on performance versus learning. If immediate performance benefits were the main goal, blocked practice would clearly be the preferred method. Unfortunately, for most situations involving structured practice environments, the instructor or therapist does not observe the learner under the conditions in which random practice conditions presumably operate best (retention and transfer), but he or she does directly observe the conditions that (falsely) suggest blocked practice to be superior.

Summary Regarding Cognitive Effort. Different lines of evidence indicate that manipulations leading to cognitive effort seem to challenge and depress immediate performance but enhance motor learning. The evidence points to three qualities of mental operation underlying cognitive effort in motor learning: self-generated cognitive operations that presumably activate full neural traces for target behaviors; relational processing involving self-generated mental regression plots associating initial performance conditions, motor program parameters, and performance outcomes, which are further relevant for broad trace development; and repeated activation of the full trace from baseline. As a convenient heuristic, these operations can be seen in terms of a Hebbian connectionist model of learning in which repeated activation of a full set of neurons associated with a task increases the likelihood that the whole set will fire under similar stimulus conditions at a later time (Hebb, 1949). Maximizing learner effort appears to enhance this process. From a cognitive viewpoint, findings associated with cognitive effort indicate that motor learning not only involves relatively low-level, data-driven sensory processes—as discussed previously and also in the following text—but also higher level, relational cognition.

Interestingly, although initial stages of motor learning appear to require cognitive effort, such effort does not involve intentional, conscious information retrieval, or "trying," as occurs successfully in the declarative/explicit domain. This concept is addressed next.

Skill Acquisition Processing

Skill acquisition belongs to a general type of processing family that is triggered rather than intentionally retrieved. Most of us who have undertaken any kind of motor learning enterprise, be it skiing or golfing or learning to sing, have heard from some trainer, in some form, that we shouldn't "try so hard." General models of learning and memory tell us something about the theoretical basis for this suggestion. Although cognitive effort appears to benefit skill acquisition in early stages, this effort is of a special type. It involves attention, or mentally "showing up," and it appears to require self-generated hypotheses, relational processing, and repeated trace activation from baseline. However, in concert with the idea that motor learning does not consistently require awareness of mechanical principles, much of the critical effort appears to occur outside of awareness. What is colloquially known as *trying* involves *conscious* cognitive effort to retrieve and implement information. In motor learning situations, this type of trying appears to "bark up the wrong neural tree." It evokes declarative or explicit memory processes, when the procedural, implicit ones are best suited for the job.

For now, the relevant data have been reported for procedural (or implicit) learning in the verbal domain. Perhaps the most striking example is a study in which amnesic subjects were asked to study a list of words during a training phase (Schacter & Graf, 1986). Subsequently, study participants received two types of tests in counterbalanced order. One test required them to fill in word stems with the first word that came to mind. Reliably, they tended to complete the stems with studied words, even though they did not even vaguely remember that they had studied those words. The other test required participants to use the same word stems to purposefully remember the earlier, studied words. At this task, they tended to fail miserably. In other words, when given stimuli that were used "nonchalantly," they *triggered* evidence of prior exposure or practice implicitly. When the same stimuli were used to *intentionally* retrieve the same information explicitly, they failed.

Equating word stem completion with implicit—or procedural— memory, this experiment elegantly demonstrated that this memory type is characterized by triggered rather than intentionally retrieved memory manifestations. Assuming that procedural/ implicit memory is uniform across verbal and motor learning, a theoretical explanation for not trying during motor learning is provided. A further implication is that declarative (explicit) and procedural (implicit) mental representations may be one and the same for some tasks. The difference may lie not with their literal structural representation but rather with the ways in which they are evoked.

Motor behaviors may be more stereotypic than sometimes is assumed. The motor learning literature is replete with descriptions of generalization that was transfer of a skill from trained to untrained situations. This phenomenon has been described not only for limb training, but has also been a central concern in speech and language training (Ballard & Thompson, 1999; Elbert, Dinnsen, Swartzlander, & Chin, 1990; Elbert & McReynolds, 1978; Elbert, Powell, & Swartzlander, 1991; Geirut, 1999; Goldstein & Hockenberger, 1991; Jacobs & Thompson, 2000; Kiernan & Snow, 1999; Powell & Elbert, 1984; Powell, Elbert, & Dinnsen, 1991). The predominant theory of motor learning proper, schema theory, centers on explanations of cognitive mechanisms involved in generalization (Schmidt, 1975). This focus is curiously at odds with the theoretical view of motor learning as a type of experientially based learning that results in stereotypic, relatively inflexible behavior (see Table 13.2). How can the views be reconciled? Is one wrong?

We don't believe so. Let us start with a review of some of the data on experiential learning and stereotypicity. We again will borrow from the literature on verbal implicit learning. Several studies have demonstrated that implicit (nonconscious) learning in the verbal domain is resistant to transfer across modalities (visual vs. auditory) and across physical environments. One example is a study by Jacoby and Dallas (1981). In that study, participants visually studied a series of words during an initial training phase. In a later test phase, they were asked to identify (name) words that were presented in degraded form, either visually (same modality) or auditorily (different modality). Some of the words had been studied previously and some were new. Implicit memory would be seen through a performance benefit on the word-identification task for previously studied—but unremembered—words, as compared to new words. Same-modality training-test conditions produced strong evidence of implicit memory. Different-modality training-test conditions produced little evidence of it. That is, implicit memory was disrupted by a change in the physical properties of the stimuli across training and test conditions.

In another experiment, participants studied words in either a pool or a games arcade environment (Graf, 1988). In a later test phase, they were asked to complete word stems, some of which could be completed with previously studied words and some of which could not. Half of the participants received the test in the same environment in which they had originally studied; the other half had a switch in environment (pool to games arcade, or the reverse). In this case, implicit memory would be seen as a tendency to complete word stems with previously studied words at a rate greater than chance, especially if the participants did not remember the studied words. Individuals whose test occurred in the same environment as the one in which they studied tended to display implicit memory. Participants whose test occurred in a different environment from the one in which they studied showed weaker evidence of implicit memory for the studied words. The results of this experiment indicated that implicit memory is sensitive not only to changes in physical modality but also to changes in physical environment.

The implication from both studies, and others like them, is that implicit learning is sensitive to the specific sensory properties of trained stimuli, including contextual properties. Implicit learning does not easily survive a change in modality or physical environment. Again assuming parallel characteristics across types of implicit memory, namely, implicit learning in verbal and physical domains, the implication is that physical motor learning must be a relatively rigid, stereotypic phenomenon. How can this view be reconciled with discussions of generalization as central to motor learning (e.g., Schmidt, 1975)?

The most obvious reconciliation is that theories of motor learning and studies of it have focused on generalization because it is not necessarily easy to come by. Perhaps variable practice is required for generalization to occur *because* motor learning is relatively rigid. A theoretical cognitive neuroscience view would hold that variable practice essentially institutes a large number of traces within a class of responses. Ultimately, subsequent and novel initial stimulus conditions evoke a trace that is sufficiently similar to a preceding one that competent performance ensues. In sum, motor learning does involve lower level, sensory, and stereotypic processes; generalization requires higher level cognitive effort, much of which appears to occur outside of conscious awareness.

Habit Formation

Habits are defined as behaviors that are executed with limited attentional allocation. They are identified by consistent competent performance to a given stimulus set in the face of simultaneously distracting tasks (e.g., Laberge & Samuels, 1974). If performance decrements are seen with the introduction of a secondary task, the behavior is not yet habituated, because the task still demands attention.

Habit formation is extremely relevant for all types of skill acquisition, including skiing, tennis playing, driving a car, dancing, singing, or speaking. Data on neural substrates involved in habit formation suggest a special role for the basal ganglia (for a review, see Salmon & Butters, 1995). Cognitive data are sparser, and most pertain to perceptual, rather than motor, learning.

Data on perceptual learning have indicated that the consistent application of a class of behaviors in response to given stimulus arrays is required for responding to become automatized, that is, stable in the face of distractors (Schneider & Fisk, 1982). There are good reasons to think that similar findings should be obtained for motor learning. If so, the implication is that an "each time, every time" attitude toward the application of training behaviors should facilitate the acquisition of new speech habits.

This is not a trivial issue for speech therapy. In most training situations—skiing, tennis, golf, driving a car, dancing, swimming, singing, even learning to walk again after injury—the learner is engaged in the task largely during training sessions or other situations in which there are no inherent diversions. The learner thus can fully attend to the task and repeatedly practice the new response. In speech therapy, however, full attentional allocation is possible only during practice or therapy sessions. The moment the learner walks out the clinician's door to make his or her next appointment or speak with a family member, a "secondary" task is introduced: communication. The learner's attention is diverted to the communicative task, and little is left for paying attention to *how* to speak. If the behavior is not yet automatized, which it cannot be early in learning, by definition the new speech task must suffer. At that point, for days or week(s), the learner will repeatedly engage in inconsistent responding; he or she will speak in the "new" mode during practice or therapy sessions, but in the old, "available" mode during most other situations. This situation may explain why many of our therapy notes indicate, week after week, that the client does well during therapy sessions but that there appears to be little carryover between sessions. He or she is incurring inconsistent responding—sometimes the "old" way and sometimes the "new" way—between and within training sessions. The new behaviors therefore fail to become habituated.

If the perceptual literature transfers to the motor literature on this point, for the speech client to acquire not only a new speech behavior but, moreover, a new *automatized* speech behavior, at some point he or she will somehow have to manage to use the new behavior in all or most communicative situations. For some learners, this may require an actual "contractual" arrangement with the clinician. Two or 3 weeks of consistent responding is required for a new behavior, according to some mythical standard. Unfortunately, we are not aware of any dosage studies that have established the amount of time, or amount of practice, needed to establish speech automaticity.

Habit Change

Habit change involves the suppression of a habituated behavior that is evoked extremely rapidly, without conscious awareness or control, and its substitution by another novel behavior that itself eventually becomes habituated. An example is the substitution of a barely abducted vocal fold configuration for a tightly adducted one during conversational speech (Berry et al., 2001; Verdolini, 2000).

Habit change may require inhibition. Habits appear to involve minimally the establishment of new neural links and possibly transfer from cortical to basal ganglia control. A cognitive view is that in habituated behaviors, input stimulations lead to a "wildfire" spread of neuronal activation to neuron sets that have fired off together in the past in response to the stimulus. In this mode of responding, the time from stimulus to response is typically very rapid and occurs without awareness or conscious control (Neely, 1977). Stated differently, habits belong to a class of behaviors in which predictable responding is facilitated by rapid, uncontrolled, and established neural connections.

The speed issue is not a small one for our discussion here. When a behavior has been habituated—for example, vocal hyperfunction—given a stimulus to respond ("speak!"), the habituated behavior will be neurally available within milliseconds (Neely, 1977). A new behavior, which has not yet been established, is not available at this short latency. Instead, the new behavior, which still comes under attentional control, may require several hundred milliseconds or even seconds to become available following stimulus onset (e.g., "speak!"; Neely, 1977). Two things must happen for the new behavior to have a chance to be activated, and to be practiced, to become a habit itself. First, a time lag must be introduced between stimulus and response to allow the new behavior to have a chance to build sufficient activation to "fire." Second, the old behavior may need to be actively inhibited by some means in the interim, lest it trigger automatically. Neely (1997) clearly documented that whereas automatic, habituated behaviors involve only facilitated responding, conscious operations can either facilitate or inhibit responses. Conscious inhibition therefore may be required to override existing habits, such as speech habits, so that new ones may be developed.

We are aware of only one approach to any domain within speech–language pathology that expressly utilizes conscious inhibition as part of the retraining paradigm. This is the Alexander Technique (Alexander, 1974). Alexander specifically described preparing to start a speech behavior, and then stopping and consciously commanding inhibition of the emerging behavior, followed by instituting a new one. Verbal inhibition may make particular sense, given the intuitive link between much conscious activity and inner verbalization.

Conclusion

A review of the different literature traditions in motor learning research has suggested a series of apparent paradoxes. Principal ones are listed in Table 13.3. Motor learning does not necessarily involve awareness of what is learned, specifically, mechanical principles, but attention to sensory substrates, which presumably drive motoric principles, apparently is relevant. Verbal processes associated with mechanical aspects of learning may occur spontaneously during early learning phases, but there is some possibility that they are irrelevant to learning or sometimes even harmful to it. Cognitive effort appears required in the form of hypothesis generation, relational processing, and repeated activation from a nonactive baseline. Conscious "trying" may be counterproductive, however. Information about performance relative to the target is necessary for motor

Table 13.3

Factors That Appear Helpful Versus Irrelevant or Harmful to Motor Learning, and Practical Suggestions for Applications

Irrelevant or harmful	Relevant and helpful	Practical suggestions
Verbalizable awareness of mechanical principles	Attention to sensory information	Leave learner space to process sensory information
Conscious "trying"	Covert cognitive effort	• Provide augmented feedback, but limited • Structure practice on variable stimuli • Randomize rather than blocking practice on various treatment goals
Frequent posttrial or continuous augmented feedback	Sparing use of augmented feedback	Provide posttrial augmented feedback, but sparingly
—	Lower-level sensory processes	Practice using stimuli and physical environments relevant to the learner
—	Higher-level cognitive processes	Variable practice using multiple stimuli and physical environments
Inconsistent use of target behavior in response to given class of stimuli ("Speak!")	Consistent use of behaviors in new response class in all contexts and environments	Encourage consistent use of behaviors in new response class in all contexts and environments
—	Conscious inhibition of old habits	Lag between stimulus ("Speak") and response ("Speak in new way"); conscious, verbal inhibition of old, habituated response

Note. Cells are not orthogonal.

learning, but less appears to enhance learning more. Lower level sensory processes appear relevant, and motor learning may belong to a class of fundamentally stereotypic, rigid processes; however, generalization, which is dependent on flexible, abstract processes, is central to most training models. Practice on variable stimuli is critical for generalization, whereas consistent responding to a class of stimuli (e.g., "speak!") may be important for habituation to occur. Inhibition may be required to suppress existing habits, allowing for a relative facilitation of emerging behaviors.

A general, theoretical view of information processing can reconcile many of the apparent contradictions and point to some good choices for training strategies (see Table 13.3). Although much empirical research remains to be conducted, especially in the speech domain, clinicians and instructors need to make decisions about training strategies now. We emphasize caution in our recommendations, but at the same time hold that it is better to base choices on informed and theoretically and empirically grounded reports rather than casual, personal intuitions. With these disclaimers in mind, some suggestions for training follow (see also Table 13.3). (Note that suggestions are not all orthogonal to each other; some of the same suggestions apply to different principles.)

First, verbal instructions about the mechanics of learning are not strongly recommended. "Discovery" approaches emphasizing sensory processes may be relatively more facilitatory. Conscious "trying" to learn or perform well may not be helpful, but placing "desirable difficulties" in the learner's path, such as limited post-performance augmented feedback, practice on variable stimuli, and randomized stimulus presentation, may enhance learning (while depressing performance) by increasing covert cognitive effort (Bjork, 1998). In fact, trainers should provide learners with clear information about the goals of training and their progress relative to those goals, but that information should be given sparingly. Although an emphasis on lower level sensory processes is critical, generalization should be emphasized through the introduction of training conditions facilitating higher level relational processing, such as variable practice. Once a new target behavior can be produced, the learner should use that behavior in place of the old one as often as possible. Finally, while new behaviors are being trained, competing habits may need to be suppressed through conscious efforts, including delay before a response and verbal commands to inhibit the old habit.

In sum, as suggested by Bjork (1998), recommendations about the introduction of desirable challenges strike closest to home in convincing instructors, teachers, therapists, and other professionals to implement these ideas. Individuals who facilitate the learning process in formalized environments usually only see the learner for a limited period of time. It therefore is natural that they might prefer to directly observe as much progress in their learners as possible, as well as learners' enthusiasm about the perceived usefulness of training strategies. Difficulties that could be introduced through practice variability and augmented feedback conditions, which tend to impede immediate progresses in performance, might not be seen as highly desirable. Imposed strategies that learners "like" may in turn be seen as positive. Both impressions are wrong with respect to motor learning. One of the most important challenges in the use of motor learning principles in practice is the education of persons who facilitate the learning process.

Finally, throughout this chapter, we have assumed that the client is motivated and is adhering to clinical recommendations as a substrate for learning. This is no small assumption. There is some evidence that the client's perception of the clinician as warm positively influences compliance with the clinician's recommendations (Francis, Korsch, & Morris, 1969). In the end, as with most training paradigms, a balance must be struck between learner and teaching variables.

References

Adams, J. A. (1987). Historical review and appraisal of research on learning, retention, and transfer of human motor skills. *Psychological Bulletin, 101*, 41–74.

Aidley, D. J. (1998). *The physiology of excitable cells* (4th ed.). Cambridge, England: Press Syndicate of the University of Cambridge.

Alexander, F. M. (1974). *The Alexander technique*. London: Thames and Hudson.

Anderson, J. R. (1976). *Language, memory, and thought.* Hillsdale, NJ: Erlbaum.

Anderson, J. R. (1982). Acquisition of cognitive skill. *Psychological Review, 89,* 369–406.

Ballard, K. J., & Thompson, C. K. (1999). Treatment and generalization of complex sentence production in agrammatism. *Journal of Speech, Language and Hearing Research, 42,* 690–707.

Beatty, W. W., Scott, J. G., Wilson, D.A., Prince, J. R., & Williamson, D. J. (1995). Memory deficits in a demented patient with probable corticobasal degeneration. *Journal of Geriatric Psychiatry and Neurology, 8*(2), 132–136.

Berry, D., Verdolini, K., Montequin, D., Hess, M., Chan, R., & Titze, I. R. (2001). New indications of an optimal glottal half-width in vocal production. *Journal of Speech, Language and Hearing Research, 44,* 29–37.

Bilodeau, E. A., Bilodeau, I. M., & Schumsky, D. A. (1959). Some effects of introducing and withdrawing knowledge of results early and late in practice. *Journal of Experimental Psychology, 58,* 142–144.

Bjork, R. A. (1998). Assessing our own competence: Heuristics and illusions. In D. Gopher & A. Koriat (Eds.), *Attention and performance: Vol. 17. Cognitive regulation of performance: Interaction of theory and application* (pp. 435–459). Cambridge, MA: MIT Press.

Broadbent, D. E. (1958). *Perception and communication.* London: Pergamon Press.

Broadbent, D. E., FitzGerald, P., & Broadbent, M. H. P. (1986). Implicit and explicit knowledge in the control of complex systems. *British Journal of Psychology, 77,* 33–50.

Bruner, J. S. (1986). *Actual minds, possible worlds.* Cambridge, MA: Harvard University Press.

Cherry, C. (1953). Some experiments on the recognition of speech with one and with two ears. *Journal of the Acoustic Society of America, 25,* 975–979.

Cleave, P. L., & Fey, M. E. (2000). Two approaches to the facilitation of grammar in children with language impairments: Rationale and description. *American Journal of Speech Language Pathology, 6,* 22–32.

Cohen, N. J., & Squire, L. R. (1980). Preserved learning and retention of pattern-analyzing skill in amnesia: Dissociation of knowing how and knowing that. *Science, 210,* 207–210.

Damasio, A. R. (1989). Time-locked multiregional retroactivation: A systems-level proposal for the neural substrates of recall and recognition. *Cognition, 33*(1–2), 25–62.

Deutsch, J. A., & Deutsch, D. (1967). Comments on selective attention: Perception or response? *Quarterly Journal of Experimental Psychology, 19,* 362–363.

Elbert, M., Dinnsen, D. A., Swartzlander, P., & Chin, S. B. (1990). Generalization to conversational speech. *Journal of Speech and Hearing Disorders, 55,* 694–699.

Elbert, M., & McReynolds, L .V. (1978). An experimental analysis of misarticulating children's generalization. *Journal of Speech and Hearing Research, 21,* 136–150.

Elbert, M., Powell, T. W., & Swartzlander, P. (1991). Toward a technology of generalization: How many exemplars are sufficient? *Journal of Speech and Hearing Research, 34,* 81–87.

Epstein, S. (1994). Integration of the cognitive and the psychodynamic unconscious. *American Psychologist, 49,* 709–724.

Eslinger, P. J., & Damasio, A. R. (1986). Preserved motor learning in Alzheimer's disease: Implications for anatomy and behavior. *Journal of Neuroscience, 6,* 3006–3009.

Fey, M. E., Cleave, P. L., Long, S. H., & Hughes, D. L. (1993). Two approaches to the facilitation of grammar in children with language impairment: An experimental evaluation. *Journal of Speech and Hearing Research, 36, 141–157.*

Fiske, S. T. (1981). Social cognition and affect. In J. Harvey (Ed.), *Cognition, social behavior, and the environment* (pp. 227–264). Hillsdale, NJ: Erlbaum.

Fitts, P. M. (1964). Perceptual-motor skills learning. In A. W. Mellon (Ed.), *Categories of human learning* (pp. 243–285). New York: Academic Press.

Francis, V., Korsch, B. M., & Morris, M. J. (1969). Gaps in doctor-patient communication. *New England Journal of Medicine, 280,* 535–540.

Freud, S. (1953). The interpretation of dreams. In J. Strachey (Ed. & Trans.), *The standard edition of the complete psychological works of Sigmund Freud* (Vols. 4 & 5). London: Hogarth. (Original work published 1900)

Geirut, J. A. (1999). Syllable onsets: Clusters and adjuncts in acquisition. *Journal of Speech, Language and Hearing Research, 42,* 708–726.

Goldstein, H., & Hockenberger, E. H. (1991). Significant progress in child language intervention: An 11-year retrospective. *Research in Developmental Disabilities, 12,* 401–424.

Graf, P. (1988). Implicit and explicit memory in same and different environments. *Science, 218,* 1243–1244.

Graf, P., Mandler, G., & Haden, P. E. (1982). Simulating amnesic symptoms in normal subjects. *Science, 218,* 1243–1244.

Graf, P., & Schacter, D. L. (1985). Implicit and explicit memory for new associations in normal and amnesic subjects. *Journal of Experimental Psychology: Learning, Memory, and Cognition, 11,* 501–518.

Hebb, D. O. (1949). *The organization of behavior.* New York: Wiley.

Hodges, N. J., & Lee, T. D. (1999). The role of augmented information prior to learning a bimanual visual-motor coordination task: Do instructions of the movement pattern facilitate learning relative to discovery learning? *British Journal of Psychology, 90,* 389–403.

Izquierdo, I., Quillfeldt, J. A., Zanatta, M. S., Quevedo, J., Schaeffer, E., Schmitz, P. K., et al. (1997). Sequential role of hippocampus and amygdala, entorhinal cortex and parietal cortex in formation and retrieval of memory for inhibitory avoidance in rats. *The European Journal of Neuroscience, 9*, 786–793.

Jacobs, B. J., & Thompson, C. K. (2000). Cross-modal generalization effects of training noncanonical sentence comprehension and production in agrammatic aphasia. *Journal of Speech, Language and Hearing Science, 43*(1), 5–20.

Jacoby, L. L., & Dallas, M. (1981). On the relationship between autobiographical memory and perceptual learning. *Journal of Experimental Psychology: General, 110*, 306–340.

Kaushall, P. I., Zetin, M., & Squire, L. R. (1981). Single case study: A psychological study of chronic, circumscribed amnesia. *The Journal of Nervous and Mental Disease, 169*, 383–389.

Kiernan, B. J., & Snow, D. P. (1999). Bound-morpheme generalization by children with SLI: Is there a functional relationship with accuracy of response to training targets? *Journal of Speech, Language and Hearing Research, 42*, 649–662.

Kime, S. K., Lamb, D. G., & Wilson, B. A. (1996). Use of a comprehensive programme of external cueing to enhance procedural memory in a patient with dense dementia. *Brain Injury, 10*(1), 17–25.

Knowlton, B. J., Mangels, J. A., & Squire, L. R. (1996). A neostriatal habit learning system in humans. *Science, 273*, 1399–1402.

Laberge, D., & Samuels, S. J. (1974). Toward a theory of automatic information processing in reading. *Cognitive Psychology, 6*, 293–323.

Labouvie-Vief, G. (1989). Modes of knowledge and the organization of development. In M. L. Commons, J. D. Sinnott, F. A. Richards, & C. Armon (Eds.), *Adult development* (Vol. 2, pp. 43–62). New York: Praeger.

Labouvie-Vief, G. (1990). Wisdom as integrated thought: Historical and developmental perspectives. In R. J. Sternberg (Ed.), *Wisdom: Its nature, origins, and development* (pp. 52–83). New York: Cambridge University Press.

Lee, T. D., & Magill, R. A. (1983). The locus of contextual interference in motor-skill acquisition. *Journal of Experimental Psychology: Learning, Memory, and Cognition, 9,* 730–746.

Lee, T. D., White, M. A., & Carnahan, H. (1990). On the role of knowledge of results in motor learning: Exploring the guidance hypothesis. *Journal of Motor Behavior, 22,* 191–208.

Luria, A. R. (1961). *The role of speech in the regulation of normal and abnormal behavior.* Oxford, England: Pergamon Press.

Magill, R. A. (1993). *Motor learning: Concepts and applications* (5th ed.). Madison, WI: Brown & Benchmark.

Magill, R. A., & Hall, K. G. (1990). A review of the contextual interference effect in motor skill acquisition. *Human Movement Science, 9,* 241–289.

Marley, T. L., Ezekiel, H. J., Lehto, N. K., Wishart, L. R., & Lee, T. D. (2000). Application of motor learning principles: The physiotherapy client as a problem-solver: II. Scheduling practice. *Physiotherapy Canada, 52,* 311–316.

Martone, M., Butters N., Payne, M., Becker, J. T., & Sax, D. S. (1984). Dissociations between skill learning and verbal recognition in amnesia and dementia. *Archives of Neurology, 41,* 965–970.

McClelland, D. C., Koestner, R., & Weinberger, J. (1989). How do self-attributed and implicit motives differ? *Psychological Review, 96,* 690–702.

McCracken, H. D., & Stelmach, G. E. (1977). A test of the schema theory of discrete motor learning. *Journal of Motor Behavior, 9,* 193–201.

McGaugh, J. L. (2000). Memory—a century of consolidation. *Science, 287,* 248–251.

Milner, B. (1962). Les troubles de la memoire accompagnant des lesions hippocampique bilaterales [Memory problems that accompany lesions of the bilateral hippocampus]. In P. Passouant (Ed.), *Physiologie de l'hippocampique.* Paris: Centre National de la Recherche Scientifique.

Neely, J. H. (1977). Semantic priming and retrieval from lexical memory: Roles of inhibitionless spreading activation and limited-capacity attention. *Journal of Experimental Psychology: General, 106,* 226–254.

Nisbett, R. E., & Wilson, T. D. (1977). Telling more than we can know: Verbal reports on mental processes. *Psychological Review, 84,* 231–259.

Nissen, M. J., Willingham, D., & Hartman, M. (1989). Explicit and implicit remembering: When is learning preserved in amnesia? *Neuropsychologie, 27,* 341–352.

Norman, D. A. (1969). Memory while shadowing. *Quarterly Journal of Experimental Psychology, 21,* 85–93.

Paivio, A. (1986). *Mental representations: A dual encoding approach.* New York: Oxford University Press.

Paivio, A. (1991). *Images in mind: The evolution of a theory.* New York: Harvester Wheatsheaf.

Piaget, J. (1973). The affective unconscious and the cognitive unconscious. *Journal of the American Psychoanalytic Association, 21,* 249–261.

Posner, M. I. (1986). *Chronometric explorations of mind.* New York: Oxford University Press.

Posner, M. I., & Snyder, C. R. R. (1975). Facilitation and inhibition in the processing of signals. In P. M. A. Rabbit & S. Dornic (Eds.), *Attention and performance* (Vol. 5, pp. 669–682). London: Academic Press.

Powell, T. W., & Elbert, M. (1984). Generalization following the remediation of early- and later-developing consonant clusters. *Journal of Speech and Hearing Disorders, 49,* 211–218.

Powell, T. W., Elbert, M., & Dinnsen, D. A. (1991). Stimulability as a factor in the phonological generalization of misarticulating preschool children. *Journal of Speech and Hearing Research, 34,* 1318–1328.

Ramig, L., Countryman, S., Thompson, L., & Horii, Y. (1995). A comparison of two forms of intensive speech treatment for Parkinson disease. *Journal of Speech and Hearing Research, 39,* 1232–1251.

Reber, A. S. (1993). *Implicit learning and tacit knowledge.* New York: Oxford University Press.

Rumelhart, D. E., McClelland, J. L., & The PDP Research Group (Eds.). (1986). *Parallel distributed processing: Explorations in the microstructure of cognition* (Vol. 1). Cambridge, MA: Bradford.

Salmon, D. P., & Butters, N. (1995). Neurobiology of skill and habit learning. *Current Opinion in Neurobiology, 5,* 184–190.

Salmoni, A. W., Schmidt, R. A., & Walter, C. B. (1984). Knowledge of results and motor learning: A review and critical reappraisal. *Psychological Bulletin, 95,* 355–386.

Schacter, D. L., & Graf, P. (1986). Preserved learning in amnesic patients: Perspectives from research on direct priming. *Journal of Clinical and Experimental Neuropsychology, 8,* 727–743.

Schmidt, R. A. (1975). *Motor skills.* New York: Harper & Row.

Schmidt, R. A. (1991). Frequent augmented feedback can degrade learning: Evidence and interpretations. In J. Requin & G. E. Stelmach (Eds.), *Tutorials in motor neuroscience* (pp. 59–75). Dordrecht, the Netherlands: Kluwer.

Schmidt, R. A., & Lee, T. D. (1999). *Motor control and learning: A behavioral emphasis* (3rd ed.). Champaign, IL: Human Kinetics.

Schmidt, R. A., & Wulf, G. (1997). Continuous concurrent feedback degrades skill learning: Implications for training and simulation. *Human Factors, 39,* 509–525.

Schneider, W., & Fisk, A. D. (1982). Concurrent automatic and controlled visual search: Can processing occur without resource cost? *Journal of Experimental Psychology: Learning, Memory, and Cognition, 8,* 261–278.

Schneider, W., & Shiffrin, R. M. (1977). Controlled and automatic information processing: I. Detection, search, and attention. *Psychological Review, 84*(2), 1–66.

Scoville, W. B., & Milner, B. (1957). Loss of recent memory after bilateral hippocampal lesions. *Journal of Neurology, Neurosurgery, and Psychiatry, 20,* 11–21.

Shadmehr, R., Brandt, J., & Corkin, S. (1998). Time-dependent motor memory processes in amnesic subjects. *Journal of Neurophysiology, 80,* 1590–1597.

Shea, C. H., & Kohl, R. M. (1990). Specificity and variability of practice. *Research Quarterly for Exercise and Sport, 61,* 169–177.

Shea, C. H., & Wulf, G. (1999). Enhancing motor learning through external-focus instructions and feedback. *Human Movement Science, 18,* 553–571.

Shea, J. B., & Morgan, R. L. (1979). Contextual interference effects on the acquisition, retention, and transfer of a motor skill. *Journal of Experimental Psychology: Human Learning and Memory, 5,* 179–187.

Snoddy, G. S. (1926). Learning and stability: A psychophysical analysis of a case of motor learning with clinical applications. *Journal of Applied Psychology, 10,* 1–36.

Squire, L. R. (1986). Mechanisms of memory. *Science, 232,* 1612–1619.

Swinnen, S. P. (1996). Information feedback for motor skill learning: A review. In H. N. Zelaznik (Ed.), *Advances in motor learning and control* (pp. 37–66). Champaign, IL: Human Kinetics.

Swinnen, S. P., Schmidt, R. A., Nicholson, D. E., & Shapiro, D. C. (1990). Information feedback for skill acquisition: Instantaneous knowledge of results degrades learning. *Journal of Experimental Psychology: Learning, Memory, and Cognition, 16,* 706–716.

Thompson, W. F., Balkwill, L. L., & Vernescu, R. (2000). Expectancies generated by recent exposure to melodic sequences. *Memory and Cognition, 28,* 547–555.

Tolman, E. C. (1932). *Purposive behavior of animals and men.* New York: Century.

Tranel, D., Damasio, A. R., Damasio, H., & Brandt, J. P. (1994). Sensorimotor skill learning in amnesia: Additional evidence for the neural basis of nondeclarative memory. *Learning and Memory, 3,* 165–179.

Tulving, E. (1984). How many memory systems are there? *American Psychologist, 40,* 385–398.

Tversky, A., & Kahneman, D. (1974). Judgment under uncertainty: Heuristics and biases. *Science, 185,* 1124–1131.

Tversky, A., & Kahneman, D. (1983). Extensional versus intuitive reasoning: The conjunction fallacy in probability judgment. *Psychological Review, 90,* 293–315.

Vakil, E., Grunhaus, L., Nagar, I., Ben-Chaim, E., Dolberg, O. T., Dannon, P. N., et al. (2000). The effect of electroconvulsive therapy (ECT) on implicit memory: Skill learning and perceptual priming in patients with major depression. *Neuropsychologia, 38,* 1405–1414.

Vander-Linden, D. W., Cauraugh, J. H., & Greene, T. A. (1993). The effect of frequency of kinetic feedback on learning an isometric force production task in nondisabled subjects. *Physical Therapy, 73*(2), 79–87.

Verdolini, K. (1997, February). *Skill acquisition principles applied to speech-language pathology.* Presentation at Brigham and Women's Hospital Cognitive Neuroscience Group, Harvard Medical School, Boston, Massachusetts.

Verdolini, K. (2000). Case study: Resonant voice therapy. In J. Stemple (Ed.), *Clinical cases in voice therapy* (pp. 46–62). San Diego: Singular.

Verdolini, K., Schacter, D. L., Kobler, J., Eigen, C., Conversano, F., Brown, C. K., et al. (2003). *Dissociation of item-specific and generalized learning for a voice task.* Manuscript in preparation.

Verdolini-Marston, K. (1991). *Processing characteristics of perceptual-motor memories with and without awareness.* Unpublished doctoral dissertation. Washington University, St. Louis.

Verdolini-Marston, K., & Balota, D. A. (1994). Role of elaborative and perceptual integrative processes in perceptual-motor performance. *Journal of Experimental Psychology: Learning, Memory, and Cognition, 20,* 739–749.

Victor, M., Adams, R. D., & Collins, G. H. (1971). *The Wernicke-Korsakoff syndrome.* Philadelphia: F. A. Davis.

Vygotsky, L. (1962). *Thought and language.* Cambridge, MA: M.I.T. Press. (Original work published 1934)

Winograd, T. (1995). Frame representations and the declarative/ procedural controversy. In D. Bobrow & A. Collins (Eds.), *Representation and understanding: Studies in cognitive science.* New York: Academic Press.

Winstein, C. J., & Schmidt, R. A. (1990). Reduced frequency of knowledge of results enhances motor skill learning. *Journal of Experimental Psychology: Learning, Memory, and Cognition, 16,* 677–691.

Wulf, G., Höb, M., & Prinz, W. (1998). Instructions for motor learning: Differential effects of internal versus external focus of attention. *Journal of Motor Behavior, 30,* 169–179.

Wulf, G., & Weigelt, C. (1997). Instructions about physical principles in learning a complex motor skill: To tell or not to tell ... *Research Quarterly for Exercise and Sport, 68,* 362–367.

Yamashita, H. (1993). Perceptual-motor learning in amnesic patients with temporal lobe lesions. *Perceptual and Motor Skills, 77*(3, Pt. 2), 1311–1314.

Zola-Morgan, S., Squire, L. R., & Mishkin, M. (1982). The neuroanatomy of amnesia: Amygdala-hippocampus versus temporal stem. *Science, 218,* 1337–1339.

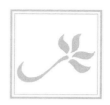

AUTHOR INDEX

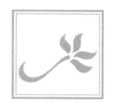

SUBJECT INDEX

recurrent laryngeal nerve (RLN) and,
149–151
research on, 148, 152–153, 156–157
respiratory function and, 359
stimulus treatment for, 158
surgical procedures and, 149, 152
theoretical/empirical knowledge about,
147–149
treatment for, 149–153, 156–160
Specificity, definition of, 355
Speech disorders. *See* Voice disorders
Speech–language pathologist
GERD and, 317
health-care delivery and, 2
as multidiscipline profession, 2–6
respiratory function and, 349
tracheoesophageal fistulization/puncture
training, 3
Speech–language pathology treatment,
189–191
Speech therapy
for Parkinson's disease, 229–242
PVFM/EPL and, 173
SSRI, 398
Starling hypothesis, 72
Stimulus control, 201
Stimulus treatment, 158
Stress, 296, 314
Stress reflux, 296
Stroboscopic examinations, 178, 194, 317
Subcutaneous drug administration, 367
Subepithelial edema, 89–90
Sublingual drug administration, 368
Substantia nigra pars compact (SNpc),
210, 213, 216
Substantia nigra pars reticulata (SNpr),
213, 227
Subthalamic nucleus procedures, 227–228
Sucralfate, 308
Superior laryngeal artery, 70
Superior thyroid artery, 70
Support, definition of, 350
Suppression, 432
Surgery
amyloidosis and, 274–275
BMZ and, 16
death and, 308
gastroesophageal reflux disease (GERD)
and, 301, 305, 308–309
microvascular lesions and, 92–96

Parkinson's disease and, 214, 222–223
scarring and, 24
spasmodic dysphonia (SD) and, 149,
152
Wegener's granulomatosis (WG) and,
276–277
Symptomatic PD, 210, 211
Systemic illness
amyloidosis, 272–275
relapsing polychondritis, 284–286
rheumatoid arthritis, 283–284
sarcoidosis, 277–280
systemic lupus erythematosus (SLE),
280–282, 285
treatment of, 274
Wegener's granulomatosis (WG), 275–
277
Systemic lupus erythematosus (SLE),
280–282, 285

TA. *See* Thyroarytenoid (TA)
TA muscle
apoptosis and, 116–117
fiber loss and atrophy and, 111–112, 122
gene therapy and, 119–120
motor unit remodeling, 117–118
muscle fiber regeneration and, 112–113
muscle use and misuse and, 118–119
myonuclei and, 114–116, 118
remodeling of, 111–120
satellite cells and, 115–116, 118
spasmodic dysphonia (SD) and, 151
treatment and prevention of muscle
fiber loss, 114–115
Task distribution, 424–426
Task variability, 422
Technology, 3–5, 7, 8
Temporomandibular joint dysfunction,
315
Tension dysphonia, 348
Tetracyclines, 399
Thalamotomy, 223–224
Thalmus, 409
Thyroarytenoid (TA), 71, 83, 214
Tobacco and smoking, 26, 127, 295, 311,
312, 316, 320
Topical drug administration, 368
Tracheoesophageal fistulization/puncture,
3, 169, 188
Traditional speech pathology, 3

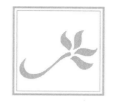

About the Editors and Contributors

Janina K. Casper, PhD, received her bachelor of arts degree from the University of Michigan, a master of science degree from The Pennsylvania State University, and a doctorate from Syracuse University. She recently retired from the Department of Otolaryngology and Communication Sciences at the SUNY Upstate Medical University in Syracuse, New York. Dr. Casper has served on numerous boards and committees of the American Speech-Language-Hearing Association (ASHA), as an associate editor of the *American Journal of Speech-Language Pathology,* and on the editorial boards of numerous journals. She is a Fellow of ASHA. She has had extensive clinical and research experience in various professional areas; however, her main focus is the voice and its disorders. She has presented short courses, seminars, workshops, and professional papers throughout the United States and internationally. Dr. Casper's research has focused on clinical issues in voice therapy and on basic phonatory physiology. She has many publications to her credit, including the widely used text *Understanding Voice Problems: A Physiological Perspective for Diagnosis and Treatment,* which she co-authored with Dr. Raymond Colton. She and Dr. Colton also co-authored *Clinical Manual for Laryngectomy and Head/Neck Cancer Rehabilitation.*

Christine M. Sapienza, PhD, is an associate professor and associate chair at the University of Florida in the Department of Communication Sciences and Disorders. Her areas of research include the study of adult normal and disordered voice and neuromotor disorders. Her publications can be found in the *Journal of Speech, Language, and Hearing Research; The Journal of the Acoustical Society of America; Journal of Applied Physiology; The Journal of Voice; American Journal of Speech–Language Pathology;* and others. She is current editor of the *Special Interest Division 3, Voice and Voice Disorders* newsletter and was an associate editor of the *Journal of Speech, Language, and Hearing Research.* She maintains an active research laboratory with seven doctoral students. She was elected an ASHA Fellow in 2003.

Contributors

Mary Andrianopoulos, PhD, is an associate professor at the University of Massachusetts–Amherst and a clinical consultant at the Center for Language, Speech, Voice and Hearing in Amherst, Massachusetts. She completed a postdoctoral fellowship at the Mayo Clinic in Rochester, Minnesota, under Drs. Aronson and Duffy. Her expertise is in the areas of neurogenic speech and voice disorders; differential diagnosis of speech, voice, and cognitive–linguistic functions; paradoxical vocal fold movement; irritable larynx syndrome; and the effects of venterolateral thalamotomy on speech, voice, and cognitive–linguistic functions. She has published and presented her research in national and international forums.

Julie Barkmeier-Kraemer, PhD, is an assistant professor in the Department of Speech and Hearing Sciences at The University of Arizona. She has extensive clinical experience with individuals diagnosed with benign vocal fold pathology, laryngeal cancer, professional voice issues, and neurogenic voice disorders. Dr. Barkmeier-Kraemer's research addresses neurologic controls of the larynx for voice and swallowing function. She is currently investigating anatomic factors that may lead to spontaneous recurrent laryngeal nerve dysfunction resulting in vocal fold paralysis.

Savita Collins, MD, is currently an assistant professor in the Department of Otolaryngology and Head and Neck Surgery at the University of Florida. Her clinical interests include laryngology, bronchoesophagology, pediatrics, and rhinology. Her residency training was completed at the University of Wisconsin–Madison. Dr. Collins completed a postdoctoral fellowship with the National Center for Voice and Speech in Iowa City, Iowa, and Madison, Wisconsin. She currently serves as medical director for the Otolaryngology Head and Neck Surgery Clinics and is the director of the junior medical student clerkship. Her research interests include spasmodic dysphonia, recurrent respiratory papillomatosis, Parkinson's disease and dysphonia, and web-based learning.

Pamela Davis, PhD, is an associate professor at The University of Sydney in Australia and has been qualified as a speech pathologist and specialist in voice since the late 1970s. She completed a PhD in respiratory and laryngeal neurophysiology in the School of Physiology and Pharmacology at the University of New South Wales in Sydney in 1986 and lectured in the School of Communication Disorders at The University of Sydney until 1996. In 1985, she was a founding member of the National Voice Centre, which was established as a Research Centre of The University of Sydney in August 1997, and was its first director. Dr. Davis is the author of more than 50 research papers, abstracts, chapters, and edited books and has been a keynote or invited speaker at 13 international conferences. Her research interests include the neural control of voice and breathing, respiratory and laryngeal control during speech and singing, and emotional influences on voice. She has supervised a number of doctoral and master's degree research students in the areas of voice, respiration, and neurophysiology.

Paul Davenport, PhD, is a professor of physiology in the Department of Physiological Sciences at the University of Florida. He received a bachelor of arts degree in chemistry from Greenville College in 1973 and his doctorate in respiratory physiology from the Department of Physiology and Biophysics at the University of Kentucky in 1980. Dr. Davenport completed a postdoctoral fellowship with Dr. Giuseppe Sant'Ambrogio in the Department of Physiology and Biophysics at the University of Texas Medical Branch in Galveston. He has been a faculty member at the University of Florida since 1981. His course teachings include respiratory physiology and general graduate physiology. He has performed research on the neural reflex control of respiration and the transduction of respiratory forces into a neural signal processed by the central nervous system. Dr. Davenport has worked extensively in the area of conscious perception of respiratory stimuli and the role of the cerebral cortex in the sensory-motor control of breathing.

Cynthia Fox, PhD, received her master's degree in communication disorders and speech science from the University of Colorado–Boulder. She is currently a doctoral candidate in the Department of Speech and Hearing Sciences at the University of Arizona–Tucson, where her emphasis is on speech motor control, with a minor in neuroscience. She has substantial experience in evaluating and treating individuals with neurological voice disorders, with a specialty in Parkinson's disease. In addition, Dr. Fox has experience treating a variety of neurological voice disorders associated with different etiologies, such as stroke and cerebral palsy. As part of the *Lee Silverman Voice Treatment* (LSVT) clinical research team, she functions as a clinician, researcher, writer, and workshop leader.

Gregory Gallivan, MD, FACS, FCCP, "The Singing Surgeon," is an internationally acclaimed operatic baritone who has combined music and medicine as a career. He specializes in thoracic/airway surgery and voice care in the greater Springfield/Palmer, Massachusetts area; is an assistant professor of clinical surgery at the University of Massachusetts School of Medicine; and is a faculty member of The Voice Foundation, a diplomate of The American Board of Thoracic Surgery and The American Board of Surgery, a member of The Society of Thoracic Surgeons, and a Fellow of the American College of Surgeons, American College of Chest Physicians, and American Society for Laser Medicine and Surgery. Dr. Gallivan is a member of the Board of Directors of the American Cancer Society–Western Massachusetts unit, medical director of the Laser Program at Mercy Medical Center, and an editorial manuscript reviewer for the journal *Chest.* Dr. Gallivan is the author of more than 100 scientific publications and presentations. A classical pianist since age 7, he studied piano, organ, voice, harmony, theory, and composition at Hartt College of Music while an undergraduate student and medical student at Tufts University. He performed the first of 18 major operatic roles on his 20th birthday and is a founding member of Project Opera/Commonwealth Opera.

Glendon M. Gardner, MD, is a graduate of Kalamazoo College and Wayne State University School of Medicine. His otolaryngology residency was completed at the Albany (New York) Medical College. He was a fellow in laryngology and care of the professional voice at the Vanderbilt University Voice Center in Nashville, where he learned state-of-the-art care of voice disorders and microlaryngeal surgical techniques. He is now a senior staff physician in the Department of Otolaryngology at the Henry Ford Health System in Detroit and a member of the system's Medical Center for the Performing Artist. He regularly cares for touring singers performing with the Michigan Opera Theater and the Detroit Symphony Orchestra, for singers performing and at the Fisher Theater and other venues in the metro Detroit area, and for locally based singers and other voice professionals. He conducts research, lectures nationally, and publishes regularly on topics related to the larynx and voice. His own direct contribution to the musical world is as a blues harmonica player.

Leslie Glaze, PhD, is director of clinical programs in the Department of Communication Disorders at the University of Minnesota. She teaches courses in voice disorders, cleft palate/craniofacial anomalies, head and neck cancer, counseling, and professional issues. Her research interests focus on clinical and instrumental measures of voice and resonance, including biofeedback as a primary treatment tool. She established two endoscopy teaching labs for velopharyngeal imaging and laryngeal videostroboscopy. Dr. Glaze collaborates with the University of Minnesota Cleft Palate, Craniofacial, and Prosthedontics Clinic. She is co-author of the textbook *Clinical Voice Pathology* and has contributed articles and chapters in areas of voice disorders, laryngectomy rehabilitation, and cleft palate. She is a current coordinator of ASHA's Special Interest Division 3, Voice and Voice Disorders.

Steven Gray, MD, was employed at the University of Utah, Division of Otolaryngology—Head and Neck Surgery and was a professor of surgery. He held the Alice and Charles B. Hetzel Presidential Endowed Chair. Dr. Gray received his residency training at the University of Iowa. His research focused on tissue engineering of the vocal folds, biologic mechanisms of vocal senescence, and voice phenotypes. Credit for any success in these areas needs to be given to his co-investigators and colleagues. Through all of their help, and especially the support of his wife, he served as president of the American Society of Pediatric Otolaryngology for 2001–2002, while enjoying research and teaching. Dr. Gray passed away in 2002, but his work will be remembered by all.

Bari Hoffman Ruddy, PhD, received her doctorate from the University of Florida in 2001. She is currently an assistant professor in the Department of Communicative Disorders at the University of Central Florida and works clinically at the Ear, Nose, Throat, and Plastic Surgery Associates Voice Care Center. Her areas of specialties include voice science and the clinical treatment of neurogenic, pediatric, and professional voices. Dr. Hoffman Ruddy's research focuses on the physiologic study of voice disorders using methods of endoscopy, aerodynamics, and acoustic measures. She is currently associate editor of the ASHA *Perspectives* publication for Special Interest Division 3 (Voice Disorders) and co-author of the book *Excellence in Singing: Managing Vocal Health.* She serves as consultant to the Walt Disney theme parks, Actors Equity, the Florida Neurological Association, and the public schools of Orange and Seminole Counties.

Barbara Jacobson, PhD, is director of the Division of Speech–Language Sciences and Disorders at Henry Ford Medical Center. Prior to that appointment, she was director of the Speech Production Laboratory. She is the author, with her colleagues Alex Johnson and Cindy Grywalski, of the *Voice Handicap Index.* Her areas of research interest include laryngeal function in neurologic disease for voice and swallowing, outcomes measurement, assessment of quality of life for patients with communication and swallowing disorders, and competency development. She is co-editor of *Medical Speech–Language Pathology: A Practitioner's Guide.*

Timothy D. Lee, PhD, is a professor in the Department of Kinesiology at McMaster University in Hamilton, Ontario, Canada. He received his doctorate from Louisiana State University in 1982. Dr. Lee's research interests include the study of theoretical issues in motor control and learning and the application of these issues in ergonomics, sport, and various populations in which motor control has been compromised. He is currently an executive editor of the *Journal of Motor Behavior* and co-chair of the Integrative Animal Biology grant selection committee of the Natural Sciences and Engineering Research Council of Canada. He has also served as president of the Canadian Society for Psychomotor Learning and Sport Psychology and was honored in 1999 as an International Fellow in the American Academy of Kinesiology and Physical Education. Dr. Lee is an avid golfer and plays right wing on the Millgrove Muskies Oldtimer Ice Hockey Team in his spare time.

Michael Lyon, PhD, attended Bridgewater State College in Massachusetts, where he earned a bachelor of arts degree in 1971 and a master of arts degree in 1975. During this period, he was employed as a research assistant in the department of Otolaryngology, Massachusetts Eye and Ear Infirmary, Harvard Medical School, studying the neuronal connectivity of the vestibular system. This work continued following a move to the department of Otolaryngology at the University of Massachusetts Medical School until 1977. He then moved to SUNY Upstate Medical Center in Syracuse, where he worked as a research associate and attended graduate school. Dr. Lyon received his doctorate from the Department of Anatomy at SUNY Health Science Center in 1986. In 1990, he was a guest researcher at the Laboratory of Cerebral Metabolism, National Institute of Mental Health, where he studied cerebral blood flow and metabolism under Louis Sokoloff. He is an associate professor in the Department of Otolaryngology at SUNY Upstate Medical University, with a joint appointment in the Department of Cell and Developmental Biology, where he has been studying blood flow for the past 12 years. Dr. Lyon is currently co-investigator of a National Institute of Aging grant to examine age-related changes to the vasculature and blood flow control mechanisms of the human posterior cricoarytenoid muscle.

Thomas Murry, PhD, is currently a professor of clinical audiology and speech pathology in the Department of Otolaryngology—Head and Neck Surgery at Columbia University College of Physicians and Surgeons in New York. Dr. Murry received his doctorate from the University of Florida Communication Sciences Laboratory, his bachelor of science degree from Indiana University of Pennsylvania, and his master of arts degree from Ohio State University. He completed his postdoctoral fellowship in experimental phonetics and speech physiology at the University of Florida in

Gainesville. Dr. Murry has published more than 100 peer-reviewed manuscripts in professional journals and has presented more than 200 lectures, courses, or seminars on swallowing disorders, laryngeal physiology, voice disorders, motor speech disorders, and the professional voice at local, national, and international meetings and symposia. Recently, Dr. Murry has been a visiting faculty member of the Clinical Rehabilitation and Research Center at Shanghai ENT Hospital, the No. 1 ENT Society of South Africa, the Tanta Medical Center in Egypt, and the Prince Phillip Hospital and Medical Center in Hong Kong. He serves on the scientific advisory board of the Voice Foundation and review boards of the *Journal of Speech and Hearing Research*, the *Journal of Medical Speech-Language Pathology*, and the *Journal of Voice*. Dr. Murry's current research involves the study of treatment outcomes in the performer's voice; factors associated with vocal aging; fatigue in the performer's voice; voice disorders; treatment of voice disorders with acupuncture; and long-term changes in the voice following medical, surgical, pharmacological, and behavioral treatments.

Lorraine Olson Ramig, PhD, is a professor at the University of Colorado–Boulder, a research associate at the Wilbur James Gould Voice Center, and an adjunct professor at Columbia University Teacher's College. She received her bachelor's degree from the University of Wisconsin–Oshkosh, her master's degree from the University of Wisconsin–Madison, and her doctorate from Purdue University. She has published numerous articles and chapters on the voice in individuals with neurological disorders and the aging voice. Together with her colleagues, she has developed the *Lee Silverman Voice Treatment* (LSVT) for Parkinson's disease. She is a Fellow in ASHA.

Robin Samlan, MS, earned her bachelor of arts degree at Indiana University and a master of science degree at the University of Wisconsin–Madison. She was a clinical fellow and staff member at the University of Wisconsin Voice Clinic. Ms. Samlan is currently a speech–language pathologist at Johns Hopkins University, where she is a faculty member in the Department of Otolaryngology—Head and Neck Surgery. She is an adjunct faculty member at Loyola College in Maryland, where she teaches a course in communication and swallowing disorders associated with head and neck cancer. Her clinical practice and research focus on the assessment and treatment of voice disorders, resonance disorders, and communication disorders associated with head and neck cancer.

Edythe A. Strand, PhD, is a consultant in the Division of Speech Pathology, Department of Neurology, at the Mayo Clinic and an associate professor in the Mayo Medical School. Dr. Strand's research has focused on developmental and acquired apraxia of speech and issues related to both speech and voice in degenerative dysarthria. Her primary clinical interests include assessment and treatment of children and adults with neurologic speech, language, and voice disorders. She is a coauthor of *Management of Speech and Swallowing in Degenerative Disease* and *Clinical Management of Motor Speech Disorders in Children and Adults* and is co-editor of *Clinical Management of Motor Speech Disorders in Children*.

Susan L. Thibeault, PhD, is a research assistant professor in the Division of Otolaryngology—Head and Neck Surgery and in the Department of Communication Disorders at the University of Utah. She has recently completed a master's of clinical investigation in genetics. Her research areas of interest include molecular and genetic mechanisms of vocal fold vibration, vocal fold injury, and wound repair. Dr. Thibeault's clinical areas of interest include voice disorders, dysphagia, and cleft lip and palate.

Kiran Tipirneni, MD, FACS, received his undergraduate and medical school training at The Ohio State University from 1986 through 1994. A general surgery internship and an otolaryngology residency were completed at The Pennsylvania State University Medical Center from 1994 through 1999. He is presently a board-certified practicing surgeon in otolaryngology—head and neck in Florida. Dr. Tipirneni is an active member of the American Academy of Otolaryngology and is a Fellow of the Academy of College Surgeons.

Monica Nindra Tipirneni, RPh, graduated from The Ohio State University School of Pharmacy in 1992 with a bachelor of science degree in pharmacy, emphasis on managemental pharmacy. Presently she is a licensed pharmacist in Ohio, Pennsylvania, and Florida. Her work experiences include a manufacturing internship with Roxane Laboratories and several years with the Veterans' Administration hospital system as a hospital staff pharmacist and outpatient pharmacist. She is working as a retail pharmacist for a major drugstore chain. Ms. Nindra Tipirneni is an active member of the Central Florida Pharmacy Association.

Katherine Verdolini, PhD, is an associate professor of communication science and disorders in the School of Health and Rehabilitation Sciences at the University of Pittsburgh. She completed her doctorate in experimental psychology and cognitive science at Washington University in St. Louis in 1991. Her general area of professional interest is clinical voice science. Dr. Verdolini's research has focused on a variety of issues pertinent to models of voice therapy, including the influence of hydration on vocal fold function and structure, vocal fold biomechanics aimed at optimizing voice output and limiting vocal fold impact stress, voice disorder epidemiology, voice therapy efficacy, and cognitive mechanisms in skill acquisition. A current interest is the role of exercise in wound healing in the larynx. Dr. Verdolini holds a 5-year K23 Award from the National Institute on Deafness and Other Communication Disorders. Her studies from that grant have explored the cognitive neurophysiology of skill acquisition for voice tasks using both cognitive studies and neurological imaging. She is a member of ASHA, the American Psychological Association, the Voice and Speech Trainers Association, the National Association of Teachers of Singing, and the Cognitive Neuroscience Society. She was recently honored with recognition as a Fellow of ASHA.

Gayle E. Woodson, MD, is professor of otolaryngology at the Southern Illinois University School of Medicine. She attended Baylor College of Medicine, served 2 years as a surgical resident at the Johns Hopkins hospitals, and completed her otolaryngology residency at Baylor College of Medicine. She spent just over 1 year as a fellow in laryngology at the Royal National Throat, Nose, and Ear Hospital in London, England. She has previously had faculty appointments at Baylor College of Medicine, the University of California–San Diego, and the University of Tennessee–Memphis. Dr.

Woodson has served on the National Institutes of Health Sensory, Language, and Speech Disorders Study section. She is the exam chair for the American Board of Otolaryngology and chair of the American Academy of Otolaryngology Home Study Course. Her clinical interests include voice disorders and reconstructive laryngeal surgery. Her basic research addresses responses to laryngeal nerve injury.

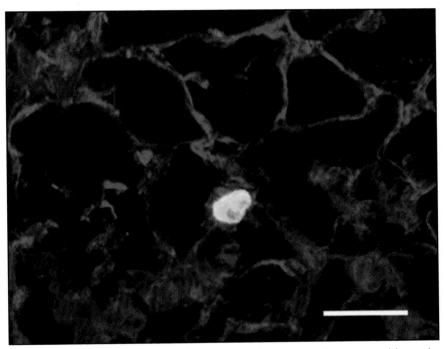

Figure 5.1. Confocal laser scanning micrograph of human thyroarytenoid muscle. Immunocytochemical staining detects slow twitch (Type 1) muscle fibers using a CY3 (indocarboryancine) fluorochrome label (red) for the slow myosin heavy chain isoform, and fast twitch (Type 2) fibers are imaged using an FITC (fluorescein isothiocyanate) label (green) for the fast myosin heavy chain isoform. Calibration bar = 50 μm.

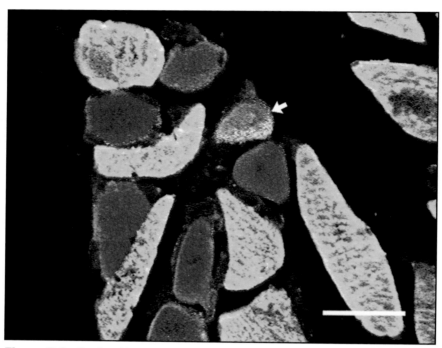

Figure 5.2. Confocal laser scanning micrographs of human thyroarytenoid muscle. Concanavalin A (red fluorochrome) images the extracellular matrix and surface of unstained muscle fibers. Small regenerating muscle fibers express the developmental myosin heavy chain isoform (green fluorochrome) in isolated regenerating fiber (arrow). Calibration bar = 50 μm.

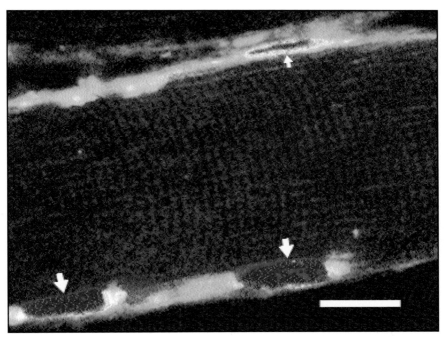

Figure 5.3. Muscle fiber in human thyroarytenoid muscle. Note the FITC (fluorescein isothiocyanate) concanavalin A fluorescence at the interface between the surface of the muscle fiber and the satellite cell (small arrow, top). This interface is seen as a gradation from green fluorescence, where there is no overprojection from the red fluorescence of the nuclear stain, to a yellow fluorescence, where overprojection combines the red ethidium homodimer emission with the green FITC emission. Note that this green/yellow fluorescent interface is not present on the inner surface of the myonuclei (large arrows, bottom). This staining difference was used to distinguish satellite cells from myonuclei. Calibration bar = 20 μm.